SURGEONS AT WAR

Recent Titles in
Contributions in Military Studies

Toward a Revolution in Military Affairs?: Defense and Security at the Dawn of the Twenty-First Century
Thierry Gongora and Harald von Riekhoff, editors

Rolling the Iron Dice: Historical Analogies and Decisions to Use Military Force in Regional Contingencies
Scot Macdonald

To Acknowledge a War: The Korean War in American Memory
Paul M. Edwards

Implosion: Downsizing the U.S. Military, 1987–2015
Bart Brasher

From Ice-Breaker to Missile Boat: The Evolution of Israel's Naval Strategy
Moshe Tzalel

Creating an American Lake: United States Imperialism and Strategic Security in the Pacific Basin, 1945–1947
Hal M. Friedman

Native vs. Settler: Ethnic Conflict in Israel/Palestine, Northern Ireland, and South Africa
Thomas G. Mitchell

Battling for Bombers: The U.S. Air Force Fights for Its Modern Strategic Aircraft Programs
Frank P. Donnini

The Formative Influences, Theories, and Campaigns of the Archduke Carl of Austria
Lee Eysturlid

Great Captains of Antiquity
Richard A. Gabriel

Doctrine Under Trial: American Artillery Employment in World War I
Mark E. Grotelueschen

Ordered to Die: A History of the Ottoman Army in the First World War
Edward J. Erickson

SURGEONS AT WAR

Medical Arrangements for the Treatment of the Sick and Wounded in the British Army during the Late 18th and 19th Centuries

Matthew H. Kaufman

Contributions in Military Studies, Number 205

GREENWOOD PRESS
Westport, Connecticut • London

Library of Congress Cataloging-in-Publication Data

Kaufman, Matthew H.

Surgeons at war : medical arrangements for the treatment of the sick and wounded in the British Army during the late 18th and 19th centuries / Matthew H. Kaufman.

p. cm.—(Contributions in military studies, ISSN 0883–6884 ; no. 205)

Includes bibliographical references and index.

ISBN 0–313–31665–1 (alk. paper)

1. Great Britain. Army—Medical care—History—18th century. 2. Great Britain. Army—Medical care—History—19th century. 3. Medicine, Military—Great Britain—History—18th century. 4. Medicine, Military—Great Britain—History—19th century. I. Title. II. Series.

UH25818th.K38 2001

355.3′45′094109033—dc21 00–034079

British Library Cataloguing in Publication Data is available.

Library of Congress Catalog Card Number: 00–034079
ISBN: 0–313–31665–1
ISSN: 0883–6884

First published in 2001

Greenwood Press, 88 Post Road West, Westport, CT 06881
An imprint of Greenwood Publishing Group, Inc.
www.greenwood.com

Printed in the United States of America

The paper used in this book complies with the Permanent Paper Standard issued by the National Information Standards Organization (Z39.48–1984).

10 9 8 7 6 5 4 3 2 1

Copyright Acknowledgment

Every reasonable effort has been made to trace the owners of copyright materials in this book, but in some instances this has proven impossible. The editor and publisher will be glad to receive information leading to more complete acknowledgments in subsequent printings of the book, and in the meantime extend their apologies for any omissions.

CONTENTS

PREFACE

Numerous texts were written during the 18th and early part of the 19th century on all aspects of military medicine and surgery. These were written by men who had often achieved high rank in the service of their country, and felt the need to convey their knowledge to others who might one day be exposed to similar experiences either in the field of battle or in home or foreign postings. Many dealt with the treatment of the various types of military trauma to which troops were commonly exposed, such as gunshot injuries, compound fractures, and damage to major blood vessels.

Relatively few texts discussed the treatment of bayonet or saber injuries, although these constituted a significant proportion of the injuries sustained in hand-to-hand fighting and when cavalry harried infantry. Although as commonly encountered as gunshot injuries, penetrating wounds involving the body cavities were generally left untreated, as the prognosis was said to be hopeless. All but the simplest of surgical procedures were fraught with danger. Death not infrequently resulted from hemorrhage, infection, or gangrene. Even if survival occurred, all but a few of the men had to be invalided out of the service. This clearly applied to the majority of the amputees, very few of whom would be able to return to active service as front-line infantrymen.

Many texts were written on the diseases that troops encountered in barracks at home and in foreign postings, because the morbidity and mortality involved were usually far higher than the losses incurred during combat. In many foreign campaigns, it was not unusual for 20–30%, or occasionally even 40%, of an army to be incapacitated or hospitalized at any one time. The various types of venereal diseases that were a common cause of chronic debility were also commonly considered, and appropriate forms of treatment discussed in great detail. Losses from all of these causes were numerically an important problem for commanders wishing to maintain the efficiency of their fighting force.

Standards of hygiene in barracks and in military hospitals both at home and abroad were often poor, and many died due to the rapid spread of infectious diseases. The greatest advances in reducing the high rates of mortality and morbidity commonly encountered in the army almost invariably came about with the appointment of competent medical administrators. In the absence of knowledge of the principles of asepsis and antisepsis, and lack of blood transfusions and antibiotics, the only means of improving the conditions of service came about through general improvements in military hygiene and through effective public health measures. Because so little was known about the cause and spread of infection, little effort was made to isolate those who were contagious. Apart from maintaining strict standards of hygiene and, where possible, improving the diet of the men, little else could be done to reduce the spread of disease.[1]

The lack of suitable medication, especially antibiotics, invariably meant that the drugs that were available to the medical staff were almost nonexistent, and those that were prescribed, such as rhubarb, calomel, cantharides, julap, and ipecacuanha, were untested, and were almost certainly useless and often dangerous. Quinine was widely available from the early part of the Crimean War, so that malaria did not prove to be a particular problem as it had undoubtedly been during the Peninsular War and on the Continent during the earlier part of the century.[2] In the Crimea, cholera, for which no suitable treatment was then available, nearly destroyed the British force. Opiates were also widely available, but could only be palliative in relieving rather than curing the worst manifestations of the wide range of clinical conditions to which the men were exposed, and for the acute treatment of the wounded.

During the 18th century, the majority of individuals who practiced military medicine and surgery could enter the medical service of the army with only minimal qualifications. In times of war, the academic standard of the medical intake was often even poorer, with some candidates having only served apprenticeships of a few months' duration. Specialist knowledge invariably had to be acquired on the job, or more often on or close to the battlefield. Even during the early part of the 19th century, only about 20%, and during the second quarter of the 19th century only about 40% of the doctors that entered the service possessed a medical degree. Over 80% of those with a medical degree had graduated from a Scottish University, and of these, about half had graduated from the University of Edinburgh.

Despite John Hunter's policy, when he was surgeon general in the 1790s, of appointing physicians only from among the most experienced men, whether they were apothecaries, or surgeons, or from civilian practice, the members of the Army Board,[3] which succeeded him, devised an extremely divisive policy. The members of the Board had minimal military experience, and had the mistaken view that an Oxbridge medical education was likely to be of greater value to a military clinician than possibly many years of practical military experience. Accordingly, they initially appointed only recent Oxbridge graduates who also possessed a diploma from the London College of Physicians to senior clinical posts, despite the fact that they often had no previous military or administrative experience. This arbitrary rule effectively excluded nearly every regular medical officer then serving in the army, but was later amended to include medical graduates from other "acceptable" universities, despite the fact that they also often had no former military experience. As they were invariably placed over men with considerable military experience, this inevitably led to bad feeling and a breakdown in the administration in the service. Its only long-term advantage was that it stimulated some of the more senior officers to retire on half-pay in order to acquire the necessary qualification to allow them to offer themselves for promotion to the rank of physician.

It had also long been appreciated that there were no appropriate medical schools in Britain to specifically train medical officers for the army and the navy. One of the most vociferous individuals who drew attention to this deficiency was an Edinburgh surgeon, John Bell, who had attended the severely injured sailors after the Battle of Camperdown in 1797, following their repatriation to the Naval Hospital at Yarmouth. Bell indicated his concerns in a brief but important *Memoir on the Present State of Naval and Military Surgery*[4] to Earl Spencer, First Lord of the Admiralty. Bell recommended the establishment of "one great School of Military Surgery" where all of the subjects encountered by a medical officer during the course of his duties would be taught by professionals.

During the early post-Waterloo period, large numbers of incompetent or elderly medical officers were immediately retired or put on half-pay. Of those retained in the service, James McGrigor, who in 1815 had been appointed director general of the Army Medical Department by Wellington and held this post for 35 years, insisted that advancement would be awarded only on the basis of merit. He also became personally involved in the selection of medical candidates for the service, and his principal efforts were directed toward improving the academic standard of candidates intending to join the army.

One of the consequences of the public concern at the poor medical treatment of the sick and wounded during the Crimean War was the establishment of the army medical school at Fort Pitt, Chatham, in 1860. This functioned along similar lines to those proposed by John Bell 60 years earlier. During the early post–Crimean War period, a corps of attendants, termed the Army Hospital Corps, was formed. Other reforms during the latter part of the 19th century led eventually to the establishment of the Royal Army Medical Corps in 1898,[5] but the factors that led to its establishment are beyond the scope of the present volume.

Where quotations from various sources have been cited, these have been provided either to give a contemporary description of the conditions under which the men fought or the medical officers worked, or to give insight into the attitude of the doctors toward the system under which they practiced. In the case of the West Indies campaign and in the Peninsula the plan was to shed light on their attitude toward the senior members of the Army Medical Board. In the case of officers serving during the Crimean War this was to shed light on what they perceived to be the incompetence of the system under which they worked. These are provided for the benefit of the general reader who may not have ready access to a reference library but who nevertheless may be interested in gaining this additional insight. While some of these quotations have been included in the text, others have been relegated to the appropriate Notes section associated with each chapter.

It is appropriate in this section to record the author's indebtedness to those individuals such as Miss Jean Archibald, Dr. Michael Barfoot and the other members of staff of the Special Collections Section of Edinburgh University Library for their invaluable assistance during all stages of the gestation period of this volume, and Dr. Malcolm Nicholson for his most helpful editorial comments on the entire manuscript. Thanks are also due to Dr. Helen Dingwall, Mr. Allan Carswell and Mr. Owen Dudley Edwards for their advice and support, and Marianne Eastwood for meticulously preparing the camera-ready version of the text. Particular thanks are also due to my academic colleagues in the Section of Anatomy, Department of Biomedical Sciences, University of Edinburgh and to my wife, Claire, and sons, Simon and David, for their tolerance during the preparation of this manuscript.

NOTES

1. "Success in war depends upon preserving military force in health and vigour. Disarmed by sickness the most intrepid warrior becomes a prey of the most pusillanimous adversary. Fleets and armies moulder away by diseases." See: Dr. Miller, cited by N. Cantlie, 1974. *A History of the Army Medical Department.* 2 Volumes (Edinburgh & London: Churchill Livingstone), Volume 1, p. 175.

2. The expedition to the Scheldt in July 1809, known as the Walcheren expedition, was a military disaster in which over a period of about 4 months 4,000 soldiers died of disease and many others had to be discharged from the service. The disease was a form of malaria. See: Cantlie, *History of the Army Medical Department*, Volume 1, pp. 395–405.

3. The Army Medical Board was established by the government after Hunter's death, in 1793, and functioned until it was disbanded in 1809 following maladministration associated with the Walcheren expedition (for details, see Chapter 1).

4. J. Bell, 1798. *Memoir on the Present State of Naval and Military Surgery. Addressed to the Right Honourable Earl Spenser [sic], First Lord of the Admiralty.* [21 pp. Yarmouth, January 20, 1798].

5. F. Smith, 1929. *A Short History of the Royal Army Medical Corps.* (Aldershot: Gale & Polden Ltd.); J.S.G. Blair, 1998. *Centenary History of the Royal Army Medical Corps (1898–1998)* (Edinburgh: Scottish Academic Press).

1

INTRODUCTION

MILITARY MEDICINE AND SURGERY DURING THE 18TH AND EARLY 19TH CENTURIES

While there were excellent schools of military medicine and military surgery on the continent of Europe that had been established during the eighteenth century, no courses of instruction were available in Britain for those who planned to enter as medical officers in the army.[1] Nor were any courses of instruction available to them once they had entered the service. This is not to say that there were no skilled medical practitioners in the army, only that any specialized knowledge that they may have acquired during their career had probably been gained on the battlefield.

Blair[2] has drawn attention to the changes in military medicine brought about as a result of the introduction of gunpowder during the 13th and 14th centuries, and the terrifying effect of injuries on armies due to the propulsion of metallic missiles.[3] The realities of the situation were particularly graphically conveyed in the writings of Ambroise Paré during the mid-16th century.[4] The continued and universal use of Latin toward the end of that century allowed a free communication between doctors in different European countries, and was instrumental in attracting Scottish doctors in particular into the service of the kings of France and Spain. The fact that Britain became a great sea power from the beginning of the 17th century provided additional scope for colonial conquests in the East and West Indies and elsewhere. This clearly necessitated the presence of competent doctors to administer to armies and navies both in shore stations and in barracks at home, and in an increasing number of stations abroad.

The principal consequences of wounding were pain, blood loss, and infection. While pain might be debilitating for a finite period of time, and excessive blood loss, if not staunched, could be fatal, it was the consequences of infection that resulted in the lingering death of many men. The greatest risk to armies in foreign parts was from tropical diseases, which spread rapidly and often caused much greater mortality and morbidity than the effects of hostile forces. In campaigns abroad, many times more troops fell victim to contagious infections, and were consequently rendered incapable of fighting, than were wounded in action. Even diseases that are now encountered only in tropical climates, such as malaria, cholera, typhoid, and typhus fevers, were encountered in all parts of Europe during the 18th and early 19th centuries. The plague had decimated whole populations, even in Britain, as recently as the middle of the previous century.[5]

Blair also reminds us that it was Charles I who was an early innovator with regard to the medical care of British sailors, with the provision of hospital ships, a free allowance of drugs, and rather short-lived courses of postgraduate lectures given by the Company of Barber-Surgeons in London. Charles II instituted changes associated with the reduction of the Standing Army, but more particularly the commissioning of medical officers to attend to the welfare of the troops.[6]

The New Model Army had been established by Oliver Cromwell in 1645 during the Civil War, and was the precursor of the Standing Army. It consisted of 12 regiments of foot and 11 regiments of horse with artillery and engineers, in all some 30,000 strong. Each regiment was allocated one regimental surgeon. A barber-surgeon was allocated to each company, and acted as a first-aid dresser in the absence of the surgeon. The Company of Surgeons had the authority to impress their members to serve in the army, and also organized the supply of medicines and surgical materials for the surgeons' chests.[7]

MEDICINE IN THE NAVY

The situation in the Naval Medical Service during the late 18th and early 19th centuries was in many regards worse than that in the army during this period. Attention is briefly drawn to the arrangements for the selection of candidates for the navy, to provide a contemporary backdrop against which the situation in the Army Medical Department may be compared.

During the first half of the 18th century, the majority of naval surgeons had to be examined by the Court of Examiners of the Company of Barber-Surgeons. By the middle of the century, however, due to irreconcilable differences between the barbers and the surgeons, this union was formally dissolved by an Act of Parliament in 1745. The surgeons founded their own Livery Company, which in 1800 became transformed into the College of Surgeons. From 1745, prospective candidates who intended entering the navy were now examined for their suitability exclusively by the Company of Surgeons at their hall in Monkwell Street, and this arrangement was confirmed by subsequent Acts of Parliament.

Lectures and dissections were undertaken under the authority of the Company of Barber-Surgeons, but as these were generally of such a poor standard, rival schools opened up in London with far more competent teachers, leading to the establishment of a number of extramural schools in that city. It should be noted that these extramural schools catered to a wide range of individuals, not all of whom were students who planned to become medical practitioners.[8] What few accounts remain of the examinations to which the candidates were subjected would seem to indicate that they were fairly superficial, and as the need for medical officers in the navy increased, particularly during times of war, so the standard of the entry fell. The examinations at Surgeons' Hall generally lasted for about fifteen minutes, after which a fee of five shillings was demanded. The successful candidate was then expected to purchase his surgeon's chest from a recognized supplier, and his drugs at Apothecaries' Hall.

The list of recommended surgical instruments and other items for the chest, in 1812, was certainly comprehensive, and would have probably occupied a large cabin trunk. The items are those recommended by the College of Surgeons, and are as follows:[9]

2 amputation knives; 1 amputating saw with spare blade; 1 metacarpal saw with spare blade; 2 catlins [double-edged amputating knives]; pair of artery forceps; 2 dozen curved needles; 2 tenaculums [hooks for holding parts]; 6 Pettit's screw tourniquets; pair of bone nippers and turnscrew; 3 trephines; saw for the head [Hey's saw for enlarging cranial orifice made by trephines]; rugins [raspatories or files]; pair of forceps; elevator; brush; 2 trocars [tube for withdrawing fluid]; 2 silver catheters [tube for drawing off urine]; 2 gum-elastic catheters; 6 scalpels; 1 small razor; key tooth instrument [for extracting teeth by torsion]; gum lancet [for lancing gum boils]; 2 pair tooth forceps; punch; 2 Seton needles [for drawing silk through the skin to leave a tract for drainage]; pair of strong probe scissors; curved bistory with button [bistoury or scalpel]; long probe; pair of bullet forceps; scoop for extracting balls; 2 probangs [throat sponges]; 1 pound ligature thread; 1 paper of needles; case, with lift out; apparatus for restoring suspended animation; set of pocket instruments; 6 lancets in a case; 2 pint pewter clyster syringes [enema syringes]; 2 sets common splints; set of Japanned iron splints for legs; 12 flannel or linen rollers; 2 18-tailed bandages; 20 yards of cloth for tourniquets; 60 yards of tape; cupping apparatus, consisting of 1 scarificator and 6 glasses.

The Court of Examiners of the College of Surgeons indicated that the following items should be expunged from the list: the lenticular, from the apparatus for restoring suspended animation, because it was "not only useless, but also a very dangerous instrument." This equally applied to tobacco, because far from restoring animation it "must always have a deadly tendency." Similarly, the probe scissors, which are "improper to be used in any operation of surgery".[10] It was only in 1811 that the Court condemned the practice of injecting tobacco fumes internally. This practice had been recommended by the Royal Humane Society in 1774 on the advice of Dr. Richard Mead. "It is not only the admission of kindly warmth into the internal parts of the body, which in all cases must prove advantageous, but its stimulus seems admirably adapted to excite irritability and to restore the suspended or languid peristaltic motion of the intestines." It was still recommended in Turnbull's *The Naval Surgeon*,[11] as being a particularly successful irritant.

The number of items that the Society of Apothecaries recommended should be present in the surgeon's chest was considerable, though these would have taken up less space than those required by the College of Surgeons. Lloyd and

Coulter[12] have indicated that the list from 1806 published by Turnbull[13] bears a strong resemblance to that approved by the apothecaries almost fifty years earlier. In addition to the various drugs itemized below, the surgeon was also expected to carry a range of items to be supplied to the convalescent seamen.[14] Those recommended by the apothecaries at that time were: barley; eggs, greased and put in salt; extract of spruce; lemon juice, clarified and preserved by adding to it a small proportion of ardent spirits; raisins; rice; coarse sugar; sago; salop; portable soup; tamarinds; and red and white wine.

The list of drugs recommended by the apothecaries was as follows:

Acid Vitriol. dilut.; Adip. suill. pp.; Aloes socotr.; Antimon. tartariz.; Aq. litharg. acetat.; Arg. nitrat.; Calomel; Camphor; Cera. flav.; Cerat. lap. calam.; Cinchon. pulv. et flav.; Conf. aromat.; Crem. tart. pulv.; Cret. pp.; Cuprum. vitriol.; Digital. purp. pulv.; Emp. cantharid.; Emp. creae c.; Emp. litharg.; Emp. comp.; Emp. cum hydr.: Eztra. colocy. c.; Flor. chamaem.; Flor. sulph.; Gum. arom. gutt.; Gum. arab.; Gum. guiac.; Hydr. muriat.; Hydr. nitrat. rub.; Ipecac. pulv.; Jalap. pulv.; Kali pp.; Liquor. vol. c.c.; Magnes. alb.; Magnes. vitriol. Nitr. purif.; Ol. lini.; Ol. menth. piper; Ol. olivar.; Ol. ricin.; Ol. terebinth.; Opium; Pulv. antimonialis; Pulv. ipecac. c.; Quassiae ras.; Res. flav.; Rhubarb pulv.; Sal. vol. c.c.; Sem. lini.; Senna; Sperm. cet.; Sp. lavend. c.; Tinct. ferr. muriat.; Tinct. scillae; Ung. Cerae.; Ung. hydrarg. fort.; Ung. hydrarg. nitrat.; Ung. rsin. flav.; Zinc vitriol.; Zinzibar pulv. Other items that were recommended were a Bolus knife, tile, bottles, corks, gally-pots, mortar and pestle, ditto (Wedgwood), needles, scales, spatula, funnel, sponges and tow.

As conditions in the service were so abominable, after just over three years in the cockpit (or the equivalent in the army) most left the service to enter private practice. When discussing the conditions in the navy, Turnbull, in his *The Naval Surgeon*, stated, "The consequences of these prejudices so much injured the service, that it was in general only resorted to as a matter of unavoidable necessity, by those young men who could not procure any other employment; and it was accordingly abandoned so soon as any other opening, however indifferent, permitted them to retire."[15] This they were allowed to do, because of an Act of Parliament of 1749 to this effect, and more importantly for most, they would not be subject to further examination by the Surgeons' Company, or the payment of apprenticeship fees. Conditions in the medical branch of the service were apparently so poor during the second half of the 18th century that if they were allowed to deteriorate further, no candidates would voluntarily apply to enter. Changes were eventually initiated toward the end of the century following the publication of Trotter's *Review of the Medical Department of the British Navy*.[16] Trotter indicated that the arrangement then in force whereby the Surgeons' Company continued to examine candidates for the navy should be terminated. This situation was deemed to be far from satisfactory, and it was suggested that a Board of Naval Surgeons should conduct this task. Trotter also believed that the drugs used on board ship should best be selected by a Board of Naval Physicians, rather than by the Society of Apothecaries.

A pamphlet from John Bell followed shortly afterward. His twenty-one-page *Memoir on the Present State of Naval and Military Surgery*, addressed to the

First Lord of the Admiralty, Earl Spencer, was published in 1798,[17] and again, but in an amended version, in 1800.[18] Bell suggested that a radical reform of the medical arrangements in both services was required. He recommended a formal period of training followed by periods of in-service study, all associated with a reasonable career structure. It took more than 60 years before any attempt was made by the government to institute some of these changes, although the establishment of the Regius Chair of Military Surgery in Edinburgh, with minimal expenditure of public funds, went some small way toward this aim.

Attention had also been repeatedly drawn to the fact that unless the very poor regard in which the naval surgeons were held by the executive or wardroom officers changed, and conditions of service improved, there was no possibility that well-qualified candidates would consider entering the service. Such pleas, for example by Sir Gilbert Blane in the third edition of his *Observations*,[19] and previously by Trotter in the first volume of his *Medicina Nautica*,[20] unfortunately carried little weight with their lordships. Despite Acts of Parliament, the conditions in the service continued to stagnate until after the Crimean War, when a range of improvements was introduced which went some way toward elevating the very low morale of the service.

It was only because of the renewal of hostilities, on this occasion with the French under Napoleon, that an Order in Council was put into effect on January 23, 1805, that not only accepted that changes had to be made, but also recommended means of improving the quality of the medical intake into the service.[21] It was with this Order that naval medical officers were first allowed to wear a distinguishing uniform,[22] giving them, from 1805, a comparative rank in the service suitable to their station; this was particularly important, as a similar arrangement was already in force in the Army Medical Department.

In 1806, Turnbull[23] reiterated many of the views expressed by Bell some years earlier.[24] Turnbull believed that candidates should all possess a university education, and preferably in Edinburgh,[25] and that after entry into the service naval surgeons should be offered specialist postgraduate courses,[26] possibly based at the various naval hospitals.

MILITARY SURGEONS IN THE ARMY DURING THE 18TH CENTURY

Most of the officers in the British army during the 18th century had no formal training in a military academy before entering a regiment, and looked down upon the members of the various specialist branches, such as the artillery and the engineers, who had attended such institutions. The executive branch of the service for the same reason also poorly regarded the military surgeons. There was an obvious and usually insurmountable social divide between the doctors who were attached to the regiments and the commissioned regular officers. Doctors were usually associated with regiments, as accessories, and their status was about the same as drummers. In some regiments, the doctor had a private contractual arrangement with the colonel or commanding officer. In others, the surgeon accompanied the regiment as private physician to the commanding officer, much as an aristocrat would have taken his secretary or doctor with him on the grand tour. A few doctors additionally served as combatants, and would then have received an additional stipend for their labors. The surgeons of Militia and Fencible corps, for example, all bore combatant commissions in addition to their medical ones, as occasionally did officers in the early days of the Indian Medical Service after its foundation in 1764.[27]

According to Hamilton,[28] this was unacceptable. He believed that: "In the regular service, double commissions, of late, have been forbid, . . . In the militia it is universally practised. The reason given for it is, that as this service is of a limited duration, for the war only, and surgeons there are not entitled to half pay on dismission, a second commission is granted as a kind of recompence; and properly, if it was understood as a perquisite; but, we apprehend, not for the good of the medical part of the service, . . . No two professions whatever are more opposite in their natures, than that of a military and medical gentleman: the reason has already been pointed out. . . . The engagements of an officer require not much serious reflection; the medical man's duty requires it almost constantly."

According to Gore,[29] during the 18th century: "The surgeon's appointment was then bought and sold like a military commission. From 1783, the sale of medical commissions was officially suppressed, but . . . was for a long period still carried on. The officer who obtained the appointment [by purchase] only required a certificate from a private medical teacher that he was qualified to practice surgery, a University degree or certificate from Surgeons' Hall not being necessary." The regimental surgeon had permission to sell his appointment when wishing to retire from the service. Such individuals "had no provision when superannuated and so infirm as to be no longer capable of performing his duty." According to Guthrie it was hardly necessary for a man to be a surgeon to practice in the army.

"This incapacity of some of the junior members of the profession imposed a greater share of labour on the seniors, and the dispatches of the Duke of Wellington have borne honourable testimony to their exertions in the field."[30]

However, he also noted "having seen young men sent out from England to the Peninsula, incapable of performing any operations in military surgery, become able operators, in a short time, from the practical lessons inculcated in our dissecting rooms, in our hospitals, and on the field of battle."[31]

A substantial proportion of the surgeons who entered the British army during the 18th century, if they had any formal training, received it in a Scottish university. Of these, only a relatively small proportion graduated with the M.D. degree. Some had served for a few years as an apprentice to a surgeon, an apothecary, or a country doctor before attending formal classes at a university and the wards of a teaching hospital for a few years. They then passed the licentiate examination of one of the colleges of surgeons, or the examination of the Society of Apothecaries, as these were adequate qualifications to practice as a doctor. If the country of origin of those that took the licentiate examination and successfully qualified and practiced medicine is similar to those who completed the Edinburgh M.D. degree during the 18th century,[32] then an approximately similar number of students came from England and Ireland as from Scotland.

Only those who had social connections and intended practising as physicians in communities with an adequate number of private patients would bother to take the M.D. degree. Many who did not complete their M.D. degree entered the army as a means of gaining excitement as well as escaping rural poverty. They hoped to save enough money to allow them to buy into a comfortable practice with whatever salary they possessed on their retirement. In some cases, this may have been supplemented by any bounty acquired during their years in the service, particularly if this coincided with periods of war. The majority of the medical students who trained in Scotland would have come from a lower middle-class background, very different from that of the officers they would encounter in the army. Almost all of these had private means, essential to maintain the standard of living expected of an officer and facilitate their promotion in the service.

Others who entered the army as surgeons had no medical qualifications whatsoever. A proportion may have served for a few years as an apothecary's or as a surgeon's apprentice, but entered the army as a regimental mate or hospital mate without any formal qualifications. This factor seems to have been less important than their competence to treat the range of conditions that they were likely to encounter in the service. In many regards, they were barely less qualified than those who had only recently acquired their license to practice.

The recruitment position into the junior ranks in the Army Medical Department was particularly poor in the 1780s and 1790s, principally because of the very low pay provided for the regimental mates, of only 3/6d per day.[33] By the early 1790s, the lack of appropriate staff, particularly hospital mates, was a considerable cause for concern to the regiments that were ordered to go to the West Indies, where the risk of death from yellow fever was a great disincentive for volunteers.

By 1796, with no improvement in the position, a royal warrant was issued which substantially increased the rates of pay of regimental surgeons and regimental mates. The designation of "mate" was abolished, as these were now to be termed assistant surgeons. They were also to receive 5/- per day, raised to 7/6d per day when on active or foreign service. More importantly, this Order granted the king's commission to all medical officers, and abolished the stigma of a warrant officer's rank. The positive effect of this royal warrant was dramatic, and most of the vacancies were rapidly filled. With this increase in the number of candidates coming forward for consideration, the Board was now able to insist on higher professional qualifications in the intake, and regimental surgeons now had to pass an examination before they could be promoted.[34]

All attempts to sort out the anomalies that existed in the salary structure proved ineffective and it now transpired that staff surgeons were paid less than regimental surgeons. All proposals to the Secretary at War were rejected, until 1804, with the granting of a new royal warrant in May of that year. Even the regulations introduced by Sir Lucas Pepys,[35] the physician-general shortly after his appointment to the Army Medical Board, were relaxed to mollify the feelings of the regular officers, so that medical officers who were not Oxbridge graduates but were nevertheless graduates of other British or Irish universities were now eligible to apply for promotion to the rank of physician.[36] However, they would be successful only if they were in all other regards appropriately qualified and passed an examination before the physician-general and two army physicians (see later this chapter).

THE MILITARY SURGICAL HIERARCHY DURING THE 18TH CENTURY

During the 18th century, the role of the surgeon was always subservient to that of the physician. Apart from instances that were deemed to be purely of a surgical nature, the surgeon was only rarely consulted in the normal course of clinical practice. It would certainly have been exceptional for a surgeon to be invited by a physician to give an opinion on the clinical management of a patient. This inevitably meant that a range of clinical conditions that undoubtedly had a surgical basis were either overlooked or misdiagnosed, and consequently mistreated. This should not, of course, detract from the situation as it then was, and continued well into the nineteenth century, where most troops and sailors died from conditions unrelated to enemy action. Blane in his *Observations* highlighted this, a point that he believed had previously been made by Alexander the Great.[37]

While doctors generally entered the army as regimental or hospital mates, or as assistant surgeons, and gradually rose through the ranks, others received their appointment through patronage. This arrangement was common during the 18th century, but continued to a more limited degree into the 19th century. According to Cantlie,[38] there were two distinct branches of military medical officers: those that belonged to the regimental branch and those that belonged to the medical staff branch. In the regimental branch, the medical officer was granted a commission in the regiment with the approval of the commanding officer. He wore the uniform of the regiment, and was directly responsible to his colonel for the regimental hospital and all aspects of its administration. Some medical officers spent their whole army career with the same regiment, and many never rose above the rank of regimental surgeon.

The medical staff branch, by contrast, was composed of medical officers who served in the general hospitals, or acted as garrison surgeons or as administrative officers either in hospitals or at the headquarters of military formations. There were relatively few general hospitals in peacetime, because the regimental hospitals carried out all aspects of medical treatment without referring individuals elsewhere. Accordingly, soldiers lived or died in their regimental hospitals, under the care of the regimental surgeon.

Regimental surgeons tended to have few opportunities to meet their professional colleagues. While they were theoretically encouraged to discuss their difficult cases with the local practitioners, this seldom occurred. Equally, while they were encouraged to read a wide range of medical textbooks, this also rarely occurred. Hamilton in his *Duties of a Regimental Surgeon*,[39] recommended that they should read Lind (on scurvy),[40] Pringle (*The Diseases of the Army, in Camp and Garrison*),[41] Monro (*The Means of Preserving the Health of Soldiers*),[42] Hunter (*A Treatise on Venereal Diseases*)[43] and various works on operative surgery. Unfortunately, relatively few either wished to or were able to follow Hamilton's well-meaning advice.

MILITARY SURGERY AND MILITARY SURGEONS

It is possible to consider here only a few of the important individuals whose exceptional talents led to improvements in the conditions of service of the men under their care. Brief biographical details will be provided only as a means of illustrating how their management skills led to improvements in hospital sanitation and ventilation, and the isolation of individuals with contagious diseases that occasionally led to the decimation of armies and the curtailment of military campaigns. Only from the mid-1840s did the introduction of general anesthesia and from the late 1860s the appreciation of the importance of antisepsis allow a wider range of operations to be performed than had formerly been possible.

During the 18th century the role of the military surgeon was relatively limited. The absence of anesthesia, aseptic and antiseptic techniques, blood transfusions, and antibiotics meant that the principal role of the surgeon was to provide first aid for the treatment of emergencies, rather than for the treatment of nonemergency conditions. Individuals were usually prepared to subject themselves to the surgeon's knife only when there was no other alternative. Many, no doubt, would even be in extremis before they would be prepared to consider this course of action.

The accepted wisdom was that in cases of military trauma, the immediate intervention of a surgeon might be lifesaving, whereas any delay would almost certainly lead to their death. Failure to intervene invariably had only one outcome, while intervention might just provide a small chance of survival. Accordingly, individuals often had little choice but to expose themselves to whatever the surgeon was able to offer. In cases of compound fracture involving the long bones of a limb or damage to a joint, there was no expectation that the limb could be saved, and the quicker it was removed the greater the chance of survival. It was the balance between no chance of survival, with a lingering death from wound infection almost invariably progressing to septicemia and later gangrene, secondary hemorrhage, or tetanus, against the small chance of survival if the traumatized and usually infected tissue was completely excised.

It is of critical importance to appreciate that until the availability of the various lifesaving procedures and drugs, the principal role of the military surgeon, both in peace and in war, was as a general practitioner who attended to all of the needs of the men under his care. During the 18th and for much of the 19th century, the military surgeon's first allegiance was to the commanding officer of his own regiment, his principal function being to maximize the number of those who would be fit for duty as necessary. Few military doctors had a university degree, and most had only the minimum entrance qualification necessary to enter the service. Very few had any specialist skills, particularly in surgery. If they were required to perform "capital" or life-threatening operations, such as an amputation or the treatment of gunshot wounds, the men's expectation of survival must have been very slim.

Civilian surgeons gained reputations then, as well as during the first half of the following century, because of their speed, courage, and sound knowledge of the underlying anatomy, and surgical intervention continued, as previously, to be a matter of last resort. Many, clearly, did not survive surgical intervention. This was particularly the case at sea, where men were already suffering the consequences of malnutrition, with tissues often devitalized by scurvy. Surgical advances usually resulted from the undertaking by individual surgeons of high-risk procedures that other surgeons were not prepared to contemplate, usually carried out when there was either no expectation or very little expectation of survival. John Hunter, for example, "Dissected out a tumor on the neck, which one of the best operating surgeons in the country had declared, rather too strongly, that no one but a fool or a madman would attempt; and the patient got perfectly well."[44]

The military surgeon's role on the battlefield, and if the soldier survived long enough to reach a hospital, was to perform heroic, lifesaving, procedures. Limbs or parts of limbs were removed rapidly, because they were usually so damaged that, if left alone, they would lead invariably to the death of the individual. Speed was always of the essence, because any prolonged surgical procedure would almost certainly lead to excessive blood loss, terrible pain, and death due to profound and irreversible surgical shock. Cantlie[45] provides many examples that demonstrate the stoicism of the patients who were subjected to the knife.

When wounds of the body cavities were sustained, their prognosis was generally considered to be hopeless, and surgical intervention was never undertaken. Even Ballingall, in the middle of the next century, was of the view that:

> Wounds of the small intestine are, for the most part, either primarily or secondarily fatal, while those of the large intestines sometimes heal without difficulty. . . . The older writers . . . pronounced wounds of the latter dangerous in the highest degree; those of the former, without exception fatal. . . . No man in his senses would think of enlarging the external wound, for the purpose of searching out and sewing up the wounded part of the gut—a practice, the propriety of which is not universally admitted, even when the wounded intestine protrudes externally. Extravasation of the contents of the bowels within the peritoneum is by no means so liable to occur as speculative writers would lead us to imagine, and, when it does happen . . . the case may, for the most part, be abandoned as hopeless. . . . It must ever be recollected that bleeding from the arm is the best preservative from internal bleeding and peritoneal inflammation—the two great sources of danger in wounds of the abdomen.[46]

Survival occasionally occurred if a puncture wound involving the large intestine led to the formation of a spontaneous colostomy. When penetrating wounds of the chest and abdomen occurred, the entrance and exit wounds were dressed, and, often, 16–24 ounces of blood were withdrawn from the arm. If the intestines were cut and protruding, they were usually stitched to the edge of the wound, in the hope that they might form either an ileostomy or colostomy, depending on the location of the lesion. If the protruding gut appeared to be sound, it was replaced, and the wound closed with ligatures and strapping, though survival tended to be the exception rather than the rule.

JOHN HUNTER, SURGEON-GENERAL AND INSPECTOR OF REGIMENTAL HOSPITALS, 1790–1793

During the 18th and 19th centuries, while the relatively small number of practitioners who planned to become consulting surgeons often spent long hours in the dissecting room during their training, some notable surgeons continued to do so throughout their surgical careers. They often combined the teaching of anatomy and surgical applied anatomy, while at the same time maintaining an enormous surgical and consulting practice. A particularly notable example was John Hunter (1728–1793) (see Figure 1.1). His income from private practice was said to have first reached £1,000 in 1774 and to have risen to at least £6,000 shortly before his death.[47]

John Hunter entered St. George's Hospital as a surgeon's apprentice in 1754, and was a house surgeon there in 1756 while at the same time teaching anatomy in his brother William's extra-academical school. When Hunter was 32, as a consequence of "inflammation of the lungs," he decided to join the army. He obtained a commission in 1760 due to his brother's influence, and was appointed to a surgeoncy on the staff of a military hospital. England was at war with Spain. As Portugal was friendly with England, the Spanish invaded it, and Hunter spent eighteen months with an expeditionary force that was sent to Portugal. He retired on half-pay in 1763, at the termination of the Seven Years War. It is said that his only experience of treating recent gunshot wounds was obtained on the island of Bellisle in 1761 during the two-month campaign there in which over 700 were either killed or wounded. Hunter had served throughout his tour of duty there in the general hospital at Palais. While he saw relatively little active service there, he collected a wide range of natural history specimens, most of which ended up in his museum.[48]

John Hunter's collection of comparative anatomy specimens was considered to be of national importance, and after his death the Treasury purchased it on behalf of the nation. The trustees of Hunter's museum, Dr. Matthew Baillie and Mr. Everard Home, recommended that the College of Surgeons should take over the custody of the museum, which contained both anatomical and pathological preparations, in order to promote and extend the knowledge of anatomy and surgery. The collection was accepted on certain conditions. It had to be accessible to the public at certain times each week. A course of comparative anatomy, consisting of 12 lectures illustrated by examples from the collection, would be given twice each year. The preparations had to be kept in a good state of preservation. Finally, its welfare was to be supervised by a Board of trustees made up of clinicians and scientists of the highest repute.[49]

Figure 1.1. John Hunter

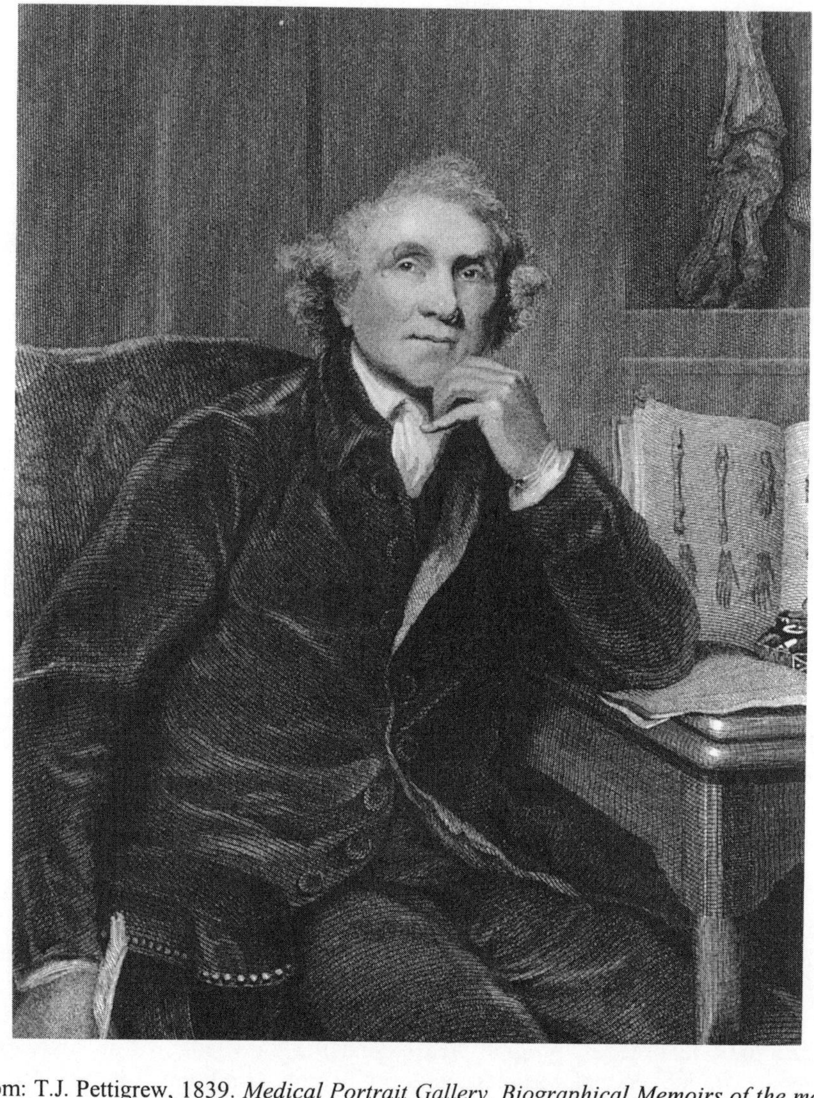

From: T.J. Pettigrew, 1839. *Medical Portrait Gallery. Biographical Memoirs of the most celebrated Physicians, Surgeons, etc. etc. who have contributed to the Advancement of Medical Science.* 4 Volumes (Volumes 1 and 2 bound together; Volumes 3 and 4 bound together) (London: Fisher, Son & Co.), Volume 2, engraving after a painting by Sir Joshua Reynolds.

It should also be noted that John Hunter's older brother, William, though far less well known these days, was an extremely distinguished anatomist, surgeon, and obstetrician. His principal claim to fame is within the field of medical education—he lectured at his extramural anatomical school in Great Windmill Street in the West End of London six days each week from October to May, for usually several hours each day, as well as spending many additional hours each day in preparing anatomical specimens and supervising students. He also carried out and supervised scientific research, and had an enormous obstetric practice. This included the appointment of physician-in-extraordinary to Queen Charlotte from 1762, and he supervised her many subsequent pregnancies.[50] He earned a great deal of money, principally from his private practice, but was also an astute collector, acknowledged antiquarian, and successful dealer on the money market. During his life, both his extensive library and his museum specimens were available to any scholars who could make use of them.[51] Much of his enormous collection of anatomical and pathological specimens, many of which relate to obstetrics, was given to the University of Glasgow, and most of these specimens are still displayed in the Museum of the Department of Anatomy.[52] What remain of his other collections formed the basis of the Hunterian Museum in Glasgow University. Most of his money was also left to the University to establish bursaries and scholarships in his memory.

The trustees of John Hunter's museum also proposed that a new building be erected to accommodate the museum, and a grant for this purpose was obtained from the government. The building was completed in 1813, at a final cost of over £49,000.[53] The collection was enormously enlarged and enhanced at various times during the 19th century by the purchase of a considerable number of private collections, including those of Liston and Sir Astley Cooper. Unfortunately, much of the collection was lost in the bombing of the College in May 1941. Of Hunter's original collection of 13,682 preparations, only 3,466 remain, of which 1,664 are included in the physiological and 1,605 in the pathological series. The College also possesses a considerable collection of portraits of Hunter.[54]

At the age of 58, in 1786, having suffered from angina for over 12 years, John Hunter was recalled from half-pay to be appointed deputy surgeon general, on the death of Mr. Middleton. This was at the height of his clinical and scientific career in London. He had been elected Fellow of the Royal Society in 1768, surgeon to St. George's Hospital in 1769, and in 1776 surgeon extra-ordinary to the King. In 1786, it was a time of peace, and Adair had been appointed surgeon general in the same year. In 1790, on Adair's death, Hunter was appointed surgeon general, and combined this post with that of inspector of regimental hospitals. It has been suggested that Hunter may have been involved from 1781 in discussions involving amending the system of promotion in the army, changes that were eventually implemented when he became surgeon general.

While Hunter's principal aim was to improve the professional standing of the regimental surgeons, the changes he recommended indicated that while he may have been a surgeon by profession, he was also an extremely able military administrator. Hunter recommended that the experience an individual gained as a regimental surgeon in all parts of the world would provide that individual with adequate training to become a military physician. He believed that the experience gained in this role more than compensated for any lack of academic medical qualifications. He also instituted the following changes, with the support of the government. He changed the system whereby commanding officers could appoint their own hospital mates to vacancies as regimental surgeons in their own regiments, insisting that only a professional person be qualified to judge an individual's suitability for such an appointment. He promoted regimental mates to hospital mates to broaden their experience, and only after hospital physicians and surgeons had recommended hospital mates would they be considered for promotion to regimental surgeons. Because of the lack of surgical experience of most candidates, Hunter was happy to promote regimental surgeons to the rank of physician, and to encourage good potential surgeons, he created the new rank of staff surgeon.

He also took steps to widen recruitment into the service. Formerly, candidates had to appear before the surgeon general in London. This arrangement was amended, in that candidates could appear in Dublin and, in special cases, in Edinburgh. The change probably encouraged many able Irish and Scottish candidates to apply for admission into the service. Many of these were well-qualified graduates, but of limited means.

He also insisted that the Treasury establish additional general hospitals to accommodate the invalids returning from the American War of Independence. In 1781, there were only three military hospitals of any size, at Portsmouth (for 60 patients), Chatham (for 60 patients), and Carisbrooke on the Isle of Wight (for a smaller number). In 1782, Adair pressed for the establishment of a larger hospital at Plymouth for 100 patients.

During Hunter's time in the service, the prospects for advancement were poor. The daily pay of a surgeon was 4/- (£73-0-0 per annum), and a surgeon in civil practice could easily earn four times this. The daily pay for a hospital mate was 2/6d, although this was increased to 3/6d (£63-17-6 per annum), because of the great difficulty encountered in recruiting suitably qualified candidates for these posts. Candidates entered the service either by purchase of a commission as a regimental surgeon or, if they did not have the appropriate funds, as a hospital mate. Candidates who could afford to pay the several hundred pounds required to purchase a commission were also required to have either a university degree or a license from one of the colleges of surgeons, and to pass an entrance examination held in the presence of the surgeon general. Those who entered as hospital mates often remained in this rank for 20 or more years, as in peacetime the opportunities for promotion were particularly poor. As warrant officers they had few rights, and could readily be dismissed from the service with no entitlement to half-pay. In times of war, the opportunities for promotion to surgeon, apothecary, or purveyor were far greater.[55]

Hunter's principal aim was to raise the status of medical officers. His sudden death in October 1793, after serving for only three years as surgeon general, deprived the army of an extremely innovative administrator. His biggest limitation was that he had been exposed only to a relatively short period of active service during war. His approach to surgery was extremely conservative, and he actively condemned what he termed "meddlesome surgery." He advocated leaving musket balls in nonlethal areas alone, and also was against the immediate amputation of limbs in all cases, preferring, where possible, to excise joints in order to preserve some limb function. His monograph *The Blood, Inflammation and Gun-Shot Wounds*,[56] published shortly after his death, was one of the most important works published at that time, and strongly advocated leaving well enough alone. Guthrie did not support many of the conservative views expressed by Hunter, particularly with regard to the treatment of gunshot injuries.[57]

GEORGE GUTHRIE, MILITARY SURGEON

George Guthrie (1785–1856) (see Figure 1.2)[58] was a particularly able and innovative military surgeon, and a contemporary of James McGrigor, a military surgeon of considerable experience (see later in this chapter) who was appointed director-general of the Army Medical Department by Wellington in 1815. Guthrie entered the army as an assistant surgeon to the 29th Regiment, in March 1801, having only one month earlier gained his membership of the Royal College of Surgeons, and while still under the age of 16. He then served in Canada for five years, before being ordered to the Peninsula where he remained, except for an interval in 1810, from 1808 to 1814. He took charge of the care of the wounded from many major battles, and was specifically commended by the Duke of Wellington for his services.

After a lengthy career in the Army Medical Department, having risen fairly rapidly through the ranks on the basis of merit alone, which included a period of active service in the Peninsula, Guthrie retired on half-pay in 1814. He then became a renowned lecturer on surgery, an activity that he pursued for almost 30 years. His lectures were particularly popular, as they were often interspersed with anecdotes from his career as a military surgeon in the Peninsula. He was also the founder and senior surgeon at the Royal Westminster Ophthalmic Hospital at Charing Cross. It was founded in December 1816 with the aid of Guthrie's friend Lord Lynedoch and under the auspices of the Duke of York and the Duke of Wellington, the latter acting as president of the hospital's board of management. He was additionally elected assistant surgeon to the Westminster Hospital in 1823 and full surgeon there in 1827; he resigned in 1843 to make way for his son who was also an accomplished surgeon.

From 1828 to 1831, he was professor of anatomy and surgery at the Royal College of Surgeons of England. From 1824, he was an active member of the College council, and was elected its president on three occasions, in 1833, 1841, and 1854. After his retirement from the army, in 1814, he attended the surgical lectures of Charles Bell and Benjamin Brodie at the Windmill Street School, where he had previously attended as a medical student, and those of Abernethy at St. Bartholomew's Hospital.

Figure 1.2. George James Guthrie

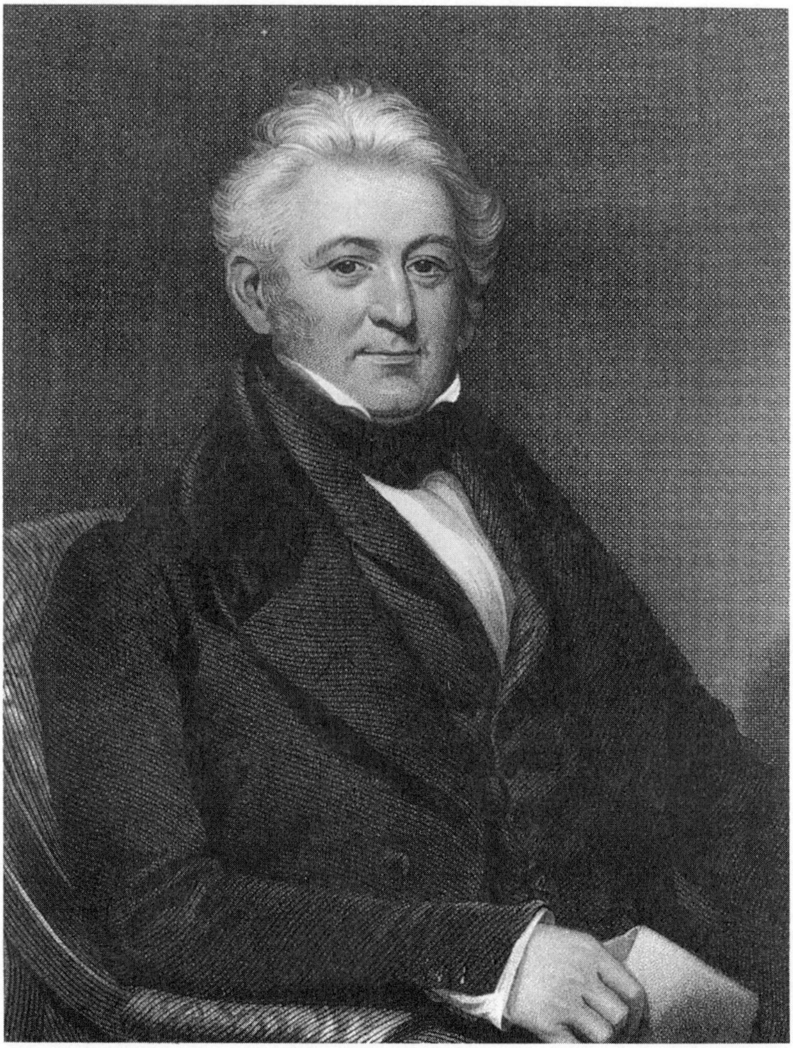

From: T.J. Pettigrew, 1839. *Medical Portrait Gallery. Biographical Memoirs of the most celebrated Physicians, Surgeons, etc. etc. who have contributed to the Advancement of Medical Science*. 4 Volumes (Volumes 1 and 2 bound together; Volumes 3 and 4 bound together) (London: Fisher, Son & Co.) Volume 4, engraving after a painting by H. Room.

Guthrie's particular skill was his ability to make considerable improvements in practical surgical procedures. He was invited by McGrigor to rejoin the Army Medical Department for six months in 1815 and by others for shorter periods of time, but he declined. He nevertheless visited Brussels shortly after Waterloo, where his advice on the management of surgical cases was greatly appreciated. While there, he is said to have operated on only two patients. On one occasion, he successfully amputated a lower limb of a French prisoner-of-war, François de Gay, through the hip joint.[59] On the other occasion, he ligated the artery of the leg by dividing the calf muscles. Both of these cases were sent to York Hospital in London to continue under his clinical care. A third man was also sent to London under Guthrie's care. A musket ball had entered the man's bladder and formed the nucleus for a bladder stone, which Guthrie successfully extracted in front of a large crowd of onlookers.

The Duke of York, who took a particular interest in the amputee, specially visited all three cases. Because the amputee (François de Gay) was French, the Duke personally wrote to Marshal Soult, and the man was transferred to the Hôtel des Invalides, and was for many years the only individual who had survived this operation in France. According to the *Lancet*,[60] Baron Larrey had performed this operation before Guthrie, "but he never had the good fortune to succeed in bringing one to France." Guthrie was later to recommend that in similar circumstances, the head and neck of the femur should be removed, to avoid amputation through the thigh, as this was likely to be a less traumatic procedure.[61]

Guthrie continued to maintain a connection with the army at York Hospital in London, where many of the wounded from the Peninsula had been sent, and for two years he was in clinical charge of two wards. He regularly demonstrated surgical cases to newly commissioned medical officers, while his lectures on surgery given over a period of almost 30 years were open to medical officers of all services without fee.[62] While at York Hospital, he was the first to use a lithotrite to crush a bladder stone in situ. During this period he was offered a knighthood by the Duke of York, but declined it because of his lack of funds.

Guthrie was also an authoritative author of some 10 books. His first definitive work was on gunshot wounds of the limbs,[63] in which he advocated immediate amputation carried out on the battlefield. This work went into three editions, and was also translated into German in 1821. In the 1820s and 1830s, he published a series of books and articles on ophthalmic surgery,[64] and these were subsequently included in his *Lectures on the Operative Surgery of the Eye*.[65] He later published a compendium of his former published works, with new comments, entitled *Commentaries on the Surgery of the War*,[66] which was sometimes termed the fifth edition of this work, and a sixth edition was later published with comments on the surgery of the Crimean War.[67]

The slim volume Guthrie published in 1838[68] consisted of the seven lectures he delivered gratis to serving medical officers. These lectures, together with others, not published in this monograph, covered the whole field of surgery. In the preamble to this book he indicated that lecture courses such as his should be supported financially by the government: "which is done so in Edinburgh [in

Britain alone at that time] and by every Sovereign in the great capitals of Europe."[69] He emphasized that the principal aim of his lectures was to provide medical officers at home on periodic leave with the opportunity to catch up on the latest trends in surgical practice.

Guthrie also recommended that the government "Should appropriate a piece of ground in Downing Street, when the old houses between it and George Street are pulled down, for the erection of a Museum to house the specimens at that time located at Chatham," particularly the specimens illustrating the "diseases of foreign climates, many of which are unknown in England, and which, from its situation [in Chatham] is comparatively of little use."

He continued that in addition to providing accommodation for a curator and other essential technical staff "Let them attach to this a Professor of Physic and another of Surgery, and they will render the country an inestimable benefit. . . . The expense need only be the difference between the half and the full-pay of these officers, and they may be otherwise employed in the public service. The saving would be that of a great number of lives. . . . It is thought proper to employ a gentleman of high character in his profession to teach the Veterinary Surgeons how to cure the Horses of the Army, and surely something of the same kind should be done for the Men."

Such views were clearly along the same lines as those espoused toward the end of the previous century by John Bell and others. It was only in Edinburgh, with the establishment of the Regius Chair of Military Surgery in 1806 and the appointment of John Thomson and his successor George Ballingall, that this recommendation had been put into practice.

A few years before Guthrie died, the fifth edition of his *Commentaries on the Surgery of the War* was published.[70] His exploits in the Peninsular War were well known and, as a result of an article in the *Lancet*,[71] almost legendary. In his *Introductory Lecture*[72] he was particularly critical of John Hunter and John Bell, both of whom he considered to be little more than amateurs, and whose views on military surgery were not supported by the experience Guthrie had gained over many years in the face of the enemy. Most of his views were expressed with the benefit of more than 25 years of hindsight. Despite their high reputation, Guthrie stated that:

> At the commencement of the war in Portugal, in 1808, there was little to depend on but the opinions of Mr. Hunter and of Mr. J. Bell. Mr. Hunter had served for a few weeks, in 1761, at the siege of Belleisle; and it was much to be regretted that his opportunities were not sufficiently numerous to enable him to draw such inferences from them as would have left but little to desire. . . . The prestige attached to his name was so great, as much to impede their progress on many essential points. Mr. John Bell had not the same opportunity of seeing an enemy, even at a distance, as was enjoyed by Mr. Hunter; and less reliance could be placed upon many of the recommendations of a man of the greatest ability, which were not supported by practical experience. . . . The confidence placed in the opinions of these, two of the greatest surgeons of the last century, was nevertheless so great, that it has cost me the labour of seven campaigns and thirty years of teaching to overcome all those which were erroneous. . . . It is only, however, during the last year I could have ventured to add, I have overcome all opposition; and that the principles and

the practice of the surgery of that war, as developed in the records I have published, are admitted by all to be, in the present state of our knowledge, correct.

Guthrie's obituary notice in the *Lancet*, though effusive, is extremely brief,[73] and needs to be read in conjunction with the biographical details of his career published in the *Lancet* some years earlier.[74] It is clear that many of Guthrie's deeds in the Peninsula, and in earlier campaigns, often, in his version at least, appeared to display the highest degree of heroism.

SIR CHARLES BELL, ANATOMIST, SCIENTIST, AND CIVIL SURGEON

Sir Charles Bell (1774–1842) (see Figure 1.3),[75] who from 1811 to 1826 co-owned and lectured at the Hunterian School in Windmill Street, was both a scientist and one of the foremost surgeons of his time. He had operated on the wounded after Waterloo, assisted by his brother-in-law, Dr. John Shaw (1792–1827). They arrived in Belgium 11 days after the battle and found many of the casualties, especially among the French, still unattended.[76] Bell is said to have attended 300 wounded principally in Brussels, a figure believed to relate to the number of operations he carried out.[77]

After Waterloo, it is recorded that in 146 primary amputations[78] there were 40 deaths (27.4%); in the three succeeding months there were 225 secondary amputations,[79] with 166 deaths (73.8%). Bell said that he could get little or no subsequent information on the result of his amputation cases after Waterloo, but that one prejudiced report had been circulated stating that only 5 survived out of 35 amputations he had performed. In reality, however, he had only performed 12 amputations in all! Dr Robert Knox, (successor to John Barclay as an extra-academical teacher of anatomy in Edinburgh), who was working in L'Hôpital de la Gendarmerie, commented on the extremely bad results of secondary amputation, saying Only one of C. Bell's lived.[80]

Both Bell and Shaw studied the effects of gunshot wounds. Bell had earlier published a monograph on this topic.[81] He had been at Portsmouth when the sick and wounded troops returned following their ignominious retreat to Corunna toward the end of January and the beginning of February 1809, with the loss of their commanding officer, Sir John Moore.

The military losses from Corunna were particularly high: 3,809 troops had died in battle, by the road or in the hospital, and 2,189 were sent as prisoners to France. Of the 28,000 that were disembarked by the English fleet, on their arrival, 4,035 men were listed as sick. Of the 2,427 of the Corunna sick hospitalized in Portsmouth, 405 died, mostly from dysentery, fever, ulcers (probably scorbutic) and pneumonia.[82]

Charles Bell's erroneous reputation as a military surgeon is principally based on his activities after the battle of Waterloo, in which he tended to the wounded in Brussels and in Antwerp. Bell also prepared an impressive series of preliminary sketches directly from his observations made at Haslar after the withdrawal from Corunna in 1809.[83] Charles Bell was a civil surgeon, and at

Figure 1.3. Sir Charles Bell

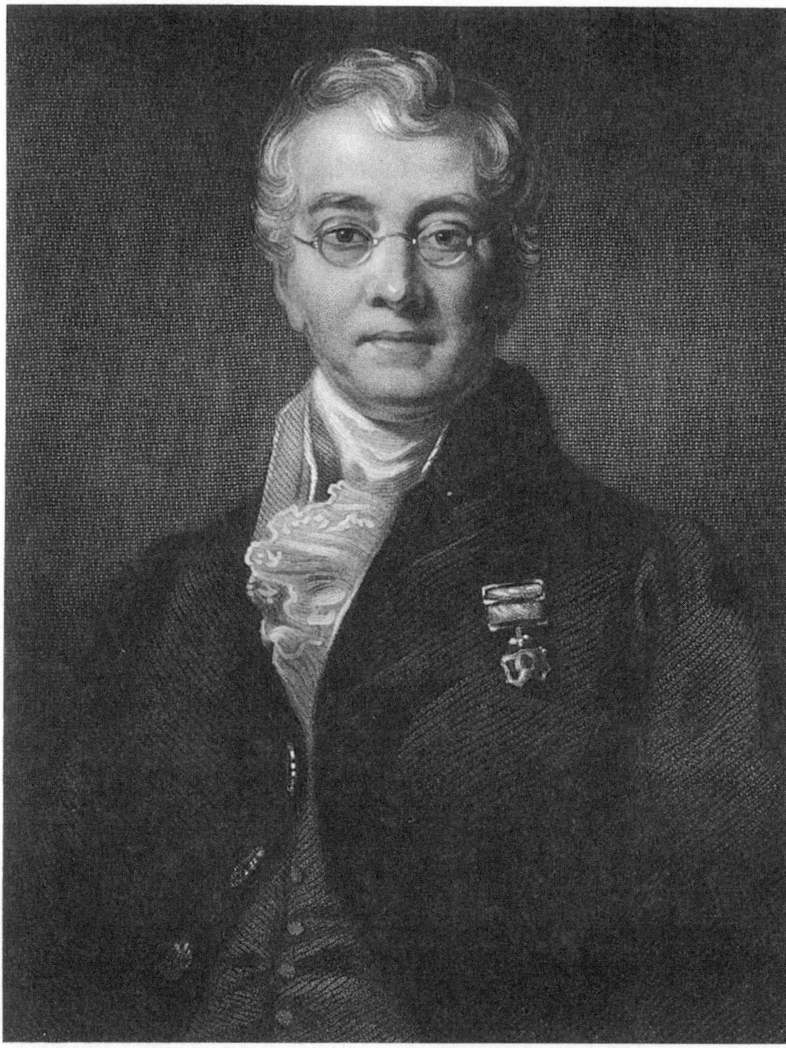

From: T.J. Pettigrew, 1839. *Medical Portrait Gallery. Biographical Memoirs of the most celebrated Physicians, Surgeons, etc. etc. who have contributed to the Advancement of Medical Science.* 4 Volumes (Volumes 1 and 2 bound together; Volumes 3 and 4 bound together) (London: Fisher, Son & Co.), Volume 3, engraving after a painting by Ballantyne.

most an individual with a keen sense of duty; he was on no account a military surgeon, and never claimed to be one. His experience in the field was extremely slight when compared with such professional military men as Dr. G. J. Guthrie, Sir John Pringle, Sir James McGrigor (1771–1858),[84] John Hennen,[85] the author of *Practice of Military Surgery*,[86] and many others.

MILITARY ADMINISTRATORS OF THE 18TH AND EARLY 19TH CENTURIES

During the second half of the 18th and early part of the 19th centuries, the army was fortunate to possess a considerable number of extremely able clinician-administrators. Two of the most notable in this regard were Sir John Pringle (1707–1782) and Sir James McGrigor (1771–1858), both of whom played important roles in improving the general conditions of service of the men. In the case of Drs. Robert Hamilton (1749–1830) and John Hennen (1779–1828), it was probably more as a consequence of their writing than of their rank in the military hierarchy.

Sir John Pringle

John Pringle (1707–1782) (see Figure 1.4)[87] played a critical role in improving the management of the military hospitals in Flanders during the war of the Austrian Succession. He attempted to eliminate overcrowding and the spread of infection principally through the segregation of men with hospital fever (i.e., typhus) and dysentery, both of which were capable of decimating whole armies, from other patients suffering from noninfectious conditions, such as fatigue, or battle casualties. He also introduced a range of relatively simple practical sanitary measures, and by this means was able to achieve a dramatic reduction in mortality rates. Not surprisingly, his books were extremely influential during his lifetime and for many years after his death, most notably his *Observations on the Diseases of the Army in Camp and Garrison*.[88] This book went to seven editions during his life, and continued to be published for almost thirty years after his death.

Many biographical accounts emphasize the value of Pringle's pioneering public health measures, particularly with regard to the management of military personnel,[89] and he has, with justification, long been regarded as the founder of modern military medicine. His research *On Substances Resisting Putrefaction*, delivered to the Royal Society several years earlier,[90] in many ways anticipated the views of Lister on the antiseptic principle. For this work, Pringle was awarded the Copley Medal of the Royal Society. His critical appreciation that jail fever was identical to hospital fever was also transmitted to the Royal Society at about this time.[91]

Pringle had been sent to Edinburgh University with the intention of entering commerce, but left after a year to study in Amsterdam, ostensibly to gain a sound knowledge of business. While there, he visited Leyden, where he attended a lecture on medicine delivered by the celebrated Boerhaave. This so impressed

Figure 1.4. John Pringle

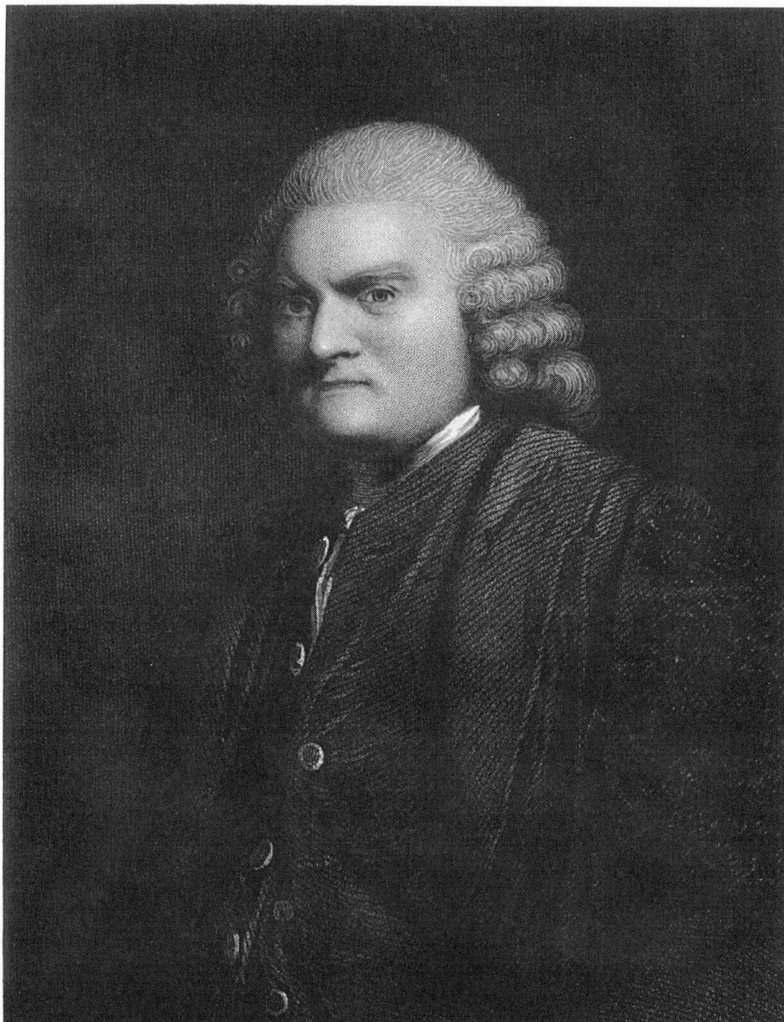

From: T.J. Pettigrew, 1839. *Medical Portrait Gallery. Biographical Memoirs of the most celebrated Physicians, Surgeons, etc. etc. who have contributed to the Advancement of Medical Science.* 4 Volumes (Volumes 1 and 2 bound together; Volumes 3 and 4 bound together) (London: Fisher, Son & Co.), Volume 2, engraving after a painting by Sir Joshua Reynolds.

Pringle that he decided to pursue a medical career, and in 1730 graduated with the M.D. degree from Leyden University. He completed his medical studies in Paris, then returned to Edinburgh and, for a few years, practiced there as a physician before being appointed in 1734 joint professor of pneumatics (i.e., metaphysics) and moral philosophy.

In 1742, Pringle was appointed both physician to the Earl of Stair, commander of the British forces on the Continent, and physician to the military hospital in Flanders. He received a salary of 20 shillings a day for the latter appointment, and was also entitled to half-pay for life.[92] Somewhat surprisingly, he was not required to resign from his professorship, and two deputies performed his lectures and other academic duties.

It has been suggested that his action in suggesting to his commanding officer, the Earl of Stair, that the military hospitals of both sides in the conflict should be regarded as neutral, and mutually protected, foreshadowed the modern Geneva Convention.[93] Unfortunately this arrangement between the British and French sides was of only brief duration.

When his patron, the Earl of Stair, retired, Pringle was promoted, by the Duke of Cumberland, physician-general to the forces in Flanders, and it was only then that he resigned from his professorship. He accompanied his commander-in-chief to Scotland, and was present, in 1745, at Culloden. For the following three years, he attended the British army on the Continent. On his return to Britain, while remaining in the army, he began practicing as a physician in London. In 1761 he was appointed physician-in-ordinary to the Queen and in 1774 physician to the King. He had, in 1766, been created a baronet. In 1772, for his services to science, he was elected president of the Royal Society, having been elected a Fellow in 1745. By this time he had gained an international reputation for his scientific research, and in 1778 he was chosen one of the eight members of the Academy of Sciences at Paris. He died in 1782.

Sir James McGrigor

James McGrigor (1771–1858) (see Figure 1.5)[94] initially attended the Marischal College, Aberdeen, where he obtained his M.A. degree in 1788. Once he had decided upon a career in medicine, he walked to Edinburgh where he attended, from 1789 to 1791, several classes in the university.[95]

Shortly after he returned to Aberdeen (in 1792), the French Revolution broke out, and then his principal wish was to become an army surgeon. He went to London, where he attended Mr. Wilson's lectures on anatomy. On September 13, 1793, he obtained, by purchase, the post of surgeon to an Irish corps, De Burgh's Regiment, later called the 88th or Connaught Rangers. He served in Flanders, and returned with the regiment to Southampton. In 1795 McGrigor was posted to the West Indies, but was shipwrecked when on the way to Grenada with a detachment of the 25th Regiment. He was rescued, and after service in Grenada and St. Vincent, returned home in 1796.

In 1798 McGrigor traveled with the 88th Regiment to Bombay and in 1801 proceeded to Ceylon. He was put in charge of a force of 8,000 European and

Figure 1.5. Sir James McGrigor

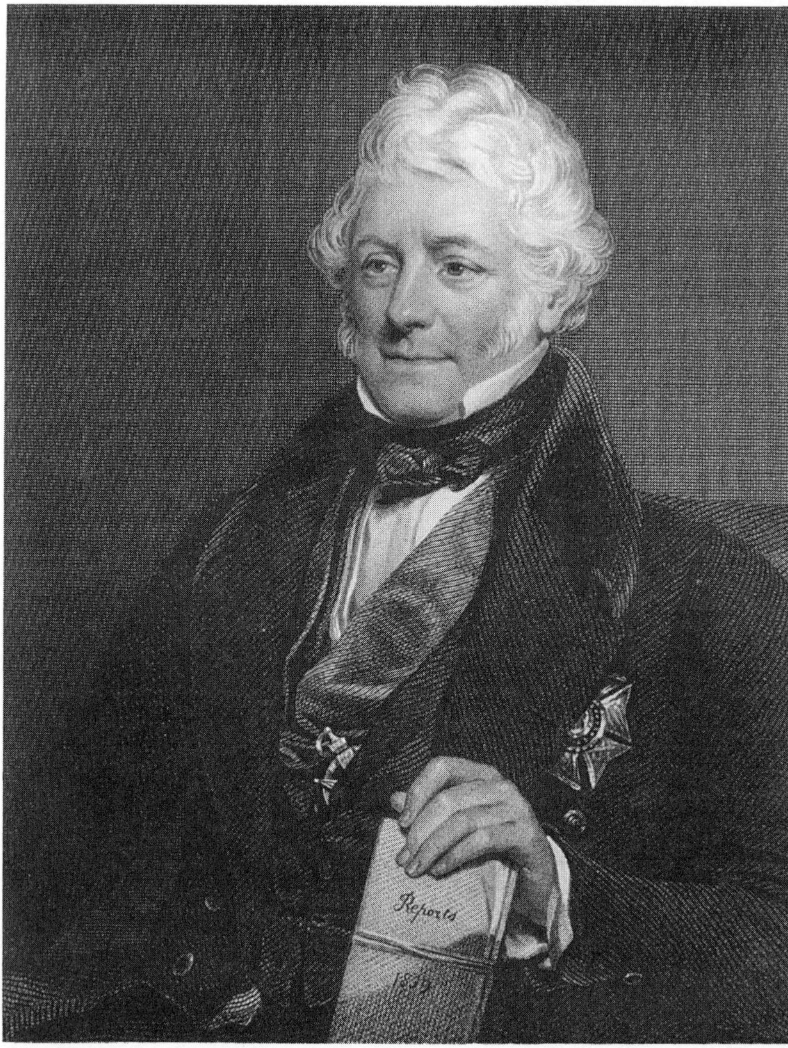

From: T.J. Pettigrew, 1839. *Medical Portrait Gallery. Biographical Memoirs of the most celebrated Physicians, Surgeons, etc. etc. who have contributed to the Advancement of Medical Science.* 4 Volumes (Volumes 1 and 2 bound together; Volumes 3 and 4 bound together) (London: Fisher, Son & Co.), Volume 4, engraving after a painting by H. Room.

Indian troops sent to the Red Sea to join the army in Egypt under the command of Major-General David Baird.

On his return to England, McGrigor transferred to the Blues (Royal Horse Guards), serving with them in Canterbury and at Windsor. At that time, Lord Melville had tried, unsuccessfully, to place McGrigor at the head of the Medical Board. In 1804 McGrigor proceeded to M.D. at Marischal College, Aberdeen, and in 1805 was promoted to one of the inspector generals of hospitals of the northern district, headquartered in York. He was then transferred to the southwest district, with headquarters at Winchester, where the Duke of York noted the improvements he introduced in the service. Later, McGrigor took charge of the Portsmouth and Isle of Wight areas. He also looked after the troops who had returned from Corunna, many of whom had typhus fever.

Before he could be appointed principal medical officer of the Portuguese army, McGrigor was dispatched to Walcheren, where many of the troops were suffering from malarial fever. By the time the island was eventually evacuated, the death toll from malaria was close to 4,000 men. On the way there in H.M.S. *Venerable*, at the mouth of the Scheldt, he was again shipwrecked. He, with others, was eventually rescued, but all were in a state of extreme exhaustion. After his work at Walcheren, McGrigor was promoted in 1809 to the rank of inspector general of hospitals, and in 1811 he returned to Portsmouth, where he was appointed physician in charge of the garrison there.

Wellington was particularly concerned about the welfare of his men, and sent a request to H.R.H. the Duke of York that "he be sent an Inspector-General of the Army Medical Department, in whose talents and judgement he could place his entire confidence, to supervise the Medical Department of the army under his command." This would be in place of Dr. Frank, who was at that time incapacitated by illness. The Duke responded in a dispatch from Frenada, dated October 30, 1811, that he "should have the most active and intelligent person that can be found to fill his station."[96]

McGrigor had previously served with Wellington in India, and was requested to proceed to Wellington's headquarters in the Peninsula. He arrived there early in 1812. With Wellington's support, as commander-in-chief, McGrigor introduced long-needed reforms into the medical service: he improved the conditions in the hospitals and the diet of the men, and introduced separate wards to stem the spread of infectious diseases. Wellington considered McGrigor, "one of the most industrious, able, and successful public servants I have ever met with."[97]

As a result of McGrigor's outstanding achievements during the Peninsular War and due to Wellington's influence, he was knighted, and in June 1815 was appointed to the newly created position of director-general of the Army Medical Department. Shortly after Waterloo, large numbers of medical officers were either permanently removed from the service or put on half-pay.

McGrigor's appointment had been made only after he had displayed his organizational skills during his period of office as Wellington's senior medical officer during the Peninsular campaign, qualities that had been recognized the previous year (1814) by the award of a knighthood (Knight Bachelor). He had been taken out of retirement to run the medical services of the army. He had been retired in 1814, with an allowance of £3 per day, then restored to active service to the newly created post of director-general of the Army Medical Department with a salary of £2,000 a year, associated with the rank of major general. During the following year he founded the Museum of Natural History and Pathological Anatomy and the great reference library at Fort Pitt, Chatham. Shortly afterward, he inaugurated "a system of medical reports and returns from all military stations, which, twenty years later, formed the basis of the 'Statistical Returns of the Health of the Army,' now perpetuated in the annual blue-books of the army medical department."[98]

One of McGrigor's principal claims to fame was his skill in organizing the efficient removal of the wounded from the battlefield. This was something Larrey had taken great pains to organize during Napoleon's various campaigns from the end of the previous century, and the benefits of which had failed to percolate through to the British high command.[99] McGrigor's action in this regard was a direct consequence of his and his medical staff's distress at seeing the delay in the rescuing, hospitalization, and treatment of the British, and even more so of the French, wounded following Waterloo. McGrigor's major reforms have been summarized by Blair,[100] and are as follows:

1. The education of medical officers, after their selection. He personally screened applicants.
2. The support of the Chair of Military Surgery at Edinburgh, and the establishment of the Chair in Dublin.
3. Assistance to widows and dependants.
4. Research into all aspects of army health.
5. Statistics—perhaps as important as any.
6. Royal Commission for medical officers.

McGrigor was particularly distressed by the lack of appreciation by the senior staff officers of the disproportionately high proportion of the casualties incurred by the junior officers compared to their relatively small numbers, when compared to the injuries sustained by the sergeants and other ranks. Similar detailed findings from the Carlist War of 1835–1837 emphasize this point.[101] McGrigor also strongly believed that the Sovereign should award some deserving army surgeons, like other meritorious serving officers, military decorations. He was subsequently, in 1831, made a baronet, but it was not until 1850, for the first time in the history of the British army, that six army surgeons were awarded the military division of the Order of the Bath. McGrigor was created a knight commander of that Order in 1850, having previously been awarded the Turkish Order of the Crescent, the Commander's Cross of the Portuguese Tower and Sword, and the Peninsular War Medal with five clasps. McGrigor was for 35 years director-general of the Army Medical Department, during a lengthy period of peace. He was eventually allowed to retire from the army in 1851, and died in London in 1858, aged 87.[102]

McGrigor's Attempts to Improve the Academic Standard of Medical Officers in the Army

Shortly after his appointment as director-general, McGrigor made vigorous efforts to improve the academic standard of those personnel who remained in the service. Many medical officers had been retired from the service because of their age, due to infirmity, or because of evidence of incompetence. He was insistent that advance in the service would henceforth be achieved only on evidence of merit. One way of demonstrating a willingness to improve was by gaining a university degree. It was recommended that those intending to become a specialist surgeon or physician should pass the fellowship examination of one of the Royal Colleges of Surgeons, or an equivalent examination of one of the Colleges of Physicians. An article dated September 30, 1816 published in the *Edinburgh Medical and Surgical Journal* recommended:

The Army Medical Board, solicitous for the improvement of the department in its various branches, and considering the present a favourable opportunity for the selection and encouragement of well educated persons, have thought it advisable to promulgate the courses of instruction, and the qualifications required from gentlemen entering the medical department of the army, and during the progress of advancement in the service.

For Hospital Assistant.

The candidates for this first commissioned appointment in the medical department, must produce certificates of regular study . . . at an established school of eminence.

The practice of medicine and surgery in an hospital or infirmary at least one year, with a regular apprenticeship, or three years without an apprenticeship; in which case a certificate of having studied practical pharmacy will be required. Regimental medical officers should also be acquainted with midwifery [as well as having evidence of attending] public establishments for diseases of eyes, and mental derangement.

A liberal education is indispensably requisite; and the greater the attainments of the candidate are in the various branches of science, in addition to competent professional knowledge, the more eligible will he be deemed for promotion.

Promotion to Regimental Surgeon.

Every gentleman must have served five years at least in the junior appointments, before he can be promoted to the rank of regimental surgeon; and he who gives the best proofs of diligent exertions in the performance of his public duty, and of attention in the acquirement of practical knowledge, will be noted as the most eligible candidate for advancement.

Gentlemen already in the service are earnestly recommended to avail themselves of every opportunity to adding to their knowledge, by attending universities or schools: for which purpose, every facility will be offered by the Director-General. They are especially desired to transmit to this Office, certificates of such classes as they may have attended subsequently to their examinations before this board, either on professional or other branches of science, that the same may be duly registered.

Medical officers are encouraged and recommended to look forward to the appointments of surgeon [or physician] to the forces; and to endeavour especially to qualify themselves for either, according to the bent of their inclinations, and to their previous study.

Advancement to either Surgeon or Physician to the Forces.

For commission of Surgeon to the Forces, it will hereafter be expected that the candidate shall have attended a public hospital three years, one of which must have been passed in London; and a diploma from the Royal College of Surgeons of London will always be respected.

The rank of Physician to the Forces requires, in addition to the knowledge and experience to be gained in the regular progress of study and of service, that the candidate should be a licentiate of the Royal College of Physicians of London, or a graduate of the University of Oxford, Cambridge, Edinburgh, Dublin, or Glasgow. The licence of the London College of Physicians will always be considered a great recommendation to those who have the other requisite qualifications.

It is to be understood that candidates who have received regular education in foreign universities, or other schools of acknowledged celebrity, will be admitted to examination.[103]

A considerable number of the medical officers took up the challenge. Of just over 1,300 men who entered the service between 1806 and 1823 without either a university degree or a fellowship diploma, just under 200 (about 15% of this group) gained a university degree or a fellowship of one of the Royal Colleges of Surgeons after entering the service. Out of over 900 men in the 1823–1854 group who entered the service with the minimal entrance qualification over this period, only just over 9% followed this route, and obtained a university degree or fellowship diploma.

Attendance at either Thomson's or Ballingall's three-month winter lecture course of military surgery in Edinburgh was also accepted as evidence of commitment, and considerable numbers of men were given leave to attend these sessions. In order to justify this leave of absence, it is likely that they would have been expected to pass the examination at the end of the course, possibly at a higher level than might have been expected of the average undergraduate.

For those gentlemen who aspired to a career in the Army Medical Department, the relatively few places available in the post-Waterloo army meant that McGrigor could now select only the most promising of the candidates. While formerly there were few restrictions on those who entered the service, this was no longer the case. Candidates for admission now had to sit an entrance examination and be interviewed before a board of three senior medical officers. If the candidate was accepted, he was then sent to Fort Pitt, Chatham, for a period of between four and nine months, before being sent to a regiment. The great advantage of this approach was that at Fort Pitt the young medical officers had access to an extensive library and a museum with anatomical and pathological specimens. More particularly, they had the opportunity to see patients with a wide variety of clinical conditions, including tropical diseases, not normally seen in the course of their previous hospital practice.

According to McGrigor, the young military surgeon in training: "Has an opportunity of seeing disease with their various shades from all parts of the world. He has at Chatham an admirable opportunity of studying . . . the morbid structure, the result of disease to which soldiers are subject . . . and in comparing them with the records of each case to see the causes of a fatal termination."[104]

During the inter-war period, Fort Pitt also provided McGrigor and his colleagues with an opportunity to offer the principally Scottish and Irish recruits guidance on etiquette that would allow them more easily to mingle with their combatant colleagues in the regimental messes which they would shortly be joining. It was also hoped that this would help to disguise the often humbler origin of the majority of the medical staff compared to those that they were likely to encounter in the other branches of the service.[105]

THE ARMY MEDICAL BOARD (1793–1809)

On Hunter's death in 1793, the Secretary for War established an Army Medical Board[106] to supervise all aspects of the administration of the service. Three eminent civilian clinicians were appointed. Two had no military experience whatsoever, while the third individual was a retired medical officer with minimal administrative experience. The Board got off to an unfortunate start when Sir Clifton Wintringham, their senior member, died shortly after taking up the post of physician-general. He was not universally liked, and Fergusson, for example, described him as "An old broken-down court-physician of London, upon a claim of having accompanied the expedition to Cuba, some forty years antecedently, [who] was appointed director-general."[107]

Sir Lucas Pepys, physician-in-ordinary to the King, soon replaced him. Mr. John Gunning was appointed surgeon general. He was a civilian surgeon at St. George's Hospital, and during 1789–1790 had been master of the Surgeons' Company.[108] The third appointee was Mr. Thomas Keate, a surgeon at the Royal Hospital at Chelsea, and a former regimental surgeon to the Foot Guards. He was appointed inspector of regimental infirmaries. These posts were part-time, and were paid at the handsome rate of £2 per day, despite the fact that they all spent the majority of their time attending to their other clinical activities. Keate, in addition to being a surgeon at the Royal Hospital at Chelsea, on a salary of £100 per annum, was also additional surgeon to the Queen and to the Prince of Wales.[109] He also operated at the York Military Hospital, for which he received £700 per annum in peacetime and £900 per annum during times of war. He was also inspector of the National CowPox Establishment, surgeon to St. George's Hospital and examiner to the College of Surgeons. His official emoluments were believed to amount to more than £1,800 per annum, to which must be added a great deal more received from his private practice.

The duties of the Board were extremely wide-ranging. They were expected to supervise the entire administrative machinery of the Medical Department of the Army, although otherwise they had minimal powers. Considering that their appointments to the Board were only part-time, and that they had minimal secretarial back up, it is only surprising that the Army Medical Board survived as long as it did without causing complete chaos to the system. The three members of the Board were eventually dismissed in 1809, but by this time the damage they had done to the morale of the medical officers in the medical branch of the service was considerable.

One of Sir Lucas Pepys' particularly arbitrary decisions soon after his appointment was that only men with an Oxbridge medical degree associated with a diploma from the London College of Physicians would be eligible for appointment as physicians within the service. This effectively excluded virtually every regimental surgeon in the service from applying for promotion. The only eligible candidates were recent Oxbridge graduates who had no military experience. These individuals were duly appointed to senior administrative positions over men with considerable military experience. Not surprisingly, this soon led to a great deal of bad feeling in the service and a breakdown of goodwill between the ranks. William Fergusson[110] was particularly critical of this decision. In his autobiography he noted:

> The physician general at home had pronounced his fiat against employing any other but graduates of the English Universities in treating the diseases of soldiers at the military hospitals [This same Physician-General, when at an after period he was ordered to proceed to the succour of the distressed army in Walcheren, refused to obey, putting on record his official declaration, that he had no knowledge of camp and contagious diseases]. The consequences were such as might have been foreseen. . . . The old medical officers were every where superseded by young men from the Universities, without the smallest advantage of clinical experience, or military medicine. Regimental hospitals were all but unknown, and in the general hospitals there was neither system, or code, or rule of management. . . . I verily believe no army ever exhibited in its hospitals a more lamentable spectacle of indiscipline and abuse.[111]

He continued as follows:

> The position of the young physicians . . . was pitiable and ridiculous. . . . Their station in society . . . proclaimed them to be a class far superior to what the army had commonly received. . . . To one of them I was attached in the first campaign. He could read Hippocrates in the original Greek, but he did not know the grain scales and weights when he saw them; and to have touched a bleeding wound, even while the sound of the cannon was booming in our ears, would have been to lose caste. He was my superior by at least four degrees of military rank, but I had to teach him what I myself was taught in the early days of my apprenticeship. . . . To have placed such a man over the heads of all who were experienced in military medicine and diseases, while he was not fit for any work, was as stupid and gross an abuse as could have been imposed on an army.[112]

The inspector of regimental infirmaries, the junior of the three appointments, had no authority to interfere with the administrative side of the regimental hospitals, as these were exclusively within the domain of the commanding officer of the regiment concerned, and regimental surgeons owed their exclusive allegiance to their commanding officers. He was principally concerned with the standard of medical care provided to the patients, their diet, and the quality of the medicines prescribed to them. By contrast, when the army was abroad on active service, it was the Board that selected which medical officers should serve in the general hospitals and supplied them with free medicines and their surgical equipment.[113]

Once an expedition had left British shores, the surgeon general took over, though there were invariably difficulties encountered in controlling the situation at such a great distance. Normally, the principal medical officers on the spot acted autonomously, promoting their own medical officers to vacancies as these arose, as these men were known entities with proven ability. Consequently, the medical officers appointed by the Board were often returned home, because there was no longer a role for them to play.

In times of war, the position was particularly difficult in that it was soon apparent that the Board was completely unable to cope with the administrative load imposed on them, even when the members of the Board worked together amicably. The Board was also expected to oversee the medical activities of the militia, and to organize the establishment of depots for the storage of hospital equipment and medicines in numerous centers throughout the country, in case of invasion.

They were also expected to organize the creation of general hospitals at each of the chief ports of embarkation. Such hospitals had already been established during the American War of Independence, in 1781, in Portsmouth and at Chatham. A new general hospital was built at Gosport near Portsmouth in 1796, and another was completed in Deal in 1797. Other hospitals, at Southampton and at Plymouth, were established in temporary accommodation, but were found to be far from satisfactory. Additional hospitals were subsequently opened, such as the York Hospital at Chelsea, which by 1799 could accommodate 500 patients, and others at Newport on the Isle of Wight, at Chatham, and at Eling, near Southampton. While some members of the Board were in favor of general hospitals, many senior medical officers, including McGrigor and Jackson, were against them. This was principally on the grounds that the mortality rates in these large hospitals tended to be considerably higher than in the smaller regimental hospitals, and that the men would behave better when subject to regimental discipline. Many also believed that they served a useful purpose only during active service.

When Gunning died in 1798, Keate was appointed surgeon general, and he in turn was replaced as inspector of regimental infirmaries by Mr. John Rush, previously a surgeon with the Horse Grenadier Guards. From 1798, the physician-general, the surgeon general, and the inspector of regimental infirmaries were each given a different remit, which meant that they could function entirely independently. As a result, while they previously used to meet on a regular basis, this was now no longer necessary and set the seed for the Board's final dissolution. The physician-general, as the senior of the three members of the Board, appointed the physicians, while the surgeon general controlled the appointment of the regimental and assistant surgeons, as well as overseeing all medical arrangements for overseas expeditions. The inspector of regimental infirmaries, as the junior appointee, nominated all apothecaries, purveyors, and hospital mates. This division of labor, even with regard to the appointment of medical staff, proved unrealistic, as all appointments were necessarily inter-dependent. As might have been expected, military experience counted for little and many appointments resulted from influence or through nepotism.

Rush died in 1801, and was replaced by Francis Knight, previously a regimental surgeon in the Guards who, like his other colleagues, had never held senior administrative rank in the service. He was appointed inspector of regimental infirmaries, and considered that his principal role was to save the government money by whatever means possible and, because of his bullying personality, he frequently attempted to exercise excessive control over the activities of the Board. Acting on his own initiative, between 1802 and 1806, he closed the general hospitals at Gosport, Plymouth, and Deal. While this action was supported by many regimental surgeons, it proved to be a particularly disastrous decision, for in 1809, when over 4,000 soldiers arrived at Portsmouth from Spain with typhus, the medical officers were unable to find adequate accommodation for them except in the local civilian hospitals. This disaster was averted only by the prompt actions of McGrigor, who was then inspector general of hospitals of the South-West District. The only reason the York Hospital was not closed was because it was where the recently commissioned medical officers were sent to receive their initial instructions in military practice.

Knight was overbearing, ambitious, and discourteous to his colleagues on the Board, and the rivalry between them only increased their inefficiency. Pepys and Keate, the two longest-serving members of the Board, both blamed Knight for not acting in the best interests of the soldiers. All of these differences of opinion were brought to a head in 1809 by the medical and administrative problems associated with the expedition to the island of Walcheren. Neither the physician-general nor the surgeon general wished to visit the island to see the conditions that led to the death of over 4,000 men, and the invaliding out of the army of a further 11,000 men, from what was termed polder or Walcheren fever, a type of malaria. At about the same time, thousands of fever cases, including many with typhus, were disembarked in Portsmouth after the retreat to Corunna.

According to Fortescue:

> The Duke of York could find no words hard enough for the Medical Board; and the climax came when, amid all the anxiety and wretchedness caused by the fatal epidemic during the expedition to the Scheldt, the three members remained comfortably in London and refused to transport their precious bodies to the front. It may indeed be pleaded for them that they were not young, and would have been absolutely useless even if they had repaired to Holland; but their attitude of helpless yet complacent expectation was not calculated to endear them to the Army or to the public.[114]

As a direct consequence of the maladministration of the Board during the Walcheren affair, the government set up a Commission of Enquiry. This had a particularly wide remit, and was also empowered to investigate the involvement of patronage and favoritism in medical appointments. The Commission noted that the financial savings achieved by Knight had been made only because of the provision of inadequate and poor food for the sick and wounded men. Equally, the medical staff had insufficient quantities of good quality medicines at their disposal. The Commission concluded that the gross inefficiency of the Board was directly responsible for the unnecessary loss of thousands of soldiers' lives each year. This clearly complements the oft-quoted contemporary view of Napier:

> Nay, many even of the well-educated surgeons sent out were for some time of little use, for superior professional skill is of little value in comparison of experience in military

arrangement; where one soldier died for want of a delicate operation, hundreds perish from the absence of military arrangement. War tries the strength of the military frame-work; it is in peace that the frame-work itself must be formed, otherwise barbarians would be the leading soldiers of the world; a perfect army can only be made by civil institutions, and those, rightly considered, would tend to confine the horrors of war to the field of battle, which would be the next best thing to the perfection of civilization that would prevent war altogether.[115]

The Board's position was indefensible. It was impossible to justify their extravagance in the provision of medicines and surgical instruments that were held in the army stores at Porchester. Over 1,100 cases of surgical instruments and 1,300 sets of pocket instruments were held in stock there. Since regimental surgeons had to purchase their own instruments, the items in stock could only be for the general hospital system. The Commission argued that there was no good reason why staff surgeons employed in the general hospitals should not, like the regimental surgeons, provide their own surgical instruments.

The Commission reported that the members of the Board had shown a lack of proper control in many of their activities, that unnecessary appointments had been made, and that their criteria for making some of these appointments were irregular. They indicated that general hospitals had been opened unnecessarily, and that wastage had occurred in relation to the accumulation of medical stores. This argument was difficult to sustain, because the Board was only acting under instructions they had received from the War Office. While the War Office was supportive of the closing of the various general hospitals indicated above, because of the financial savings involved, it actively supported the establishment of temporary general hospitals, particularly when the fear of invasion was at its greatest.

The antagonism that existed among the different members of the Board clearly had a detrimental effect on its efficiency. Only one solution was available to the Commission; they immediately dissolved the Board. The secretary of the Board had been dismissed for accepting fees from candidates, and it had even been suggested that Mr. Keate had accepted bribes. All the documentation relating to these adverse criticisms of the members of the Board had, conveniently, been lost in a fire in 1803.

A new Board was established in 1810, consisting entirely of senior regular military medical officers, all of whom had both substantial military and administrative experience. It was also decided that in the future there would be no more part-time civilians appointed to the Board.

With the dissolution of the Medical Board and its damning report, it might reasonably have been expected that the wastage of medical supplies, the tremendous loss of life, and even higher number of those invalided out of the service might have had a deep impact on the authorities. Medical transport was in all regards inadequate, and the hospital facilities to receive the sick were grossly inadequate. If changes were instituted, the memory of the errors made during this debacle was short-lived.

The first chairman of the new Board was John Weir, shortly afterward to be elected director-general of the Army Medical Department. He had seen active service in North America (1776) and Jamaica (1784), later becoming purveyor of hospital medicines and stores in Jamaica (1790). He rose to inspector general in 1795, and went on half-pay in 1798. He returned to full-pay as director-general in February 1810, and finally retired in 1815. He acquired the M.D. degree (honorary) from King's College, Aberdeen, in 1794.[116] When Weir died in 1819, McGrigor succeeded him as director-general.

Weir had two very able and experienced assistants, Dr. Theodore Gordon and Dr. Charles (later Sir Charles) Ker (died 1837).[117] He became an assistant inspector of hospitals in 1799, but went on half-pay the same year. Over the next six years, he alternated between being on full-pay and half-pay on an almost annual basis. In 1805 he was appointed inspector of hospitals, and in February 1810 was appointed principal inspector in the Army Medical Department. He retired on half-pay in 1815, and was created a knight bachelor in 1822. He acquired his Edinburgh M.D. degree in 1787.

ANOMALOUS ARRANGEMENTS WITHIN THE ARTILLERY AND ENGINEER ARMS OF THE SERVICE—THE ORDNANCE MEDICAL DEPARTMENT

From as early as 1727, the artillery appointed its own medical officers. Because of the increasing importance of the artillery and the engineers, both of whom were under the direction of the master general of the ordnance, this led to the establishment of a separate medical department with its own surgeon general. The medical establishment for the Military Department of the Ordnance was formally established in 1797, and its arrangements were regularized by royal warrant in 1801. Because of the higher-than-average number of candidates who wished to enter this branch of the service, the medical establishment was able to select only those medical officers who possessed a license from the College of Surgeons, and who were of good moral character. The surgeon general, Dr. John Rollo, had sole authority over the administration of his men, and was assisted by his own inspector general of hospitals and a deputy inspector. In 1804, Rollo became both surgeon general and inspector of hospitals.

A new hospital was built at the Royal Artillery headquarters at Woolwich for the special needs of this branch of the service, and its facilities were significantly better than those in the other general hospitals in Britain at that time. The wards were small and were designed to accommodate only five or six patients, and each possessed excellent ventilation, vapor baths, showers, and even portable water closets. The hospital also had its own convalescent unit where the men were sent after release from the main hospital so that they did not need to return directly to duty.

During the Peninsular War, the first general hospital for the exclusive use of the Ordnance was established in Lisbon, with a staff of 18 medical officers, the most senior of whom also supervised the local battery hospitals. Despite its small size, the Ordnance Medical Department survived as an independent entity until 1853. It had been agreed with the War Office that the Army Medical Department would eventually absorb them, but only after the retirement of their director-general, who had been in their service for 55 years. This amalgamation with the much larger Army Medical Department was inevitable. Due to their small size, the prospects for promotion were extremely limited, and its administrative infrastructure excessively heavy. Despite this, the medical officers within the Ordnance Medical Department were reticent to amalgamate with the Army Medical Department. They believed that they would lose their identity and esprit de corps, and would have to serve under officers considerably junior to themselves, as the chances of promotion in the larger department were so much greater.

The total number of medical officers in the Ordnance Medical Department in 1806 was 30, and this rose to a maximum in 1814 of 103. In 1822, the number fell to 28, reflecting the government-imposed reduction in the size of the military establishment. It rose slowly to 38 in 1841 and to 47 in 1850, shortly before its amalgamation with the Army Medical Department.[118]

NOTES

1. J. Bell, 1800. *Memorial Concerning the Present State of Military and Naval Surgery. Addressed Several Years ago to the Right Honourable Earl Spencer, First Lord of the Admiralty; and now Submitted to the Public* (Edinburgh: Longman & Rees; London: Cadell & Davies) [41 pp.], pp. 39–40; K. MacLeod, 1906. Netley. *Caledonian Medical Journal* **6**, 379–390, p. 382; G. Ballingall, 1843. Instruction for medical officers of the army and navy. *Lancet* **I**, 268–270.

2. J.S.G. Blair, 1988. The Scots and military medicine. In: *The Influence of Scottish Medicine: An Historical Assessment of its International Impact.* Editor: D. E. Dow (Carnforth, Lancs.: Parthenon Publishing Group Ltd.), pp. 17–30.

3. E. D. Lowry, 1968. *Interior Ballistics: How a Gun Converts Chemical Energy into Projectile Motion* (New York: Doubleday & Company).

4. G. Keynes, 1968. *The Apologie and Treatise of Ambroise Paré, containing the Voyages made into Divers Places, with Many of his Writings Upon Surgery* (New York: Dover Publications).

5. According to Pepys in his diary entry of September 27, 1665: "Here I saw this week's Bill of Mortality, where in, blessed be God, there is above 1,800 decrease, being the first considerable decrease we have had." According to the footnote to this item, 5,553 deaths from the plague occurred in the week of September 19–26, and 7,615 had died in the previous week. See: R. Latham and W. Matthews, Eds. 1972. *The Diary of Samuel Pepys* (London: Bell & Hyman), Volume 6, pp. 243–245.

6. Blair, *The Scots and military medicine*, pp. 20, 21.

7. N. Cantlie, 1974. *A History of the Army Medical Department.* 2 Volumes (Edinburgh and London: Churchill Livingstone), Volume 1, pp. 32–58.

8. In Edinburgh, for example, a very broad spectrum of individuals attended Robert Knox's extramural classes: "The benches of Knox's class-room were occupied by a scholarly, earnest, and appreciative class; the majority were strictly medical students, but mingling with these were English barristers, Cambridge scholars and mathematicians, Scottish advocates and divines, scions of the nobility, artists, and men of letters." See: H. Lonsdale, 1870. *A Sketch of the Life and Writings of Robert Knox the Anatomist. By His Pupil and Colleague* (London: Macmillan & Co.), p. 131.

9. C. Lloyd, and J. L. S. Coulter, 1961. *Medicine and the Navy 1200–1900.* Volume 3. 1714–1815 (Edinburgh and London: E. & S. Livingstone Ltd.), pp. 16–17.

10. J. Dobson, 1957. The pernicious remedy of the naval surgeon. *Journal of the Royal Naval Medical Service* **43**, 23–28.

11. W. Turnbull, 1806. *The Naval Surgeon; Comprising the Entire Duties of Professional Men at Sea. To Which are Subjoined, a System of Naval Surgery, and a Compendious Pharmacopoeia. The Whole Illustrated by Plates* (London: Richard Phillips & B. McMillan).

12. Lloyd and Coulter, *Medicine and the Navy*, pp. 54–56.

13. Turnbull, *The Naval Surgeon*, p. 393.

14. These were termed "necessaries," or "medical comforts" in the army.

15. Turnbull, *The Naval Surgeon*, p. viii.

16. T. Trotter, 1790. *A Review of the Medical Department in the British Navy* (London: Admiralty) (cited by Lloyd and Coulter, *Medicine and the Navy*).

17. J. Bell, 1798. *Memoir on the Present State of Naval and Military Surgery. Addressed to the Right Honourable Earl Spenser [sic], First Lord of the Admiralty* [21 pp. Yarmouth, January 20, 1798].

18. Bell, *Memorial.*

19. G. Blane, 1799. *Observations on the Diseases of Seamen.* 3rd Edition (London: Murray & Highley) [The 1st edition was published in 1785, the 2nd in 1789, and the 3rd edition is the much enlarged version].

20. T. Trotter, 1797. *Medicina Nautica: An Essay on the Diseases of Seamen: Comprehending the History of Health in His Majesty's Fleet, under the Command of Richard Earl Howe, Admiral* (London: T. Cadell Jun. & W. Davies). [This represents Volume 1 in the series; Volume 2 was published in 1799 under the following title: T. Trotter, 1799. *Medicina Nautica: An Essay on the Diseases of Seamen: with an Appendix Containing Communications on the New Doctrine of Contagion and Yellow Fever, by American Physicians; Transmitted to the Admiralty by Sir John Temple, Bart. His Majesty's Consul-General* (London: T. Longman & O. Rees; Portsea: T. Whitehead Jun.); Volume 3 was published in 1803 under the following title: T. Trotter, 1803. *Medicina Nautica: An Essay on the Diseases of Seamen: Comprehending the History of Health in the Channel for the Years 1799, 1800, and 1801* (London: T. N. Longman & O. Rees)].

21. In 1802, all officers in the navy except surgeons and chaplains had their pay raised. See Lloyd and Coulter, *Medicine and the Navy*, Volume 3, p. 32. Reforms to the pay structure were recommended by the Sick and Hurt Board "to induce well-qualified and respectable persons to enter the service." By this Order, surgeons' mates were to be called assistant surgeons and be paid 8/6d a day, hospital mates were to receive 6/6d a day, those unqualified to be paid 4/- a day, and were to receive an allowance and lodging money at a rate of 10/6d a week when not accommodated in the hospital. The surgeons on active service were to be paid 11/- a day, and 15/- a day when in hospital ships, and 20/- a day after serving in a hospital for 10 years. The surgeons not provided with a residence in a hospital were to be allowed 15/- a week lodging money. After 10 years of service, physicians were to be paid 2 guineas a day.

22. The naval surgeon's uniform consisted of a captain's undress uniform with stand-up collar. A physician in the service was to be distinguished by the presence of gold lace on his sleeves.

23. Turnbull, *The Naval Surgeon*, pp. xxix–xlv.

24. Bell, *Memorial;* Bell, *Memoir.*

25. Turnbull, *The Naval Surgeon*, p. xxxiii: "One advantage, however, attends the regular commencement of study at a university, namely, that the student is there taught to entertain enlarged and scientific views of his subjects, which, in the more confined situation of an inferior seminary, he has neither the opportunities to do, nor is he so apt to

imbibe them. It is for this reason that the University of Edinburgh has been so deservedly distinguished for the scientific acquirements of its medical pupils; and though in the metropolis a great display of abilities prevails among the teachers, still the course of study is seldom so beneficial to the student, from the want of that connexion among the different professional branches, which a university so happily possesses."

26. Turnbull, *The Naval Surgeon*, pp. xxxiv–xxxv: "Would it not, therefore, after a student has acquired some general knowledge of the extent of the service, be proper to limit his views, in the finishing part of his studies, to the Naval Department alone; and, instead of wasting his time in attending on the common Medical and Surgical Lectures, that an institution should be formed, by the appointment of Government, for completing the instruction of all such whose practice is afterwards to be devoted to the Naval Department?"

27. D. G. Crawford, 1914. *A History of the Indian Medical Service 1600–1913*. 2 Volumes. Volume 1, 529 pp.; Volume 2, 535 pp. (London: W. Thacker & Co.; Calcutta and Simla: Thacker, Spink and Co.), Volume 1, pp. 223–247. Such men (p. 222) "held commissions as combatant officers, in addition to their warrants as Assistant Surgeons, entering the service as Ensign or Lieutenant and as Assistant Surgeon. When a man's turn came for promotion, either to Captain or to Surgeon, he was obliged to make his choice between the two branches, either taking the promotion which came to him, and permanently relinquishing the other branch, or once for all declining it, if he preferred to wait for promotion in the other branch."

28. R. Hamilton, 1788. *The Duties of a Regimental Surgeon Considered: with Observations on his General Qualifications; and Hints Relative to a More Respectable Practice, and Better Regulation of that Department. Wherein are Interspersed many Medical Anecdotes, and Subjects Discussed, Equally Interesting to every Practitioner*. 2 Volumes (London: J. Johnson, J. Murray, T. Longman; Ipswich: J. Shave), Volume 1, pp. 146–147.

29. A. Gore, 1879. *The Story of Our Services under the Crown. A Historical Sketch of the Army Medical Staff* (London: Ballière, Tindall & Cox), pp. 104–105.

30. G. J. Guthrie, 1815. *On Gun-Shot Wounds of the Extremities, Requiring the Different Operations of Amputation, with their after-treatment: Establishing the Advantages of Amputation on the Field of Battle to the Delay usually recommended, &c. &c. With Four Explanatory Plates* (London: Longman, Hurst, Rees, Orme & Brown), p. x.

31. Guthrie, *Gun-Shot Wounds*, pp. v–vi.

32. D. Hamilton, 1981. *The Healers: A History of Medicine in Scotland* (Edinburgh: Canongate), p. 119.

33. Cantlie, *Army Medical Department*, Volume 1, pp. 173, 180.

34. Cantlie, *Army Medical Department*, Volume 1, pp. 198–199.

35. Physician-in-ordinary to King George III. In 1804, he was elected president of the Royal College of Physicians.

36. Cantlie, *Army Medical Department*, Volume 1, p. 181. The exact date of this change of policy by Pepys is not stated. The situation was formally relaxed in 1811 when Weir allowed any surgeon who held the degree of M.D. to attain the appointment of physician. See: Cantlie, *Army Medical Department*, Volume 1, p. 422.

37. G. Blane, 1799. *Observations on the Diseases of Seamen*. 3rd Edition (London: Murray & Highley) [The 1st edition was published in 1785, the 2nd in 1789, and the 3rd edition is the much enlarged version], p. 183.

38. Cantlie, *Army Medical Department*, Volume 1, pp. 418–453.

39. Hamilton, *Duties of a Regimental Surgeon*, Volume 1, Chapter 9, entitled: "Of the perusal of books, and of some which should form part of his library," pp. 306–341.

40. J. Lind, 1753. *A Treatise of the Scurvy. In Three Parts. Containing an Inquiry into the Nature, Causes, and Cure, of that Disease. Together with a Critical and Chronological View of what has been Published on the Subject* (Edinburgh: Sands, Murray and Cochran; London: A. Millar) [456 pp.].

41. J. Pringle, 1752. *Observations on the Diseases of the Army, in Camp and Garrison. In three parts. With an Appendix, Containing some Papers of Experiments, Read at Several Meetings of the Royal Society* (London: A. Millar, D. Wilson & T. Payne).

42. D. Monro, 1780. *Observations on the Means of Preserving the Health of Soldiers: and of Conducting Military Hospitals. And on Diseases Incident to Soldiers in the Time of Service, and on the same Diseases as they have appeared in London.* 2 Volumes. Volume 1 and Volume 2 bound together. 2nd Edition. Vol. 1, 374 pp., Vol. 2, 304 pp. (London: J. Murray and G. Robinson).

43. J. Hunter, 1786. *A Treatise on the Venereal Disease* (London: No publisher details) [The explanation for the lack of a publisher is provided in Hunter's biography written by his brother-in-law, Everard Home. He states in J. Hunter, 1794, *A Treatise on the Blood, Inflammation and Gun-Shot Wounds, by the late John Hunter. To which is prefixed, a short account of the author's life, by his Brother-in-Law, Everard Home* (London: George Nicol) (The account of John Hunter's life appears on pp. xiii–lxvii) that "It is to be considered among the peculiarities of his character, that he chose to have his works printed and published in his own house, where they were also sold; but finding this measure to bear hard upon the booksellers, in a way which had not been emphasised, and which was not intended, the second editions were sold by Mr. Johnson in St. Paul's Churchyard, and Mr. Nicol in Pall-Mall."]

44. Hunter, *Inflammation*, p. xxxi.

45. Cantlie, *Army Medical Department*. Three examples are presented where men appeared to be indifferent to the pain inevitably associated with the operation of amputation. Volume 1, p. 329: "Dr Bell...was going to take off the thigh of a soldier . . . and he requested I would hold down the man for him . . . he seemed insensible to the scene that was passing around him, and with much composure was eating almonds out of his waistcoat pocket. . . . The operation was the most shocking sight I ever witnessed." In another case, Volume 1, p. 344, a man had been severely wounded by a shell, and it was necessary to amputate an arm and both legs. After removing the arm and then one leg, the surgeon suggested that the man have a rest before the second leg was removed. The man insisted "It's no use to make two bites at a cherry, what use in making so much fuss about a leg that would be of no service to me or anyone else again." As a third example, Volume 1, p. 388, the Hon. Fitzroy Somerset . . . arrived with a shattered elbow and Gunning decided on immediate amputation. Only after the operation was he recognized by his characteristic voice "Hullo, don't carry that arm away till I have taken off the ring. Not a groan, not a sigh, not a remark had been extorted either by the wound or the operation."

46. G. Ballingall, 1833. *Outlines of the Course of Lectures on Military Surgery, delivered in the University of Edinburgh* (Edinburgh: Adam Black; London: Longman, Rees, Orme, Brown & Green) [This is the 1st edition of Ballingall's *Outlines of Military Surgery*; 589 pp.], p. 339.

47. Anon., 1908. John Hunter 1728–1793. *Dictionary of National Biography* **10** (London: Smith, Elder & Co.) pp. 287–293.

48. Hunter, *Inflammation*, pp. xxv, xxvi, xxxviii; H. A. L. Howell, 1912. John Hunter, F.R.S., Surgeon-General and Inspector-General of Hospitals. *Journal of the Royal Army Medical Corps* **19**, 143–150; Z. Cope, 1959. *The Royal College of Surgeons of England. A History* (London: A. Blond), p. 274.

49. Cope, *Surgeons*, pp. 22–26, 274–306.

50. R. Porter, 1985. William Hunter: a surgeon and a gentleman. In: *William Hunter and the eighteenth-century medical world,* eds. W. F. Bynum and R. Porter (Cambridge: University Press), pp. 7–34.

51. C. H. Brock, 1985. The happiness of riches. In: *William Hunter and the eighteenth-century medical world,* eds. W.F. Bynum and R. Porter (Cambridge: University Press), pp. 35–54.

52. A. J. Marshall, 1970. *Catalogue of the Anatomical Preparations of Dr. William Hunter in the Museum of the Anatomy Department* (Glasgow: University Press) [Preface and Introduction, pp. vii–lxxvii].

53. Cope, *Surgeons*, pp. 30–31.

54. S. Taylor, 1993. *John Hunter and his painters: a lecture given at The Royal College of Surgeons of Engand on 11 May 1993* (London: Royal College of Surgeons of England), pp. 1–8.

55. Cantlie, *Army Medical Department*, Volume 1, pp. 172–173.

56. Hunter, *Inflammation*.

57. Hunter, *Inflammation*, pp. 521–565.

58. Anon., 1959–1960. Guthrie, George James 1785–1856. *Dictionary of National Biography* **8** (Oxford: Oxford University Press), pp. 818–819.

59. This patient was a private in the 45th Regiment of the French Infantry, who had been wounded at the Battle of Waterloo by a musket-ball that fractured the neck of his femur. He was admitted to the Elizabeth Hospital in Brussels on July 5, and Guthrie performed the operation on July 7, 19 days after he had received his injury. On November 19, he was transferred to York Hospital, London, under the care of Guthrie. The case is briefly described in the 2nd edition of his book *On Gun-Shot Wounds* (Guthrie, *Gun-Shot Wounds of the Extremities*, 1820, pp. 332–340); Plate II, Figure 1, shows the appearance of his thigh region after the wound healed, and Figure 2, shows the appearance of the neck of the femur with the ragged fracture through the intertrochanteric region.

60. Anon., 1850. Biographical Sketch of G. J. Guthrie, esq., F.R.S., Late President of the College of Surgeons. *Lancet* **I**, 726–738, p. 733.

61. G. J. Guthrie, 1838. *Clinical Lectures on Compound Fractures of the Extremities, on Excision of the Head of the Thigh-Bone, the Arm-Bone, and the Elbow-Joint: On the Diseases of the Peninsula, and on Several Miscellaneous Subjects. Delivered at the Westminster Hospital* (London: John Churchill).

62. This followed the tradition established in Edinburgh by Thomson, and continued by Ballingall, where members in the medical service of the army, navy and Honourable East India Company could attend their lectures gratis. It is difficult to believe that many full-time medical officers could attend Guthrie's lectures other than on a very intermittent basis, while those who were retired on half-pay were probably fully occupied in establishing themselves in full-time clinical practice. The situation in Edinburgh was slightly different, in that many medical service personnel took time off to obtain their M.D. degree, following the advice of Sir James McGrigor. This was one means of demonstrating their commitment to expanding their knowledge, and in this way keeping abreast of medical advances, while at the same time increasing their prospects for promotion within the service.

63. Guthrie, *Gun-Shot Wounds of the Extremities*, 1815 [2nd edition, 1820, 3rd edition, 1827].

64. G. J. Guthrie, 1819. *A Treatise on the Operations for the Formation of an Artificial Pupil; in which the Morbid States of the Eye requiring them, are considered; and the Mode of Performing the Operation, adopted to each peculiar Case, fully explained; with an account of the opinions and practice of the different Foreign and British authors who*

have written on the subject (London: Longman, Hurst, Rees, Orme & Brown; Callow; Burgess & Hill; Anderson; Cox & Co.; Highly; Underwood; Edinburgh: Constable & Co.; Dublin: Hodges & McArthur).

65. G. J. Guthrie, 1823. *Lectures on the Operative Surgery of the Eye: being the substance of that part of the Author's Course of Lectures on the Principles and Practice of Surgery which relates to the Diseases of that Organ: Published for the Purpose of Assisting in Bringing the Management of these Complaints within the Principles which Regulate the Practice of Surgery in General* (London: Burgess & Hill).

66. G. J. Guthrie, 1853. *Commentaries on the Surgery of the War in Portugal, Spain, France, and the Netherlands, from the Battle of Roliça, in 1808, to that of Waterloo, in 1815, Showing the Improvements made during and since that period in the great art and science of surgery on all the subjects to which they relate.* 5th Edition (London: Henry Renshaw).

67. G. J. Guthrie, 1855. *Commentaries on the Surgery of the War in Portugal, Spain, France, and the Netherlands, from the Battle of Roliça, in 1808, to that of Waterloo, in 1815, with Additions Relating to those in the Crimea in 1854–55, Showing the Improvements made During and Since that Period in the Great Art and Science of Surgery on all the Subjects to which they Relate.* 6th Edition (Revised to October 1855) (London: Henry Renshaw).

68. Guthrie, *Clinical Lectures.*

69. Guthrie, *Clinical Lectures*, Preamble, no page number.

70. Guthrie, *Commentaries on Surgery*, 1853.

71. Anon., *Biographical Sketch of Guthrie.*

72. Guthrie, *Commentaries on Surgery*, 1853, p. 5.

73. Anon., 1856. Death of Mr Guthrie. *Lancet* **I**, 500; Anon., 1856. *Lancet* **I**, 519–520 [Obituary notice of George James Guthrie]; Anon., 1856. Marble Bust of Mr. Guthrie. *Lancet* **I**, 556.

74. Anon., *Biographical Sketch of Guthrie.*

75. A. Pichot, 1860. *The Life and Labours of Sir Charles Bell K.G.H., F.R.S.S., L. & E.* (London: Richard Bentley); J. Struthers, 1867. Sir Charles Bell. In: *Historical Sketch of the Edinburgh Anatomical School* (Edinburgh: Maclachlan & Stewart). pp. 44–55; Anon., 1963–1964. Bell, Sir Charles 1774–1842. *Dictionary of National Biography* **2** (London: Oxford University Press, 154–157).

76. H. Ellis, 1994. Sir Charles Bell: Haemorrhage from a cut throat 1828. In: *Surgical Case-Histories from the Past* (London: Royal Society of Medicine Press), 144–148, p. 145; J. Thomson, 1816. *Report of observations made in the British Military Hospitals in Belgium, after the Battle of Waterloo; with some remarks upon amputation* (Edinburgh: W. Blackwood; London: T. Cadell & W. Davies). [While the British wounded were collected within a few days after the battle, many of the French casualties lay on the battlefield for far longer. According to Thomson (pp. 7, 8): "Even those of the wounded who had been necessarily left, some for one, two, or even three days did not appear to have suffered in any respect from the privations and exposure to which they had been subjected." He continued (p. 9): "Several thousands of the French, most of them severely wounded, were left behind upon the field of battle, or in the route of their flight . . . the wounds were generally in a bad condition, and those who had suffered them, affected with fevers. These circumstances, joined to the great depression of spirits which was the natural consequence of so signal a defeat, tended much to increase the number of deaths which occurred among the wounded French."]

77. G. Gordon-Taylor and E. W. Walls, 1958. *Sir Charles Bell: His Life and Times* (Edinburgh and London: E. & S. Livingstone), p. 272.

78. Primary, or immediate, amputation: one performed after the period of shock, and before the development of inflammation see: Anon., 1957. *Dorland's Illustrated Medical Dictionary*. 23rd Edition (Philadelphia and London: W. B. Saunders Co.). According to Guthrie, the primary operation should be performed as soon after the initial period of shock had passed, and certainly within 48 hours after receipt of the injury. See: G. J. Guthrie, 1827. *A Treatise on Gun-Shot Wounds, on Inflammation, Erisipelas, and Mortification, on Injuries of Nerves, and on Wounds of the Extremities Requiring the Different Operations of Amputation; in which The Various Methods of Performing these Operations are Shown, Together with their After-Treatment; and containing an account of the author's successful Case of Amputation at the Hip-Joint. Being a Record of the Opinions and Practice of the Surgical Department of the British Army, at the Termination of the Wars in Spain, Portugal, France, and the Netherlands, in 1814 and 1815*. The 3rd Edition (London: Burgess & Hill), pp. 231–239. This was also the view of Mr. Gunning, who was the senior surgeon on the British medical staff during the Peninsular War, as well as Baron Larrey, the most senior French military surgeon. See: Cantlie, *Army Medical Department*, Volume 1, p. 344.

79. Secondary amputation: one performed during suppuration. See: Anon., *Dorland*. Also defined as one that is performed during a period of healing. See: Anon., 1989. *Churchill's Illustrated Medical Dictionary* (New York: Churchill Livingstone). Amputation in these cases was performed when no cure was achieved following conservative treatment of the wound. According to Guthrie, "those performed from the third week to a later period . . . are by no means performed by military surgeons with such confidence or success [as primary amputations], as those done on the field of battle . . . they are found to be attended with considerable danger . . . and to be followed frequently by greater evils than those operations performed on the field." See: Guthrie, *Gun-Shot Wounds* 1827, p. 252.

80. Gordon-Taylor and Walls, *Bell*, p. 94.

81. C. Bell, 1814. *A Dissertation on Gunshot Wounds* (London: Longman, Hurst, Rees, Orme & Brown) [This book is entirely illustrated by the author's engravings, many of which are based on the series of sketches in oil displayed in the Playfair Hall of the Royal College of Surgeons of Edinburgh. His drawing of a soldier, wounded at Corunna, suffering from lockjaw, entitled "opisthotonos," was used as an illustration in his *Anatomy of Expression* (3rd Edition); C. Bell, 1844. *The Anatomy and Philosophy of Expression as Connected with the Fine Arts*. 3rd Edition (London: John Murray) (p. 160, where the author notes: "I took it from soldiers wounded in the head, at the Battle of Corunna. Three men were similarly hurt, and in short successive intervals similarly affected, so that the character could not be mistaken")].

82. Gordon-Taylor and Walls, *Bell*, pp. 41–42.

83. Gordon-Taylor and Walls, *Bell*, p. 42.

84. Anon., 1959–1960. McGrigor, Sir James, M.D. 1771–1858. *Dictionary of National Biography* **12** (Oxford: Oxford University Press), 546–549; R. Blanco, 1971. Sir James McGrigor and the Army Medical Corps. *History Today* **21**, 132–140; R. L. Blanco, 1974. *Wellington's Surgeon General: Sir James McGrigor* (Durham, N.C.: Duke University Press).

85. Anon., 1959–1960. Hennen, John, M.D. 1779–1828. *Dictionary of National Biography* **9** (Oxford: Oxford University Press), 424.

86. J. Hennen, 1818. *Observations on Some important points in the Practice of Military Surgery, and in the Arrangement and Police of Hospitals. Illustrated by Cases and Dissections* (Edinburgh: A. Constable & Co.; London: Longman, Hurst, Rees, Orme & Brown; Dublin: J. Cumming) [Dedicated to Sir James McGrigor, Knt. M.D. F.R.S.] .

87. Anon., 1959–1960. Pringle, Sir John 1707–1782. *Dictionary of National Biography* **16** (Oxford: Oxford University Press), 386–388.

88. Pringle, *Diseases of the Army.*

89. A. Kippis, 1783. *Six Discourses, Delivered by Sir John Pringle, Bart. when President of the Royal Society; on Occasion of Six Annual Assignments of Sir Godfrey Copley's Medal. To which is Prefixed the Life of the Author* (London: W. Strahan & T. Cadell) ["*The Life of the Author*" appears on pp. i–xcvi]; H.A.L. Howell, 1909. Sir John Pringle, Bart. *Journal of the Royal Army Medical Corps* **13**, 615–620; J. D. Comrie, 1932. *A History of Scottish Medicine.* 2nd Edition. 2 Volumes (London: Baillière, Tindall & Cox), Volume 2, pp. 441–447.

90. J. Pringle, 1750a. Some experiments on substances resisting putrefaction. *Philosophical Transactions (Royal Society of London)* **46**, 480–488 [This continues as: A continuation of the experiments on substances resisting putrefaction. *Philosophical Transactions (Royal Society of London)* **46**, 525–534; and: Further experiments on substances resisting putrefaction; with experiments upon the means of hastening and promoting it. *Philosophical Transactions (Royal Society of London)* **46**, 550–558]

91. J. Pringle, 1750b. *Observations on the Nature and Cure of Hospital and Jayl-fever. In a letter to Doctor Mead, Physician to his Majesty, &c.* (London: A. Millar & D. Wilson). [52 pp.]

92. Kippis, *Six Discourses*, p. viii.

93. Howell, *Sir John Pringle*, p. 620.

94. Anon., *McGrigor.*

95. Blanco, *Wellington's Surgeon General*, p. 6 see Footnote 7, p. 185 [This information is based on McGrigor's four notebooks entitled "Monro's Anatomy Lectures," dated October 1790 to March 1791, which are now located in the Muniment Room at the Royal Army Medical College. According to the *Matriculation Album, Rolls, University of Edinburgh* 1786–1803, McGrigor matriculated only in the academic year 1790–1791 for the following subjects: anatomy and surgery a combined course given by Professor Monro secundus, and for practice of medicine (a course given by Professor William Cullen). If he attended other classes on a regular basis while at the university, there is no evidence that he paid the necessary course fee required to attend them].

96. [John] Gurwood, 1834–1838. *The Dispatches of Field Marshall The Duke of Wellington K.G during his various Campaigns in India, Denmark, Portugal, Spain, The Low Countries, and France. From 1799–1818. Compiled from Official and Authentic Documents.* 12 Volumes, and Supplement to the 1st, 2nd, and 3rd Volumes relating to India 1799–1818 (London: John Murray) [The dates are 1799–1818 in all volumes except Volume 12, where the dates are 1799–1815; the years of publication are as follows: 1834 Vol. 1, 1835 Vols. 2–4, 1836 Vols. 5 and 6, 1837 Vols. 8 and 9, 1838 Vols. 10–12, 1839 Index to The Dispatches of Field Marshall the Duke of Wellington], Volume 8, p. 365. The full quotation is as follows:

Frenada 30th October 1811.
Wellington to Lieutenant-Colonel Torrens, Military Secretary to the Commander in Chief.
My Dear Torrens
I am sorry to tell you that Dr Frank, the Inspector of Hospitals, is so unwell as to be obliged to go home; and the department under him is so important, that if, as I fear, he should not be able to come out again, it will be necessary that we should have the most active and intelligent person that can be found to fill his station.

97. Gurwood, *Dispatches of Wellington*, Volume 12, p. 79. The full quotation is as follows:

To Major-General Torrens
London 26th July 1814
Sir
I have the honor to transmit to you a memorial from Dr McGrigor, Inspector of Hospitals, which I beg you to lay before his Royal Highness the Commander in Chief, with my request that the claims of that officer be favourably considered.
I have every reason to be satisfied with the manner in which Mr McGrigor conducted the department under his directions; and I consider him one of the most industrious, able, and successful public servants I have ever met with.
I have the honor to be, &c
Wellington.

98. Anon., *McGrigor*, p. 548.

99. J. Dible, 1970. *Napoleon's Surgeon* (London: William Heinemann Medical Books Ltd.), pp. 5, 9, 16, 17.

100. Blair, *The Scots and military medicine*, p. 5.

101. During the Carlist War, 197 49.3% of 400 officers compared to 1,495 15.6% of 9,600 sergeants and rank and file were wounded in action. R. Alcock, 1838. *Notes on the Medical History and Statistics of the British Legion of Spain; Comprising the Results of Gun-Shot Wounds in Relation to Important Questions in Surgery* (London: J. Churchill); M. H. Kaufman, B. N. Purdue, and A. L. Carswell, 1996. Old wounds and distant battles: the Alcock-Ballingall collection of military surgery at the University of Edinburgh. *Journal of the Royal College of Surgeons of Edinburgh* **41**, 339–350, pp. 342–344.

102. Anon., *McGrigor*, p. 548; A. Peterkin and W. Johnston, 1968. *Commissioned Officers in the Medical Services of the British Army 1660–1960.* 2 Volumes. Volume 1, 1660–1898, 638 pp., Volume 2, 1898–1960, 452 pp. (London: Wellcome Historical Medical Library) [This volume is sometimes referred to as: "Drew, R. Editor", with the same details], Volume 2, pp. 418–453; for additional details of his life before 1815, see: T. J. Pettigrew, 1839. *Medical Portrait Gallery. Biographical Memoirs of the most celebrated Physicians, Surgeons, etc. etc. who have contributed to the Advancement of Medical Science.* 4 Volumes. Volumes 1 and 2 bound together; Volumes 3 and 4 bound together (London: Fisher, Son, & Co.), Volume 4, section entitled "Sir James McGrigor, Bart. M.D. L.L.D., F.R.S., L. & E. Physician Extraordinary to the Queen, &c., &c., &c.," 12 pp.; J. McGrigor, 1861. *The Autobiography and Services of Sir James McGrigor, Bart. Late Director-General of the Army Medical Department, with an Appendix of Notes and Original Correspondence* (London: Longman, Green, Longman, & Roberts).

103. Anon., 1817. Medical Department of the Army. *Edinburgh Medical and Surgical Journal* **13**, 124–125.

104. Blanco, *Wellington's Surgeon General,* p. 166.

105. Dr. William Johnstone Fyffe entered the Army Medical Service in 1848 and served for a few months at Fort Pitt. While commending the library and pathological museum, he was less complimentary about many of his contemporaries. He stated that:

> The medical service was then principally recruited from the Scotch and Irish schools, some of them very rough specimens, who were entirely innocent at first of the ordinary uses of a silver fork or finger-basin at dinner. And whose period of probation at a military Mess-table was not the least useful part of their education.

He was also critical of McGrigor, stating that:

> It was generally understood that Scotchmen obtained the best appointments, especially Aberdeen men, as the Director-General hailed from the granite city.

See: W. J. Fyffe, 1889. Reminiscences of an Army-Surgeon. *Collection of Army Pamphlets* **9**, 1–24 (Contemporary Medical Archive Centre, Wellcome Trust, London, RAMC 423).

106. Cantlie, *Army Medical Department*, Volume 1, pp. 170–204.

107. J. Fergusson, 1846. *Notes and Recollections of a Professional Life, by the Late William Fergusson, Esq. M.D. Inspector General of Military Hospitals. Edited by his son, James Fergusson* (London: Longman, Brown, Green & Longmans), p. 56.

108. Cope, *Surgeons*, pp. 13–15.

109. Cantlie, *Army Medical Department*, Volume 1, p. 178.

110. Fergusson joined the army as an assistant surgeon, and served in Flanders in 1794, and the West Indies in 1796 as a staff surgeon. In 1801, he accompanied an expedition to the Baltic, and was on the flagship when Copenhagen was attacked. He was a principal medical officer in the Peninsula and present at the Battle of Talavera. From 1815–1817 he was again in the West Indies, and was retired on half-pay in 1817. He planned to settle in Edinburgh as a physician, but after 4 years was invited by the Duke of Gloucester to practice in Windsor, where he remained for the rest of his professional life; Fergusson, *Notes* [Editor's Preface, see pp. xi–xiv]; Anon., 1959–1960. Fergusson, William, M.D. 1773–1846. *Dictionary of National Biography* **6** (Oxford: Oxford University Press). p. 1229; Peterkin and Johnston, *Commissioned Officers*, Volume 1, p. 79.

111. Fergusson, *Notes*, pp. 56–57.

112. Fergusson, *Notes*, pp. 57–58.

113. The basic allowance was one physician for every 2,000 soldiers, one staff surgeon for every 1,000 men, and a hospital mate for every 160 men. There was some degree of flexibility, in that the figures could vary a little according to circumstances, such as the amount of sickness that was likely to occur on an expedition.

114. J. W. Fortescue, 1899–1930. *A History of the British Army*. 13 Volumes (London: Macmillan & Co.), Volume 10, 1920, p. 195.

115. W.F.P. Napier, 1828–1840. *History of the War in the Peninsula and in the South of France, from the Year 1807 to the Year 1814* [The complete set consists of 6 Volumes. Volume 1, 1828 (London: John Murray); Volume 2, 1829; Volume 3, 1831; Volume 4, 1834; Volume 5, 1836; Volume 6, 1840; (Volumes 2–6, London: Thomas & William Boone)], Volume 5, 1836, Book 19, p. 250.

116. Peterkin and Johnston, *Commissioned Officers*, Volume 1, Reference Number 829, p. 46.

117. Peterkin and Johnston, *Commissioned Officers*, Volume 1, Reference Number 989, p. 57; in some of the early records, his surname is spelled Kerr.

118. Cantlie, *Army Medical Department*, Volume 1, pp. 205–208.

2

THE WARS AGAINST FRANCE, 1793–1815

THE WARS AGAINST FRANCE LEADING UP TO THE PENINSULAR WAR

While it is not appropriate to provide a complete chronology of the events that occurred during the two decades of war between the French and British that spanned the 18th and 19th centuries, it is important that certain key events are noted. This allows the medical problems encountered, particularly by the British forces, to be more readily understood. It is also necessary to highlight the changes that occurred in the administrative arrangements of the medical services during this period, but more importantly to note how lessons learned in previous campaigns had largely been forgotten during the intervening periods of peace and government cost-cutting. These lessons had to be relearned during the next conflict, usually at considerable cost in lives of the fighting men. While the interval of peace in this case was for only 10 years, that between the end of the Peninsular War and the War in the East was far longer, almost 40 years, and the administrative difficulties encountered during the Crimean War had even more tragic consequences.

Declaration of War in 1793

In February 1793, France declared war on Britain and Holland. William Pitt, the British Prime Minister, requested Austria and Prussia to join the Allies, to maintain the neutrality of Holland, and to allow free access to shipping in the Scheldt. Britain was in no position to undertake a full Continental war. Over the previous ten years since the end of the American War of Independence in 1783, the government had allowed the strength of the armed services to diminish to such an extent that there was now a fighting force of less than 15,000 men. There were only 28 under-strength battalions available for the defense of the country; 19 were in the West Indies to prevent an uprising of the local population there, and 9 were in India. Insufficient ablebodied men offered themselves for military service. Commissions were still available for payment, and many junior officers entered the army in this way, with no military experience whatsoever. This scheme had been introduced in the late 17th century to provide retiring officers with some finance from the sale of their commission, and avoided the government having to pay them a pension. While this system was clearly open to abuse, even during the Peninsular War, it has been suggested that probably not more than about one-fifth of commissions were obtained by this means.[1] This system also enabled gifted individuals, including Arthur Wellesley, the future Duke of Wellington, to rise to a high rank at an early age. "The army-brokers, who in the days of purchase negotiated for officers the sale of commissions, exchanges, and the like, carried on openly a most scandalous traffic. . . . Officers, who had been driven to sell out of the army by their debts or their misconduct, were able after a lucky turn at play to purchase reinstatement for themselves with the rank of Lieutenant-colonel. Undesirable characters . . . contrived to buy for their sons the command of regiments; and mere children were exalted in the course of a few weeks to the dignity of field officers."[2]

Frederick Augustus, Duke of York, second son of George III, commanded the British force. He was 28, and had been sent to Berlin at the age of 16 to study the profession of arms under Frederick the Great. He embarked to Holland with under 2,000 men of all ranks from several battalions of the Guards to join the Dutch and Austrian armies. The British force was outnumbered by the 10,000 well-equipped Hanoverian and equally well-equipped 8,000 Hessian mercenaries; both of these forces were funded by the British government. The medical arrangements were organized by the surgeon general and inspector of regimental infirmaries, John Hunter. General hospitals accompanied this force, and appropriate medical staffing and provisions were also organized by Hunter on behalf of the War Office. The selection of medical officers was based as far as was practicable on Hunter's principle that all had to be appointed on the basis of merit alone, based on their proven surgical skills. Some were selected from those on the retired list, while others came from among the ranks of the regimental surgeons. All were appointed staff surgeons.

The merits of the different components of the Allied army are discussed by Fortescue in the following terms: In relation to the Hessians, "the majority of this force had served in America, where they had learned to manoeuvre rapidly and to fight in dispersed order. . . . The Hessians were particularly good light troops, and were armed with rifles. The Hanoverians were fine soldiers but without the advantage of the Hessians in experience and training. The Dutch by contrast were hastily raised, ill organised, disciplined, trained, and equipped. The British, like the Dutch were deficient in training and discipline due to persistent neglect. . . . The British cavalry was very well mounted, but both the officers and men were so ignorant that they needed to be instructed . . . by foreigners."[3]

The Guards took their regimental hospitals with them, each able to accommodate about 40 patients, although they had no special facilities to transport either the hospital or its equipment with them when they were on the move. All wagons and carts for this purpose had to be obtained locally. No facilities were available to rescue the wounded from the battlefield, and the badly injured men often had to wait until after the fighting was over before they could be rescued. If they were fortunate, their colleagues assisted them to a local regimental hospital just beyond cannon-ball range where all the emergency surgery took place by the regimental surgeons and their assistants.

The British medical arrangements were far inferior to those of the Hanoverians and the Hessians. Both of these forces had proportionately more regimental surgeons and regimental mates than were allocated to the British force by the Army Medical Department according to the formula that they had long employed. Their hospital units were fully mobile, with specially designed wagons that could easily cope with the hospital equipment. They were also self-contained, and did not need to rely on finding local modes of transport, which were often inadequate.

By May 1793, the Allied army numbered 100,000 men, and was under the overall command of the Prince of Coburg, the Austrian commander-in-chief. The main British general hospital was based at Bruges, with a smaller hospital located at Ostend. Despite strict written rules of procedure provided by the surgeon general, difficulties soon arose between individual members of the medical staff as to who had responsibility for the various categories of patients. To circumvent these increasing difficulties, Dr. Hugh Kennedy was appointed inspector general to the Duke of York, his principal role being to act on his own initiative, as a traveling trouble-shooter.

As the Allied line was so thinly stretched, it was relatively easy for the French forces to overwhelm the Allies at particularly weak points. Allied losses at this time were particularly heavy, not helped by the high incidence of dysentery and fevers due to the marshy camping grounds and the poor quality of the water. Up to about 10% of the Allied force suffered from these conditions at this time. The hospitals at Bruges and Ostend were rapidly overwhelmed, particularly when the sick rates rose to closer to 20% slightly later in the campaign. An additional hospital was established at Menin, and more medical staff sent out from England to bridge the gap. No adequate medical facilities were available to link the regimental hospitals, located near to the front lines, and the general hospitals to the rear. Mobile hospital units were organized to cater to this need, but many of the invalids needed to be transported back to England, where beds could be found for them.

The surgeon general had heard about the discontent among the medical staff, and sent out Mr. Everard Home, his brother-in-law, to investigate the likely cause of the difficulties encountered in the war zone. Unfortunately, Kennedy took Home's presence as a personal slight, and would have nothing to do with him. The major problem recognized by Home appeared to relate to the poor administrative infrastructure within the medical system. Great hardship was encountered by the wounded when they were being transferred between the regimental and general hospitals in totally inadequate modes of transport.[4]

Little was achieved during 1793 beyond the temporary withdrawal of the French from Dutch soil. Toward the end of the year, with Hunter's death, the control of the Army Medical Department passed into the hands of the Army Medical Board. They changed Hunter's policy of appointing men based on their experience, and, not surprisingly, the discontent within the service only increased.

The members of the Board were particularly distressed by the hostile attitude toward them taken by Kennedy, who insisted in controlling all promotions of staff and regimental medical officers. Following numerous letters to Kennedy, all of which remained unanswered, the Board eventually lost patience and informed Lord Amherst of the intolerable situation regarding Kennedy. Amherst, who had the duties although not the title of commander-in-chief of the Horse Guards, immediately confirmed the Board's authority, and informed Kennedy that his powers were limited exclusively to making temporary appointments to fill vacancies. Because of the mounting pressure on hospital beds, arrangements were made for large numbers of the sick and wounded to be evacuated to Deal. As the conditions there were found to be overcrowded and otherwise unsatisfactory, the men were then sent on to London to the newly established York hospital in Chelsea. This hospital, even with temporary hutting, could still only cater to about 200 patients.

The Position during 1794

During the early part of 1794, about 30,000 recruits joined the army, and the undesirable practice of selling commissions continued. Very few of these officers had any previous military experience, and few of the recruits serving under them were properly trained. As there was a considerable fear of an invasion, many men joined the local militias and the other volunteer corps. If all of these men, as well as the foreign mercenary troops, are included, the full strength of the British army at this time was close to 265,000 men. Of those in Flanders, the Duke of York had under his command about 30,000 men. The total strength of the Allied armies was about 120,000 men, while that of the French was just over 200,000.

During 1794, the Austrians and British were each defeated on a number of occasions by superior French forces, although on May 22 the French were themselves defeated by the Austrians, with losses in the region of 6,000 men. As the year progressed, the Austrians suffered several defeats, and they were eventually forced to retreat to Brussels. The British forces were also forced to evacuate Ostend, and retreated toward Ghent. The general hospital there was closed, and the sick and wounded evacuated to Antwerp, although additional general hospitals had to be established to accommodate them. The severely disrupted functioning of the medical arrangements caused sufficient concern among the medical staff that numerous complaints about Kennedy's incompetence eventually reached the Duke of York. He was forced to establish an inquiry, but this achieved little, and eventually the surgeon general, Mr. John Gunning, was obliged to visit Flanders to investigate the difficulties encountered in the local medical arrangements. There were 3,500 sick, and Gunning immediately arranged that additional physicians and apothecaries be sent out to assist those who were already there. The conditions in the wards were deplorable, and the only assistance available to the medical staff was in the form of untrained, unwilling, and disorderly regimental orderlies and nurses, all of whom lacked the basic skills required to allow the wards to function efficiently.

Later in the year, the Austrians withdrew their forces beyond the Meuse, leaving the Duke of York's forces in an extremely vulnerable position, and he had no option but to withdraw north toward Holland. During this retreat, discipline broke down, principally because many of his senior officers had purchased their commissions and were completely deficient in military skills. Some were said to be too drunk to travel with their men. The ordinary soldiers suffered because of their inadequate clothing, and an appeal had to be made to the British public to supplement the men's clothing. Unscrupulous senior officers had misappropriated and largely squandered their clothing allowance. This long-standing arrangement, whereby colonels of regiments were given an allowance to clothe their men, was amended in 1798, but the alternative system also failed when it transpired that the government was not prepared to cover the additional cost involved. This inevitably led to the loss of many men during the winter months from the effects of cold and exposure.

In the absence of the Austrians, the British and the Dutch were left to defend Holland against the French, and had to retreat first to the river Meuse, and then to the river Waal. Because of the shortage of clothing, almost 15% of the British force were off sick in September, and this figure rose to almost 30% by the end of November. The German forces, with their better supplies of clothing, still had a sickness rate at that time of almost 20%. The hospitals were unable to cope, and the death rates rose rapidly, despite the fact that a proportion of the most severely unwell among the British were evacuated to England. By Christmas 1794, some of the infantry regiments, with many of their men now barefoot, had sickness rates approaching 40%. In the cavalry, the sickness rates were often less than 10%.

Deterioration in the Conditions in the Hospitals during 1795, and the End of the Disastrous Campaign in Flanders

During the early part of 1795, the conditions in many of the hospitals were extremely poor, with little equipment or bedding available for the patients. The Secretary for War, Henry Dundas (Viscount Melville, from 1802), had only a limited experience of the military, gained when he held a commission in the Royal Edinburgh Volunteers.[5] Fortescue did not have a high opinion of him, stating, "Dundas was honest in so far as he never sought to enrich himself with the public money; but in political matters he was little more than an unscrupulous though very successful intriguer."[6] Dundas sent out Sir Jerome Fitzpatrick[7] to investigate the situation, with the authority to offer advice to improve the conditions of the men, but particularly the conditions in which the sick and wounded were transported, and for those who were to be evacuated back to England.

This brought Fitzpatrick into constant conflict with the senior members of the medical administration. He was extremely critical of the conditions in the hospitals, as well as the indifference of many of the medical staff toward their patients. When some of the most glaring deficiencies were drawn to the attention of the commander-in-chief, these were speedily rectified, such as the deductions that the hospitalized and convalescent patients had to pay for their food.[8]

During the period between December 1794 and the end of February 1795, all of the rivers froze over, and this consequently allowed the French to attack the Allied forces on a regular basis. As they were vastly outnumbered, the Allies were forced to retreat continuously, and the 7,000 patients in the general hospitals had to be evacuated to safety behind the lines. The Allied losses, in both manpower and horses, were extremely high, mostly from exhaustion and from the effects of the extreme cold. Hundreds froze to death.[9] By the middle of February, the commander-in-chief, now Lieutenant-General Harcourt, as the Duke of York had returned to England, had no option but to leave the most gravely ill, with a few medical staff to assist them, to the mercy of the advancing French. While the Dutch treated the British sick and wounded abominably, those who were fortunate enough to fall into French hands were well treated.[10]

Leaving the most severely wounded men behind to the mercy of the enemy was occasionally inevitable, and Hennen was magnanimous in his views on the decency of combatants with regard to the treatment of enemy wounded. He observed:

> Should a reverse, however, take place, it then becomes the duty of a certain proportion of the medical staff to devote themselves for their wounded, and become prisoners of war along with them; . . . I have never witnessed an act of unnecessary severity practised either by the French or English armies on their wounded prisoners; while, on the contrary, the contending nations have, in numerous instances, vied with each other in acts of tenderness and humanity to those whom the chance of war had thrown into their hands. It is also a soothing reflection that, where the wounded are very numerous, and particularly with compound fractures, there will be a vast saving of human life by leaving them in the power of the enemy, and not dragging them with the retreating army.[11]

The medical arrangements had by now completely broken down, and the blame largely fell on Kennedy, although the standard of care offered by many of the medical staff was abominable. Many of the doctors were both apathetic and indifferent to the distress of their patients. Even the commander-in-chief had nothing good to say about the activities of the majority of the medical staff. Kennedy died of illness in Germany on April 28, 1795, and did not live long enough to defend his actions.

There were some good medical officers, and Dr. Robert Jackson was among the best of them. The commander-in-chief appointed him directly from his post as regimental surgeon to the Buffs to that of physician-in-charge of the general hospital at Bremen, much to the distress of the Medical Board. His promotion had not followed the usual procedure, as he had been appointed as a principal medical officer (PMO) above a number of physicians already serving in the campaign. He was a great believer in cleanliness, and was meticulous in the care and treatment of the sick and wounded, almost all of whom were filthy dirty and ragged. The areas where they were accommodated were regularly fumigated, the men washed daily and given regular changes of clothing and straw and a blanket for their bedding. By these measures alone the sickness rate fell dramatically, and most of Jackson's patients could eventually be repatriated back to England.

Robert Jackson (1750–1827)

Jackson was apprenticed for three years to a surgeon at Biggar, and later spent a short time at the University of Edinburgh, but had to leave his medical studies there because of lack of funds. He was largely self-taught, but acted as an assistant to a doctor in Jamaica. He then made his way to New York, where he volunteered for military service and was taken on by the colonel of the First Battalion of the 71st Regiment (Fraser's Highlanders) as an acting surgeons' mate. He was taken prisoner during the American War of Independence. Initially, he tended the British wounded but was given permission by George Washington to look after the American wounded. In recognition of these activities, he was freely repatriated to the British force without the usual exchange of prisoners. After returning to Britain, he decided to wander around Europe on foot, covering in the region of 5,000 miles in this way. He visited Leyden, and in 1786 took and passed the M.D. degree by examination. He was a gifted linguist, and went to Paris to attend the hospitals there and to study languages, including Arabic.[12] He later studied Gaelic; he had earlier vowed never to read any medical text in translation, being only satisfied when reading it in its original language.

Jackson practiced as a physician in Stockton-on-Tees for seven years, but had little relish for private practice. In 1793, he volunteered for military service and was appointed surgeon to the 3rd Regiment, or Buffs. He was sent to France, and joined H.R.H. the Duke of York who was later appointed commander-in-chief. The Duke, rather than the Army Medical Board, appointed him physician and head of the Army Depot Hospital at Chatham. His appointment was made on the strength of one of his books on the fevers encountered in the West Indies,[13] despite the fact that he was not a member of the College of Physicians and was therefore technically ineligible for the office of army physician.

The members of the Army Medical Board never forgave his unconventional mode of appointment, and did everything in their power to publicly discredit him. On one occasion, an attempt was made by members of the Medical Board to remove him from the service.[14] After an official investigation, his management of the situation was upheld, and he was completely exonerated of all blame. He was extremely bitter, and resigned from the service, because he was not allowed to press counter-charges against his tormentors and never received an apology from them.

In 1803, following the outbreak of the Peninsular War, Jackson again volunteered for service. The commander-in-chief, the Duke of York appointed him inspector of hospitals, again without consulting either the surgeon general or the physician-general to the forces. They claimed that he did not possess the M.D. degree. Jackson's claim that his diploma had been lost with the rest of his baggage on his travels was not believed, despite the fact that he had informed them that Leyden would be prepared to provide him with a duplicate copy should this be requested to confirm his medical qualification. After other acrimonious encounters with the Medical Board, he again resigned from the army. When walking in London some time later, he saw the surgeon general (Mr. Keate) and assaulted him about his shoulders with his gold-headed cane. For this offense, but principally because he was not prepared to discuss his grievances in the court, the magistrates sentenced him to six months in the King's Bench prison. Jackson had many supporters, not least Dr. McGrigor, afterward head of the Army Medical Department.

Jackson was clearly an exceptionally gifted administrative reformer and an authority on tropical fevers, but was always a fierce critic of the medical authorities, and over the years had many acrimonious encounters with the Medical Board. He had recommended the appointment of "sanitary officers" who would advise on the siting of camps and hospitals, but this suggestion was ignored and not implemented before the onset of the Crimean War. Fergusson had also made observations along similar lines in his autobiography.[15]

In all, Jackson published 23 pamphlets and books, many of which were on fevers,[16] and medical administration.[17] Throughout his career, he was unconventional, and a thorn in the side of the military medical administration. A biographical account of his unconventional life was published in the *Journal of the Royal Army Medical Corps*.[18]

The War in Flanders

The war in Flanders and Holland was a disaster both for the army and for the Army Medical Department. One of the principal weaknesses was the physician-general's policy of appointing civilian physicians, albeit well qualified, but with no previous military experience, to run the general hospitals. Hospital equipment and transport for the sick and wounded were largely deficient, and all necessary medical care had to be undertaken while the army was continuously on the retreat. There was also no continuity of command. The field officers, who were technically in command of the regimental hospitals, were changed on such a frequent basis that they never had sufficient time to understand the workings of the hospital system. General Harcourt, the commander-in-chief, recommended the establishment of a separate hospital corps with sober and honest individuals who would care for the sick and wounded on the wards, but this was not implemented.

Many among the medical staff believed that the general hospitals should be abolished because they were expensive to run, and had a significantly higher mortality than the regimental hospitals. Furthermore, they did not allow the regimental surgeons continuity of patient care, as the treatment of their patients was taken over by the staff surgeons and physicians appointed directly from civilian practice. Not surprisingly, the regimental surgeons got depressed with their lot.

In this regard, particularly in relation to McGrigor's experiences in Egypt in 1801, Fortescue stated the following: "The secret was that the regimental surgeons, proud of their corps and anxious to keep its ranks as full as possible, worked with the greatest ardour not only to restore their patients to health but to send them back to the front as disciplined soldiers. Being constantly in touch with every man, they knew his constitution and disposition, and possessed, moreover, a very keen eye for malingering. In the base-hospital at Belem, on the contrary, all was perfunctory and orderless."[19]

The higher mortality noted in the general hospitals was in part because they received the more severely ill patients, but the chronic overcrowding in them, which inevitably led to the spread of hospital gangrene and typhus, dramatically worsened the situation. The death rates in some of them were as high as 60%.[20] In the regimental hospitals, the sick were often widely dispersed in different buildings, and cross-infection was therefore minimized. General hospitals were essential; otherwise the regimental hospitals would not have been able to function as mobile units. Their value would have been considerably greater, however, had they effective mobile ambulance wagons to carry the less sick patients from one regimental hospital to another, without the need to transport them to the general hospitals where the risk of cross-infection was so much greater.

On March 8, 1795, the British Cabinet at last decided to withdraw its troops from the Continent, and on the 11th, Harcourt received information that transports for 23,000 men were on their way to him. By the 22nd, the British marched to Bremen for embarkation. Finally, on April 14, the infantry and part of the artillery took ship for England. "Thus disgracefully ended the first expedition of Pitt and Dundas to the Low Countries."[21]

After the hostilities in Europe had temporarily settled down, recriminations within the Army Medical Department began flying in all directions. The Board's policy of appointing civilians to the most senior medical posts above experienced military men served only to increase the administrative chaos during the campaign. Few among the medical staff survived the campaign with an enhanced reputation, apart from Jackson, and he was a marked man as far as the Board was concerned because of his inappropriate mechanism of promotion.

The War in the West Indies, 1793–1798, and the Enormous Losses of Life from Yellow Fever

In 1791, there was an uprising on the French Island of St. Domingo, and refugees poured into Jamaica, Dominica, and the other islands of the British West Indies. Nineteen battalions of British troops were sent out at the request of the British residents to protect them against the possibility of an uprising of the local negro population.[22] After the declaration of war in Europe, some of the

French possessions were seized. The local population of Haiti rebelled, and planned to massacre the white planters. There were 6,000 French troops and 14,000 white militia on the island, and after much fighting reinforcements eventually arrived from Britain, and the capital city was captured. Operations were mounted against each of the French territories, and after fierce fighting most of the Leeward Islands came under British control.

In 1793, the activities in the West Indies became an even greater drain on the system than the more important European campaign in terms of men lost. The government was particularly supportive of the British merchants and sugar plantation owners who were making enormous fortunes at the expense of the local populations, many of whom were stimulated to mutiny against their British masters by expatriate French citizens. According to Fortescue, cited by Cantlie,[23] during the six-year period between 1793 and 1798, there were about 100,000 casualties and 50,000 deaths, mostly from yellow fever. Supplying the reinforcements needed to maintain the campaign in the West Indies was a perpetual drain on the system, particularly in 1794, when the withdrawal of troops from Flanders almost led to the outright defeat of those who remained. While it was known for over a hundred years that tropical diseases such as malaria, dysentery, and yellow fever were endemic in the West Indies, long intervals existed when the islands were virtually infection-free. It was therefore particularly unfortunate that the troubles in the West Indies should coincide with a particularly virulent outbreak of yellow fever.

The losses among the senior hospital staff sent to the West Indies were particularly high, and it was impossible to replace them at the rate that they were being lost. The inspector general of the Ordnance Medical Department openly criticized the physician-general for his policy of appointing only Oxbridge-educated physicians as none had any experience in the treatment of tropical diseases. This undoubtedly led to the inordinately high death rates that occurred from yellow fever in the West Indies. Every effort was made to send a proportion of the convalescents to Nova Scotia or to Bermuda, to get them out of the unhealthy climate of the West Indies, although the majority were invalided to England to restore their health.

The most dangerous regions for yellow fever were the coastal plains during the rainy season, but dysentery occurred throughout the year because the flies infected the food and water. While the practice of drinking large rations of rum had long been shown to be of little value against enteritis,[24] the practice continued. Salted pork and beef were standard items of army diet, and the wearing of uniforms more suitable for temperate climates rather than the tropics led to excessive sweating, an increase in the drinking of rum, and then enteritis.

The first epidemic of yellow fever struck in June 1794, and many of the British soldiers succumbed. Despite reinforcements, the British fighting force was decimated. The French also managed to send reinforcements from France, despite the British blockades of the French ports. They promised the Negro slaves their freedom, and gained much local support. The local medical arrangements were excellent, as the Board had no wish to be criticized as they had been for their deficiencies in Flanders. Enormous consignments of hospital equipment and medicines accompanied the men during 1796 and 1797. The one great deficiency, however, was the absence of a hospital corps, and this was a view that was shared by all members of the Army Medical Service. According to Fergusson:

> In the army of St. Domingo [in 1795] . . . a hospital corps [termed the Royal Hospital Corps] was formed under the direction of Colonel Gilbert Waugh, . . . but with all his knowledge the attempt was a miserable failure, . . . The regiments of the expedition were called upon to furnish proper men, and it would indeed have been wonderful if they had sent their best. They acted as all regiments will act in similar circumstances, when left to do as they like. Had they a man among them whom they were tired of flogging, and who could neither be induced to die or to desert, he was the elect for the hospital corps, or at best he might be a simpleton, not fit to stand sentry in a position of trust, or so awkward in the ranks that he could not be trusted with a ball-cartridge. In short, such a collection of incorrigible and incapable villains I believe was never brought together; and it was a true relief to the army when their drunkenness and the yellow fever killed them off. Such will never do for an hospital corps. They should either be raised as an independent body, or be formed from the emeriti of the army, out of the old soldiers who had served their time, and then to be promoted into it as a reward and indulgence, with some trifling distinction of superior pay. This, surely, is not impracticable, even in our impracticable army.[25]

Dr. Jackson was sent out to St. Domingo as physician, and it was here that he implemented his ideas about expanding the role of the regimental hospitals. He arranged for the supply of fresh rather than salted meat and wine instead of port, and by this means saved the Treasury in the region of £80,000 each year.

The British government decided that the cost of lives of their troops was excessive, considering the duties that they had been invited by the British merchants and plantation owners to perform. Accordingly, Dundas agreed to allow the recruitment of local Negroes to form native battalions to act in a policing capacity. Because those that enlisted had been offered their freedom, large numbers volunteered, and within a short period enough men had come forward to form what was to become the West India Regiment. From 1799 the West India Regiment and one British regiment exclusively defended the islands. This policy was certainly supported by the majority of the medical staff who had seen at first hand the plight of the white soldiers in the West Indies.[26]

During the second half of 1798, the British eventually withdrew from the West Indies, leaving the islands to be policed by local militia with French or Colonial officers in charge. The local troops were relatively immune to the fevers that were endemic to the area and to the local bowel diseases that so debilitated the foreign troops. This arrangement also resulted in the saving of countless British lives and millions of pounds for the Treasury.

Resurgence of Military Activities against the French on the Continent

Once the disturbances in the West Indies had settled down, those troops who had not succumbed to one of the many conditions endemic in these parts were repatriated back to Britain. The expeditions to the West Indies had occupied large numbers of men when all activities on the Continent involving British forces had ceased. This is not to say that the Continent was not seething with activity. Holland, Spain, and Prussia had joined forces with the French, with Austria acting in isolation against them. The British took most of the Dutch colonies in Southern Africa and in the East and West Indies and Ceylon. With French-induced agitation in Ireland during 1796 and 1797, over 13,000 British troops had to be dispatched to the south of Ireland to guard against the possibility of invasion from the sea, and a general hospital was established at Clonmel to meet the needs of these men.

In 1798, the British formed a coalition with Russia, Portugal, Turkey, and the two Sicilies, and only then felt able to support an expedition to the Continent. From 1795, a massive attempt was made to rebuild the army for what was inevitably going to be a lengthy struggle with the French and her allies for supremacy in Europe.

Following the increase in strength of the army, and the treaty with Russia, Pitt decided that it was now an opportune time to invade Holland. After a lengthy bombardment from the sea, on August 27, 1799, a force of 12,000 men landed in Helder in Holland and established a land base there. Energetic fighting ensued over the next few months, with each side advancing, only shortly afterward to be repulsed. In early September, the British force had over 10% either sick or wounded, and this figure rose to over 12% by later in the month. The more seriously wounded were repatriated to York hospital, Chelsea, where Mr. Thomas Keate acted as senior surgeon. When Gunning died in 1798, Keate had replaced him as surgeon general. The losses due to sickness had now risen to over 20% of the British force, and when the dead and wounded are included, the figure was closer to one-third of the entire strength.

Jackson was sent out by the surgeon general to supervize the Russian medical arrangements. The Russian sick rate amounted to nearly 25% of their strength, and was largely due to malarial infection, which was at that time endemic in the Low Countries.

Both sides had extreme difficulty coping with their sick and wounded, and it was agreed that a cease-fire should take effect from October 18, with the proviso that Holland would be evacuated by the end of November. Thousands of British and Russian patients were evacuated to Britain. The British paid a high price for this relatively brief expedition to the Continent, which, in all, lasted for only four months. The medical arrangements worked well and the incidence of cross-infection and hospital gangrene was extremely low.

The Egyptian Campaign

The next major encounter between the British and the French occurred in Egypt during 1801–1802,[27] as the French decided that this should be a stopping-off post for their forthcoming expedition to conquer the British possessions in India. After a successful naval encounter, the French forces under Napoleon were cut off from their supplies, and their morale was low. It was planned that the British force would be joined by reinforcements from India.

Dr. James Franck, an inspector of hospitals, initially supervized the British medical arrangements.[28] He was shortly afterward replaced by Dr. Thomas Young, a principal medical officer who had earlier distinguished himself both in the West Indies and in the recent expedition to Holland in 1802,[29] though Franck remained in Egypt with the force. In early March 1801, the British force landed at Aboukir Bay near Alexandria. Because of the shallowness of the water, the ships had to anchor five to seven miles from land. As the flat boats approached the shore, they came under heavy fire. Large numbers of casualties were sustained, including the loss of a number of medical officers. Camps were set up in the coastal region, close to where the troops had landed.

Despite an intense French attempt to rout the British troops on March 21, the French having been reinforced by troops sent from Cairo, a well-trained British force under Major-General Moore, later of Corunna fame, repulsed them. The French losses were over 1,000 dead and 600 wounded, while the British losses were 243 killed and 1,793 wounded.[30] As there was no wheeled transport, a field hospital was established in a local mosque which came under fire during the battle, as did the tented accommodation for the wounded. While victory was achieved, the force lost its commander, Abercromby, who was mortally wounded by a musket-ball which shattered his upper thigh. As an amputation was considered too risky a procedure to undertake in his case, he was taken aboard a hospital ship but died a week later from gangrene.[31] General Hely Hutchinson succeeded Abercromby.

Reinforcements eventually arrived from India and the Cape, but the Indian infantry regiments under Sir David Baird arrived too late to take part in any of the operations.[32] The medical officer in charge of the Indian expedition was Dr. James McGrigor, a regimental surgeon of the 88th or Connaught Rangers. His appointment caused some concern among the Honourable East India Company (HEIC) medical staff, and he was granted a special commission in the HEIC. The majority of his assistant surgeons were in the employ of the HEIC.[33]

While over 1,000 men had been evacuated out of the war zone to stations in the Mediterranean, such as to Malta and Gibraltar, and others returned to England, the inspector of hospitals, Thomas Young, still had over 2,500 sick to cope with. Many suffered from bowel infections due to the dusty dry conditions and the innumerable flies.

This was another campaign where the Board's formula for determining the provision of hospital equipment and bedding needed, based on the assumption that 10% of the force was hospitalized at any time, was seen to be well under the actual need. The actual figure was nearer 25% by March, and over 40% of Hutchinson's force was soon ineffective due to sickness. At the end of the campaign, 16% (2,982 men) of the force were hospitalized in Alexandria due to sickness, and an additional 3,000 wounded men had to be hospitalized throughout the campaign.

While a proportion of the cases of enteritis were fairly mild, those due to bacillary and amebic dysentery were relatively common, and often had lethal consequences. Other diseases, such as the plague and ophthalmia, also put a considerable strain on the medical resources. Both of the latter conditions were endemic in the Eastern Mediterranean at that time. The mortality from the plague[34] was about 45%, and this included members of the medical staff and their orderlies, despite the fact that when it was recognized quarantine was strictly enforced. The source of the infection that involved the British troops was believed to have been the arrival of an infected ship from Smyrna, which had been boarded by some of the soldiers.

Ophthalmia, or "Egyptian ophthalmia," was justifiably referred to as "one of the plagues of Egypt," and among the British forces led to either total blindness or blindness in one eye of hundreds of troops. This condition was almost certainly trachoma, and the infective organism was *Chlamydia trachomatis*. It resulted from the unsanitary conditions then prevalent in the townships, was extremely infectious, and was carried by flies. By the end of 1810, there were over 3,000 blinded soldiers at Chelsea and Kilmainham who had suffered from this condition.

Ophthalmia was also encountered by the French troops, and over 3,000 cases were treated, but with no cases of blindness. Larrey is credited with giving the first detailed description of this disease.[35] This difference in the outcome can only be understood in terms of the different treatment of this condition in the two armies. The French avoided surgical intervention and the application of powerful drugs into the eyes, such as copper sulphate, lead acetate, and silver nitrate, as used by the British surgeons.[36]

According to Larrey: "The English on their arrival in Egypt likewise suffered from this disease [ophthalmia]. After a short time they adopted the French method of treatment, which they learnt of from a copy of my Memoir they found in our hospitals at Rosetta; from this time they, too, saved the sight of most of their patients."[37] This may have been wishful thinking on his part, as many of the British who encountered this condition suffered grave consequences because of the severity of the treatment they received from their doctors.

Larrey believed that a considerable number of cases of ophthalmia among the French troops were due to gonorrhea.[38] This was also Fergusson's view in relation to the condition seen in the children of soldiers at the Royal Military Asylum. He also believed that the Egyptian ophthalmia was far less contagious than assumed by many of his contemporaries, as he saw many examples where the wives and children of soldiers diagnosed as having this condition remained free from it despite living in close proximity to the sufferers. He also saw many examples where ophthalmia was self-induced; it was relatively commonly seen in certain regiments when the men did not wish to be sent on what were perceived to be dangerous foreign postings.[39]

Other Smaller Campaigns between 1801 and 1807

After the conclusion of the fighting in Egypt, the British army took part in campaigns in the West Indies, and captured colonies that had formerly belonged to both the French and the Dutch. Numerous garrison hospitals were established throughout the islands to cope with the considerable number of troops who invariably suffered from the various fevers that were endemic in these islands.

Other expeditions went to the former Dutch colony of Ceylon, and intermittent fighting took place there over the years, with particularly high losses due to tropical fevers. The island was eventually subjugated in 1818.

While Gibraltar had been under siege from the Spanish army and navy during the period between 1779 and 1783, the situation was stable during the late 18th and early 19th centuries. A large garrison was maintained there, and many of the convalescent patients from Egypt had been sent there to recuperate. Occasional epidemics of yellow fever led to large numbers of deaths both within the garrison and among the local population during this period. Other expeditions took place during 1807, the first to South America and the second to Egypt, once more, on this occasion to capture Alexandria. Most of these forays were to expand the boundaries of the Empire.

THE PENINSULAR WAR, 1808–1814

It is only appropriate here to provide a brief outline of the principal campaigns of the Peninsular War insofar as these shed light on the medical arrangements in force during this lengthy conflict. A number of accounts shed important light on various aspects of the military surgery of the conflict,[40] while others were written by individuals who played an important part in the organization of the medical administration during this period.[41] Reference is also made to more recent monographs and articles in which the medical arrangements during this conflict were assessed in some detail.[42] Reference is also made to accounts of the military aspects of the campaign, some of which are also contemporary,[43] including the complete correspondence of Wellington over this period.[44]

As Portugal had been one of Britain's few stalwart allies over the years it was appropriate that Britain should go to her aid when the French declared war on her in 1807. The French had insisted that Portugal should declare war on Britain, but when this suggestion was declined, the French declared war on Portugal instead, and Napoleon sent a force to occupy Lisbon. Napoleon also declared war on Spain, as he wished to put his brother Joseph onto the Spanish throne. After the French invasion of Spain, in June 1808, Joseph was declared King.

As it was becoming obvious that a continental war was looming Lord Castlereagh, the Secretary for War, actively encouraged an increase in the size of the regular army. By the end of 1808 it had reached about 200,000 men. Under the direction of the Duke of York, their commander-in-chief, and General John Moore, the army was both a well-trained and well-disciplined force.

Events in Portugal and Spain during 1808

The British government agreed to assist the Spanish patriots, and sent a force to Portugal in July 1808 under Lieutenant-General Sir Arthur Wellesley. Nineteen medical staff officers accompanied him. He disembarked with his force of 10,000 men at Mondego Bay, 80 miles north of Lisbon, during the first week of August, and General Spencer joined him with 5,000 men. The combined group marched toward Lisbon. Their first engagement took place at Roliça, about half way between Mondego Bay and Lisbon, on August 17, when the French position was successfully stormed. Guthrie was the senior regimental surgeon present, and did the majority of the operating. The wounded were later taken to the hospital ship *Enterprise*. Three days later, Wellesley was reinforced with two additional brigades, bringing his strength up to 17,000 men, with 1,500 Portuguese auxiliaries.

On August 21, Andoche Junot, the French general, marched with 13,000 men from Lisbon, and engaged Wellesley's force on the Vimeiro ridge. The French advance was halted, with the loss of 1,600 men. The hospital at Vimeiro was converted into a field hospital for both sides, and numerous emergency amputations were undertaken there. Bullock carts then evacuated the wounded to the general hospital that had recently been opened at Oporto.

While Wellesley had planned to follow up his recent victory by attacking Lisbon, his command was taken from him by Lieutenant-General Sir Harry Burrard, though the next day he was in turn superseded by Lieutenant-General Sir Hew Dalrymple, Governor of Gibraltar, with Burrard acting as his deputy. Both decided to await the arrival of further reinforcements of 14,000 men under the command of Sir John Moore. Shortly afterward, the shameful Convention of Cintra was concluded by Dalrymple and Burrard, to which Wellesley is said to have reluctantly added his signature.[45] This allowed the French to evacuate Portugal, taking with them all of their plunder and equipment. It was also agreed that the French were to be repatriated to France on British ships.

The three senior British staff officers, Burrard, Dalrymple, and Wellesley, returned to England, leaving the force of 30,000 men under the command of Sir John Moore. Because of the general feeling of disgust in England regarding the terms of the Convention of Cintra,[46] all three generals who had signed the agreement were recalled to face a court of inquiry, from which only Wellesley escaped criticism.

When Sir David Baird arrived in Corunna (La Coruña) on October 8 with 14,000 men, the Spanish, while happy to accept British arms and funding, were reluctant to allow them onto Spanish territory. With the approval of the British government, Sir John Moore joined up with Sir David Baird's force, with the aim of cooperating with the Spanish to drive the French out of their country. Ten thousand British troops were left in Lisbon to defend the city, should the need arise, while the rest of the force marched north.

The two British forces were to unite at Valladolid, about 220 miles south east of Corunna, with the principal aim of cutting the French supply line. To reach this city, Sir John Moore's force had a journey of nearly 400 miles across mountainous and largely unknown terrain, while Sir David Baird's force had to travel from Corunna over similarly mountainous and largely unknown terrain. As Moore approached Salamanca, he was unaware that the city had recently surrendered to the French. As the Treasury had omitted to supply either force with bullion, no funds were available to purchase or even hire local bullock carts to transport their equipment. This, and the early onset of dreadful winter weather, severely hampered the progress of the two forces toward each other.

As there were no lines of communication between the two commanders, or with the Spanish authorities, both groups were unaware that the French had regrouped and captured the city of Valladolid, where they were both meant to meet up. When this information eventually reached Moore, he immediately instructed Baird to withdraw to Corunna. The fortunate capture of a French dispatch updated Moore on the strength of the French force and their proposed plans. With this intelligence, Moore instructed Baird to meet him at Astorga, a town about 85 miles from Valladolid, and about 115 miles from Corunna (almost in a straight line), with the intention that their combined army would then attack the French force commanded by Marshal Soult. The two British forces met on December 20.

Just as Moore was about to attack Soult's force, he was informed that the advanced force of Napoleon's far larger army was only 20 miles to the south of him. Moore had no alternative but to withdraw to Astorga and then retreat over the western part of the Cantabrian Mountains to Corunna. The news that they were to retreat, rather than engage the French, completely dispirited the men, and discipline within the British force all but disappeared. As the British force retreated through deep snow, with the French force only 36 hours behind them, numerous drunken stragglers were left behind, and were rounded up and either killed or taken prisoner by the French cavalry. The Spanish army, under Romana, many of whom had typhus, joined up with Sir John Moore's retreating force, and spread typhus into the British ranks. The weather was dreadful, and several thousand troops, their horses and bullocks, and their accompanying families were frozen to death along the route during the 18-day withdrawal to Corunna.

While Sir John Moore's army arrived at Corunna on January 11, 1809, their transports were detained at Vigo due to inclement weather, and could not reach them until the 14th, by which time the French had arrived. The British force, now down to about 15,000 fighting men, rallied and fought off the French. During the ensuing battle, Sir John Moore was mortally wounded. His force, with over 4,000 sick, many with typhus, embarked for England, untroubled by the French who had withdrawn from the attack thus giving the British force enough time to retreat in good order to the transporters.

Sir John Moore "died after having conducted one of the most difficult retreats on record, and secured the safety of the army entrusted to him. . . . He was mounted when he was thrown to the ground by a cannon ball which struck him on the left shoulder, carrying it entirely away, with part of the collar bone. . . . His achievements extorted admiration even from his enemies; as the monument erected by the French officers over his grave at Corunna attests."[47]

In their retreat, the 35,000-strong Anglo-Spanish infantry and cavalry had suffered terribly, not only from attacks from Napoleon's forces, but also from hunger and fatigue, and by the time the majority disembarked at Portsmouth, typhus fever had spread widely among them. Because the sick and healthy were mixed together indiscriminately, the number of cases of typhus caused great alarm.

The military losses from Corunna were particularly high: 3,809 troops had died in battle, by the road, or in the hospital, and 2,189 were sent as prisoners to France. Of the 28,000 that were disembarked by the English fleet, on their arrival, 4,035 men were listed as sick. Of the 2,427 of the Corunna sick hospitalized in Portsmouth, 405 died, mostly from dysentery, fever, ulcers (probably scorbutic), and pneumonia.[48]

The inspector of regimental infirmaries had previously closed 1,200 beds at Gosport, Plymouth, and Deal. Not surprisingly, all of the normal hospital accommodation in and around Portsmouth was overwhelmed, and barracks were rapidly converted into hospitals. The unaccommodated part of the naval hospital at Haslar, calculated to be able to accommodate about 4,000 sick and wounded seamen, was entirely given up to the army. The situation was so desperate that an appeal was made for medical assistance from London. Charles Bell volunteered and administered to the wounded.[49] Charles Bell's monograph on gunshot wounds[50] relates to his experiences in the treatment and management of these men.

Return of the Main British Force to Portugal, and Events in the Peninsula during 1809

During mid-April 1809, Sir Arthur Wellesley returned to Portugal to reinforce and unite with the 10,000 men who had been left behind in Lisbon the previous autumn under the command of Sir John Cradock. While the force in Lisbon had expected to be attacked at any time, the French were preoccupied with surviving over the winter months, and only in March did they move toward the coastal city of Oporto, and sacked the city. By the end of March, Wellesley's force now comprised over 20,000 British troops, 3,000 Hanoverians, and about 16,000 Portuguese.

Wellesley decided to attack Soult's forces at Oporto, and, on May 11, took them completely by surprise.[51] Wellesley's losses were also relatively slight. The British force had previously grouped at Coimbra, about 100 miles south of Oporto, where they established a general hospital and left their 2,600 sick, about 10% of his force, in the charge of a number of assistant surgeons. A general hospital was also established at Oporto, and this hospital and that at Coimbra were put under the direction of Dr. Franck, now inspector of hospitals.

Wellesley's force moved south to Abrantes, to concentrate on attacking the French force under Victor reaching it early in June. There was no adequate supply of pack animals to transport all of the essential items needed to maintain the army, such as the heavy cooking utensils, and the surgeons' panniers. Equally, no transport was available to carry the provisions; what was needed was purchased along the route, as required. The men were additionally required to carry three days' ration of bread. The few bullock wagons that were available carried essential rations to a central supply area, from where these were distributed to regiments and brigades. Because of the very poor standard of hygiene on the march, some of the men went down with typhus. Despite guidance from the medical staff regarding improving the standard of personal cleanliness, little could be done to reduce its incidence.

Wellesley was reinforced at Abrantes, and marched with about 23,000 men and 30 guns. By July 15, his force had reached Plasencia. Here he joined forces with a Spanish army under General Cuesta, and the combined force reached Talavera on July 22. This town was just to the north of the river Tagus, and about 60 miles southwest of Madrid. Wellesley's force now consisted of 17,000 British and 3,000 Hanoverians of the King's German Legion, while the Spanish force of 32,000 men concentrated on defending the town itself. Wellesley persistently complained in his *Dispatches* about the difficulties he encountered with his Spanish allies.[52] The French had 46,000 seasoned troops under the command of Marshal Victor, and the battle of Talavera took place on July 28. Despite numerous frontal assaults by the French in the open country between the two sides, all of which were repulsed, the British line held. Toward the end of the day, the dried grass on the field of battle caught fire, and hundreds of the wounded of both sides perished where they fell. The French then withdrew, leaving 7,000 dead and wounded and 17 guns on the field. The British casualties were only slightly less, with 3,915 wounded and 1,448 killed, a high proportion belonging to the German Legion.[53] To recognize the magnitude of Wellesley's victory at Talavera,[54] he was elevated to the Peerage, and was thenceforth to be styled Viscount Wellington.[55]

The task confronting the medical staff after the battle of Talavera was an enormous one. The burden largely fell on the shoulders of Guthrie, who was acting in an administrative capacity in place of Franck who was laid low due to a bout of dysentery.[56] Regimental hospitals were established about 700 yards beyond the range of the cannons and musket fire, and it took two days before all of the wounded from both sides were removed from the field of battle. Some were carried to the hospitals while mules, horses, and bullock carts transported others.

Because the British force was in no fit state to move, all of the medical staff attended to the immediate needs of the sick, but particularly the needs of the wounded from both sides. As the food available to the British was so limited, it was arranged that those in the hospital would receive full rations, while those of the fit men were reduced to nearer one-third of their normal ration.

Much to Wellington's surprise and concern, he received news that Soult had regrouped, and with a force of 50,000 men was marching from the north to cut off his lines of communication and supply. He was then forced, on August 3, to march east to Oropesa. The fate of the casualties proved a great problem. While transport was arranged for 2,000 of them, by leaving behind the nonessential stores, 700 of the "walking wounded" had to manage as best they were able. Many of these fell into the hands of the Spanish marauders and peasants, and were killed for their few possessions. Despite promises from the Spanish general to provide transport for the wounded, nearly 1,500, with a number of medical staff, had to be left behind to the mercy of the French. Despite their agitation, the wounded and the medical staff were all treated with every courtesy and consideration. The French high command indicated that they were particularly impressed with the general condition of the casualties.[57]

It is also appropriate to quote Napier on this topic, in relation to the kindness and consideration shown by the French to his eldest brother, Major Napier, the officer commanding the Fiftieth, who was wounded and taken prisoner:

> He was returned among the killed. When the French renewed the attack at Elvina . . . being hurt, he endeavoured to return [to his own lines], but the enemy coming down, he was stabbed, and thrown to the ground with five wounds; and death appeared inevitable, when a French drummer rescued him from his assailants, and placed him behind a wall. A soldier with whom he had been struggling . . . returned to kill him, but was prevented by the drummer . . . the Duke of Dalmatia being apprised of major Napier's situation, had him conveyed to good quarters. . . . The marshal also obtained for the drummer the decoration of the legion of honour. The events of the war obliged Soult to depart in a few days from Coruña, but he recommended major Napier to the attention of marshal Ney; and that marshal also treated his prisoner with the kindness of a friend rather than the rigour of an enemy, for he quartered him with the French consul, supplied him with money, gave him a general invitation to his house on all public occasions. . . . When the flag of truce arrived . . . sent him, and with him the few English prisoners taken in the battle, at once to England, merely demanding that none should serve until regularly exchanged."[58]

Wellington crossed the river Tagus at Arzobispo, and pressed on toward the west, although the troops had little in the way of rations, and to survive they had to fend for themselves from the surrounding countryside. A general hospital was established at Truxillo, although by now the wounded had decreased to about 2,000, the rest having either died along the route or been captured by the French. The fate of the captured medical officers was not clear, and despite Wellington's proposal that they be returned to either side without exchange, the British medical officers were released only about a year later.

With the routing of all of the Spanish armies by the French, there was little value in the British remaining in Spain, so they withdrew to Badajoz, just on the Spanish side of the border. Here they were re-supplied from Lisbon and from the close-by depot at Elvas, just on the Portuguese side of the border.

Where they camped was a notorious malarial area, and as no precautions had been taken, nearly 30% of the force, just over 3,000 men, had to be hospitalized, and over 500 men died during this outbreak. The area was extremely dry, being atypical of most malarial country, but had small pools of drinking water close to the camping ground where the *anopheles* mosquitoes bred.

The general hospitals that had been established were overwhelmed with nearly 6,000 patients, 1,500 of whom had been wounded at Talavera.[59] The regimental hospitals were also overflowing, and had over 3,000 sick and wounded patients to look after.

Members of the medical staff were not consulted when decisions were made about the siting of camps, and this omission, as here, not infrequently proved disastrous, and enormous losses of life due to sickness might have been avoided. According to Fergusson:

In the West Indies I found medical opinion equally at discount. The convenience of the Engineer, the whim of the Quarter-master General, or General commanding, and the profit of the contractor, seemed alone ever to be consulted. There was not a station in the command where the health of the troops seemed ever to have been thought of, or a health opinion called for. It might be given, but it was always treated as an unauthorised assumption. . . . Let us hope, henceforward, that in peace at least no station will ever be chosen for barracks, upon which the health authorities have not previously been . . . consulted. It is their duty and their place to give opinion upon it. If incompetent, let them be superseded by abler men, but let it never be said hereafter, that Great Britain has persisted in sacrificing her best defenders in compliment to contractors, and engineers, and builders, without reference to the qualified health authorities, that could have taught them better.[60]

All of the regimental assistant surgeons, who were available in Lisbon and elsewhere, were brought in to cope with the massive numbers of sick and wounded. Wellington was well aware of the shortage of medical staff, and its effect on the morale of the men, and drew attention to this in one of his dispatches to the Earl of Liverpool, Secretary of State.

Badajos, 14th November 1809.

It is besides very necessary that some effectual measures should be taken to increase the medical staff, not with gentlemen of rank, but with hospital mates. The duty of the general hospitals in every active army ought to be done by the general Medical Staff, and the regiments ought to have their surgeons and assistants entirely disengaged for any extraordinary event or sickness that may occur. We have not now one surgeon or assistant with each regiment, instead of three, the others being employed in the hospitals instead of hospital mates, and we have always been equally deficient. Indeed, one of the reasons which induced me to cross the Tagus on the 4th August, instead of attacking Soult, was the want of surgeons with the Army, all being employed with the hospitals, and there being scarcely one for each brigade; and if we had had an action, we should not have been able to dress our wounded.[61]

The shortage of medical staff in Portugal unfortunately coincided with the difficulties that were encountered in Holland a few months after the invasion of the island of Walcheren in July 1809, and its final abandonment in December of that year. This was associated with the loss of 4,000 men from malaria, and the invaliding out of the army of a further 11,000 men.

In a supplementary letter addressed to the commander-in-chief, from Badajoz, dated November 16, 1809, Wellington again emphasized his desperate need for hospital mates. He noted:

That which this army wants, principally is an additional number of Hospital Mates. There is not a sufficient number of officers of this description to do the duties of the General Hospitals; the Regimental Surgeons and their Assistants are therefore necessarily employed in the General Hospitals; and the regiments are not attended as they ought to be at all times, but particularly at this season.[62]

A dispatch from Wellington to the Earl of Liverpool, sent one week later, informed him that the English newspapers were publishing accurate information on the state of preparedness of the Allied armies, information that would undoubtedly be invaluable to the enemy. He considered that, in his view, such editors were irresponsible in this regard, and that their enthusiasm should be curtailed. This lapse of security can only have emanated from Wellington's headquarters, and that someone there was receiving money from the press for this information.

> Badajos, 21st November 1809.
>
> I beg to draw your Lordship's attention to the frequent paragraphs in the English newspapers, describing the position, the numbers, the objects and the means of attaining them, possessed by the armies in Spain and Portugal.
>
> In some instances, the English newspapers have accurately stated, not only the regiments occupying a position, but the number of men fit for duty of which each regiment was composed; and this intelligence must have reached the enemy at the same time it did me, at a moment at which it was most important that he should not receive it.
>
> The newspapers have recently published an account of the defensive positions occupied by the different English and Portuguese corps, which certainly conveyed to the enemy the first knowledge he had of them; and I enclose a paragraph recently published, describing the line of operation which I should follow in case of the occurrence of a certain event, the preparations which I had made for that operation, and where I had formed my magazines.
>
> It is not necessary to inquire in what manner the newspapers acquire this description of information; but if the editors really feel an anxiety for the success of the military operations in the Peninsula, they will refrain from giving this information to the public, as they must know that their papers are read by the enemy, and that the information which they are desirous of conveying to their English readers is mischievous to the public, exactly in proportion as it is well founded and correct.
>
> Your Lordship will be the best judge whether any and what measures ought to be adopted to prevent the publication of this description of intelligence.[63]

By the middle of December, despite the fact that many of the men were now fit enough to be transferred into the convalescent beds, more junior medical staff were requested from England.

Situation in the Peninsula during 1810

The period in winter quarters was mostly spent in exercising the men, and it was hoped that this period of rest and recuperation would improve their general health. The percentage of sick gradually diminished during the first few months of 1810, from nearly 30% at the beginning of January to just under 20% by the beginning of April.[64] By May 1810, large numbers of reinforcements had reached Wellington, so that his force now consisted of over 30,000 men, some of whom had arrived from Walcheren, and required time to adjust to the conditions in Portugal and to achieve campaign fitness. Unfortunately, many of those who had served in Holland suffered relapses of malaria throughout the whole of 1810, and continued to suffer from this condition well into 1811. Wellington also had under his command an untried Portuguese army of 20,000 men.

The first concerted attack by the French, under the command of Marshal Ney and with an army of about 30,000 men, was against the fortress of Ciudad Rodrigo. This held out for six weeks until July 10,[65] but the town of Almeida was rapidly overwhelmed and surrendered toward the end of August. The French advanced westward into Portugal, and Marshal Massena's force confronted Wellington's army at Busaco, on September 27. Wellington now had just over 50,000 men at his disposal, and following his usual practice defended a steep ridge about 500 feet high and about 9 miles in length. While the French sent large numbers of men forward in massive columns, Wellington's force kept out of sight behind the ridge until the last moment, when they repelled the attack by volleys of musket fire. The French suffered nearly four times the casualties sustained by Wellington's combined British and Portuguese force.

The majority of the wounded were treated locally in the regimental hospitals located just beyond the ridge, although the more severely wounded had to be transported to the general hospital at Coimbra, about six miles to the south. The track over which the bullock carts had to travel was so uneven that it greatly increased the suffering of the casualties.

Wellington decided not to pursue the French, but to continue to Torres Vedras where there were reasonably safe defense positions. This encampment was reached on October 10. The countryside through which they traveled was laid waste, and would not have had adequate food to supply the pursuing French force or their animals. Marshal Massena's men were extremely low on rations, and encamped for about a month at a safe distance from Torres Vedras before they eventually decided to withdraw to Santarem, about 20 miles to the east, and remained there for several more months.

The general hospital at Coimbra was closed after functioning for only a few days and the wounded transported by river and along the coast to Lisbon. Others who were less fortunate had to make the journey to Lisbon over land, at about two miles per hour in the case of those who traveled by bullock cart, and many reached their destination in a very poor state of health.[66] The most severely injured were transported south in the newly acquired spring wagons that had recently been supplied to the staff surgeons for just such a purpose.

Apart from the 1,000 or so men retained in the regimental hospitals, the majority of the sick and wounded were now accommodated in Lisbon which, by December, was overflowing with patients. Earlier in the year, just over 11% of the force were hospitalized. During the malarial season, which lasted from June until September, the sick rate rose to 15–20%. In the late summer, from August until October, there was an increasing incidence of the various fly-borne diseases, while typhus, which was louse-borne, tended to occur during the winter months when the men were crowded together for warmth. The winter months were also associated with an increased incidence of respiratory and rheumatic diseases, due principally to exposure to the cold and damp conditions in the accommodation. Leg ulcers continued to be a problem, as were venereal diseases because of the close contact between the men and the local population.

During the winter months of 1810, an attempt was also made to ensure that the medical staff visited their patients in the general hospital on a more regular basis, to ensure that those who should be discharged were not retained any longer than was absolutely necessary on medical grounds. The convalescent patients tended to be retained on the wards to act as auxiliaries. The incidence of sickness among the Portuguese troops was always lower than that in the British force, principally because of their reduced susceptibility to malaria, and to the various local bowel diseases then prevalent.

During the early part of the year, about 5,000 men had been sent by Wellington to Cadiz, the fortress town to the west of Gibraltar, as this was considered to be a potential site of French incursion into the south of Spain. In June, the garrison there had been increased to 9,000 men, and together with a Spanish force was then besieged by the French under Marshal Victor. The siege was eventually raised in August 1812, when the French finally withdrew to face Wellington's army in the north.

Events during 1811

During March 1811, the French force under Massena decamped and retreated toward the Spanish border. The British, who found only evidence of destruction and carnage along the route, chased them. Their losses since Salamanca had been considerable, somewhere in the order of 25,000 men, due to sickness or death, and many had been taken prisoner.

In the south of Portugal, Beresford, with a force of 37,000 Allied troops, only 10,000 of whom were British, engaged Soult's force, with 23,000 men, at the battle of Albuera, in May 1811.[67] This was close to the stronghold of Badajoz. Despite the superiority of the French cavalry and artillery, they were eventually defeated because of the lethal effect of the firepower of the British infantry. The losses of life on both sides were enormous. Almost two-thirds of British infantry involved in the engagement were killed or wounded. With the very limited facilities available to remove the wounded from the battlefield, some of the 3,000 casualties remained there for more than a day despite the continuous torrential rain. When they reached the regimental hospital, they were attended to by Guthrie and his colleagues, all of whom worked almost continuously for days on end operating on the casualties.

The next action took place in September, in Coa, and lasted over a period of two days, although there were over 300 serious British casualties. From October, Wellington's army settled into winter quarters.[68] The sick rate was close to 30%, principally due to the various bowel diseases to which the men from Walcheren were particularly susceptible, while others suffered from typhus.

The British army was also involved in activities against the French and their allies in the Far East. The Government of India decided to launch an expedition against the island of Java, at that time the principal center of the Dutch Empire in the East Indies.[69] Napoleon had earlier made Java a military center from which the British settlements in the area could be attacked, and had sent out General Daendels in 1808 to place the colony in a state of readiness for that purpose; his force was said to consist of about 20,000 men. Both the British army and navy were happy with the idea of attacking such a rich commercial settlement, because of the prospect of gaining rich prize-money. Over 5,000 Sepoys from the Bengal army volunteered for the task, and the force was placed under the command of Sir Samuel Auchmuty. Because of the importance of the expedition, and presumably for the excitement, the Governor-General accompanied the expedition. The ships mostly set sail during the last two weeks of April, and intelligence reached Auchmuty on July 20 that General Daendels had left Java and been replaced by the equally competent General Janssens. The British force reached Penang by May 21, and proceeded to Malacca. The force finally disembarked off Chilingching during early August, a village situated on an island that was effectively shielded against enemy attack. The enemy force was invited to surrender, but declined to do so.

After a number of skirmishes during August, a considerable proportion of the enemy were eventually routed, and over 6,000 prisoners taken, including two generals and all of the headquarters staff, including, in all, about 250 officers. During this period, 40 enemy officers were killed, and another 63 were wounded; of the rank and file, more than 2,000 had either been killed or wounded. General Janssens escaped and regrouped, so that by September 16 he had at his command a force of about 8,000 men, only about one-tenth of whom were regulars and equipped with firearms. A full frontal attack was ordered, and the enemy was completely routed. Janssen, after some protestations, capitulated, and the last of the Dutch East Indian possessions passed into British hands. To commemorate this victory against the French, the members of the Honourable East India Company (HEIC) were awarded the Java Medal.[70]

The Return to Spain: 1812

During the early part of January 1812, Wellington stormed the fortress town of Ciudad Rodrigo. As it was still in the depths of winter, the French there were caught completely by surprise. Despite this, the British sustained over 1,000 casualties. This was Wellington's first foray into Spain for some time, and reversed the situation eighteen months earlier when a French force captured this fortress town in July 1810 after a campaign lasting six weeks. The wounded were given immediate attention nearby, then transferred to the local regimental hospitals where all emergency operations were performed. The majority of the wounded were then sent to the well-equipped general hospital at Coimbra for further treatment. Guthrie's men were the exception, in that they were retained in the nearby regimental hospitals for his personal attention, contrary to the instructions, and much to the annoyance, of the adjutant general.

Wellington's winter campaign coincided with Dr. James McGrigor's appearance on the scene as his newly appointed inspector of hospitals. McGrigor had arrived in Lisbon on January 10, 1812, to take over the duties of Dr. Franck, who had returned to England due to illness during the previous October.[71] McGrigor was very soon able to implement plans whose principal aim was to improve the administrative infrastructure of the Army Medical Department.

After his successful siege of Ciudad Rodrigo, Wellington decided to attack the strategically important fortress town of Badajoz, which had been captured by Soult during the spring of the previous year. The fortress was now in the hands of about 5,000 seasoned French troops, and, like Ciudad Rodrigo, was stormed by Wellington. This occurred in March 1812, with very substantial losses sustained by both sides. There were said to be about 1,000 dead and 4,000 wounded on the British side alone.[72]

To accommodate the casualties, McGrigor established an additional general hospital and a number of small field hospitals for the immediate treatment of the wounded. These were usually within musket range of the French, and caused additional distress to the wounded. Two spring wagons were supplied to each unit to hasten the transport of their wounded to the various hospitals, and were far superior to the bullock carts that had previously been available for this task.

At the suggestion of McGrigor,[73] the sterling work of the surgeons was first acknowledged in one of Wellington's public dispatches, dated April 8, 1812, addressed to the Secretary of State, the Earl of Liverpool.[74] The contents of this dispatch had the expected effect of raising the morale of all of the members of the Army Medical Department both in the Peninsula and elsewhere. It also had the effect of informing their brother officers that "their brethren had been publicly acknowledged in the same manner as those of the military officers."[75] The British public also duly noted the contents of Wellington's dispatch.

Following the storming of Badajoz, most of the regimental hospitals were fully occupied with the casualties. There were in addition over 14,000 sick, nearly 30% of Wellington's strength, mostly suffering from malaria, dysentery, and the various other fevers endemic in that part of Spain. In all, these occupied most of the beds in 11 general hospitals. Wellington's original plan was that he should drive out Soult's force, but this had to be abandoned when he appreciated that a greater threat was being posed by Marshal Auguste Marmont and his army, near Salamanca. Accordingly, Lieutenant-General Lord Hill, with a relatively small force, was left to prevent Soult from moving north and reinforcing Marmont.

In June, Wellington moved north with a force of about 43,000 men toward Salamanca. The two forces finally engaged on July 22, about 10 miles to the south of the city of Salamanca.[76] While the French were decisively defeated, both sides sustained heavy casualties. The French lost nearly 14,000 men, including 7,000 prisoners, while the Allies suffered over 5,000 casualties, with 250 officers and 4,000 men wounded.

Later in July, Valladolid was captured by the Allies, and soon afterward so was Madrid. Both Salamanca and Valladolid had been in French hands since the end of 1808. With the capture of Valladolid, a large number of wounded French troops became prisoners of the Allies. Shortly afterward, Valladolid was recaptured by the French under Clausel, but when Wellington returned from Madrid in September, the French force in the city surrendered. In order to protect his rear from possible attack by Soult, Wellington left a force under General Hill in Madrid.

Wellington then marched north from Madrid to Burgos, but the siege was not a success, and after five separate assaults, and with over 2,000 casualties and over a month of abortive activity, Wellington was forced to retire. The majority of the wounded had to be withdrawn to the general hospital at Valladolid, as the facilities near Burgos were so poor. As the summer progressed, the sick rate rose dramatically. During September, almost 18,000 of Wellington's force were sick and most required hospitalization. Salamanca was the busiest of the general hospitals, and over 1,000 patients died there during the three summer months, mostly from fevers and bowel complaints.

It soon became clear to Wellington that both to the south and north of him there were two powerful French armies advancing in his direction. He had no choice but to withdraw toward Valladolid. While the majority of his men were keen to fight, they were unaware that they were now outnumbered by almost 3:2. Soult was approaching Madrid from the south with 60,000 men, while another French force under Marmont was approaching Wellington from the north. Wellington was particularly distressed that he might have to leave large numbers of casualties in French hands. He was, however, reassured by McGrigor that this would not be the case, as all but the most severely wounded, who were not in any case fit to be moved, had already been transported to the general hospitals along his proposed line of withdrawal. Those 100 or so men who had to be left behind were placed under the care of two medical officers and a purveyor, the latter to provide hospital "comforts" and other extras whenever they might become available.

Wellington's withdrawal to Salamanca necessitated the transfer of all of the sick and wounded from Valladolid either to Oporto or to Celorico. The situation was getting more critical by the day, as Hill's force was clearly no match for Soult's superior numbers, and Hill had no choice but to withdraw, joining Wellington's force near to Salamanca on November 8. The sick and wounded were evacuated from Madrid to Salamanca under the direction of Guthrie, and during their journey they also gathered together a further 2,000 sick who appeared to be wandering almost aimlessly along the track. By the time they reached Salamanca, almost 1,000 of the wounded had recovered sufficiently to be able to rejoin their old regiments. The rest were sent in convoy to Ciudad Rodrigo. Of those who were too sick to move, about 60 had to remain in Salamanca, and these were left in the care of three medical officers and a purveyor.

For a contemporary account of the intolerable conditions encountered in the Peninsula in 1812, it is difficult to improve upon the bitter description provided 20 or so years later by Napier in his *History of the War in the Peninsula.* There was great dissatisfaction felt at all levels in the British army between the care and treatment of their wounded compared to the much higher standard that was believed to be provided by the French. According to Napier:

> It is a common, yet erroneous notion, that the English system of hospitals in the Peninsula was admirable, and that the French hospitals were neglected. Strenuous . . . exertions were made by lord Wellington and the chiefs of the medical staff to form good hospital

establishments, but the want of money, and still more the want of previous institutions, foiled their utmost efforts . . . Napoleon . . . furnished his hospitals with all things requisite...baron Larrey . . . organized the establishment called the hospital "Ambulance" . . . waggons of a peculiar construction, well horsed, served by men trained and incorporated as soldiers, and subject to a strict discipline . . . ready to . . . carry off wounded men; and the astonishing rapidity with which the fallen French soldiers disappeared from a field of battle attested the excellence of the institution. . . .

In the British army, the carrying off the wounded, depended, partly upon the casual assistance of a weak waggon train, very badly disciplined, furnishing only three waggons to a division, and not originally appropriated to that service; partly upon the spare commissariat animals, but principally upon the resources of the country, whether of bullock carts, mules, or donkeys. . . . Wellington complained, that when he demanded more [regular medical officers], the . . . board in London neglected his demands. . . . Shoals of hospital mates and students were . . . sent out, and . . . arrived for the most part ignorant alike of war, and their own profession . . . many . . . of the well educated surgeons sent out were for some time of little use, for superior professional skill is of little value in comparison of experience in military arrangement; where one soldier dies from the want of a delicate operation, hundreds perish from the absence of military arrangement. War tries the strength of the military frame-work; it is in peace that the frame-work itself must be formed.[77]

The difficulties associated with Wellington's retreat were worsened by the onset of torrential rain, and this, and the loss of the rations, severely tested the discipline of the force. Many stragglers who failed to keep up with the main force were rounded up by the French cavalry and either killed or taken prisoner. Eventually, after 30 days of forced marching, Wellington's army reached the fortress town of Ciudad Rodrigo, many in a state of extreme exhaustion. Of these, 19,500 men were suffering from one form of sickness or another, amounting in all to almost 30% of his strength. As the seriously ill could neither be adequately fed nor treated along the route, the condition of many of these men deteriorated, and a considerable number died shortly after their arrival at Ciudad Rodrigo. Wellington had additionally lost over 9,000 men along the route from Salamanca. Many had died from sickness or exhaustion, while the French had captured others.

The hospitals were now overwhelmed with the sick and wounded, and all of the available British doctors were rushed in to offer help. The Spanish doctors also gave assistance, as did those of the French doctors who were willing to help. The French medical officers principally served in the base hospitals, and received the standard British rate of pay for their help. Of the total complement of medical staff available in the Peninsula, a high proportion were needed to care for those troops who had retreated with Wellington from Salamanca.

Because of the crowded conditions in the hospitals, typhus again became a problem, and many died from it. This had a particularly disastrous effect on the severely debilitated and exhausted troops. The men were also vulnerable to dysentery, which caused over 2,300 deaths in 1812, compared to almost 1,000 deaths from typhus. During the same year, over 2,000 men died from typhoid. Between the middle of December 1812 and the end of January 1813, the rest of the army are said to have lost between 400 and 500 men each week from typhus and dysentery alone.[78]

Wellington was clearly extremely impressed with McGrigor's handling of the withdrawal from Salamanca. For the first time he allowed him executive authority to control the establishment of and activities within regimental hospitals, but he also provided him with the authority to transfer which patients he thought should be sent to the general hospitals. This was a critical initiative on Wellington's part, and allowed McGrigor to make decisions that had previously been within the exclusive domain of the adjutant general's office.[79]

Accordingly, the regimental hospitals were expanded and more adequately equipped, and relatively few patients were transferred to the general hospitals. McGrigor also insisted that accurate weekly, monthly, and quarterly in-patient returns be submitted from the regimental hospitals to his office, so that for the first time accurate figures were available which allowed statistical comparisons to be made on a year-to-year basis. This also allowed overall admission and discharge rates to be determined, and death rates from various conditions to be accurately established.

Activities in the Peninsula during 1813 and the Early Part of 1814

The troops in their winter quarters were kept under strict military discipline, and every effort was made to repair and rebuild the villages in which they were billeted. The men were supplied with new clothing and blankets, and their accommodation was well ventilated and not overcrowded. McGrigor also requested hutted hospital accommodation, which could be easily constructed, and could also be moved from one place to another. Wellington approved the expense involved, and the materials requested reached Oporto within a matter of weeks, and allowed the establishment of a mobile regimental hospital that could accommodate up to 4,000 patients near to the town of Castello Rodrigo.

The sick rate in the army gradually diminished, from well over 30% early in the year to about 15% by May. This halving in the number of the sick was of critical importance, in that it allowed Wellington's regiments to be maintained at maximum strength for his next offensive. By April 1813, his army contained almost 52,000 British, 28,000 Portuguese, and about 20,000 Spanish soldiers. The French, who were widely dispersed fighting the Spanish guerrillas, could only muster a force of about 50,000 men. Hundreds of British lives were undoubtedly saved by McGrigor's support of the regimental hospital system, by sparing men from the dreadful journeys by bullock carts to the general hospitals.

Additional reinforcements reached Wellington over the winter months, depleting the force retained in England to defend the country against an invasion to about 25,000 men. In order to shorten his lines of communication with England, Wellington decided to move his army in the direction of the northern coast of Spain. Supplies were shipped to him in the greatest of secrecy from England to the port of Corunna, for future use when his force eventually reached Santander. To confuse the French as to his real intentions, Wellington instructed Lieutenant-General Sir John Murray, who commanded a force of about 18,000 men in the eastern part of Spain, to attack the coastal city of Tarragona, close to the city of Barcelona. Many of the troops involved in this exercize came from Sicily, but also included men from Italy, Germany, Spain, and Portugal, but under British commanders. Some of the actions, for example, at Castalla ended in a French defeat, while the siege against Tarragona ended in an Allied defeat. This was principally due to the ineffectiveness of Murray, who was court-martialed after the war. Murray was acquitted of all charges, however, save that of abandoning his guns, for which he received only a reprimand.[80]

Wellington's army was then divided into two groups: his own force of 30,000 men which was to advance initially to Salamanca and then toward Santander, and the main force that was to march directly north through the Transmontes district of Spain. During June, as Wellington marched toward Santander, the French were forced successively to evacuate Valladolid, Palencia, and Burgos. On June 21, after a number of relatively minor skirmishes, the two armies faced each other in the valley of Vittoria.[81] They were relatively evenly matched, but the French army was forced to retreat, after abandoning all of its guns and supplies. The French losses were in the region of 7,000 men, while the Allies sustained over 5,000 casualties, about 4,200 men wounded and 800 killed. The British contingent of the force had the highest number of casualties, with over 3,000 officers and men wounded. This was one of the few decisive battles of the Peninsular War, and successfully liberated Spain from the French invaders.

After the battle of Vittoria, over 4,800 British, Portuguese, and French casualties were collected from the battlefield, and operated on continuously over a period of days by all of the surgeons working under the direction of John Hennen. General hospitals were established just to the north of Vittoria, in the various ports along the coast of the Bay of Biscay. This was much more convenient than having to transport patients the 300 or so miles to the ports along the Portuguese coast. The base hospital at Lisbon was now no longer needed, and was eventually closed in August 1813. The nearest general hospital to Vittoria, at Santander, could initially accommodate 4,000 patients. Its capacity was later increased by almost 1,000 beds, when its accommodation was supplemented by the arrival of portable wooden huts.

Within a week of the battle of Vittoria, the Allies advanced to the French border. Wellington, after two assaults, and with over 2,000 casualties, finally captured San Sebastian on August 31. On his other front, Napoleon had arranged a temporary truce with Austria, Russia, and Prussia, but this only held until September 3, because Napoleon refused to accept the river Rhine as one of the borders of France. Wellington then decided that this was an appropriate time for him to invade France. He crossed the river Bidassoa on October 7, and attacked the fortified center at Sare. In December, Wellington's force forded the river Nive, and attacked the French at Bayonne.

During Wellington's assault on Bayonne after the winter, Soult's force was surrounded and eventually compelled to withdraw to Orthez. Toward the end of March, Wellington attacked and eventually captured the city of Toulouse, this being the last British victory in the Peninsular War. During the early months of 1814, Napoleon's armies were severely defeated by the combined might of the

Russian, Austrian, and Prussian armies, and he was eventually forced to abdicate. While the news reached Wellington on April 12, the city of Bayonne did not surrender until the 26th.

Medical Arrangements during the Peninsular War

As in conflicts during the latter part of the previous century, the medical service was divided into staff and regimental branches, the former under the principal medical officer (PMO), the inspector of army hospitals, who was the adviser to the commander-in-chief, and the regimental officers whose allegiance was to their colonel. The staff officers technically were members of the Civil Department, and held only relative military rank. They covered the full range of medical specialties, but also had important administrative functions, though the most senior administrators were the deputy inspectors of hospitals. The staff officers often combined administrative and clinical posts.[82] They were also responsible for requesting the transport needed to evacuate the sick and wounded.

After the demise of the Army Medical Board in 1809–1810, it was now technically possible for all ranks to be selected on the basis of merit and experience to achieve the rank of physician. It had been clearly demonstrated during the previous 20 years that an individual could be an efficient administrator only if he had an appropriate basis of military experience. Accordingly, no physicians were appointed directly from civilian practice, and their role was now exclusively that of the senior clinician who looked after the needs of the medical patients.

Regimental mates entered the service mostly having only just obtained their license from the College of Surgeons. They, and often the regimental surgeons in times of peace, were generally considered the lowest of the low in the profession, and it was only in times of war that the essential role they played on the battlefield gave them some recognition. It was to be many years before they were to receive gallantry awards and decorations. Even in the Peninsular War the standard of the intake into the Army Medical Department was extremely poor. As the war progressed the need for more regimental and hospital mates (these individuals were subsequently termed assistant surgeons) grew, but the standard of entry declined. Those who survived during wartime gained experience on the job, and most developed into reasonably competent surgeons, although, it has to be admitted, at the expense of many patients along the way.

Hospitals were still separated into regimental hospitals, staffed by regimental mates and regimental surgeons, whose medical staff owed their allegiance exclusively to their colonel, and general hospitals where staff surgeons looked after the patients.[83] Two wives per company were allowed to accompany their husbands, and from these were selected individuals to cook and wash the linen of the men in the regimental hospitals. In the general hospitals, one ward master and six orderlies were allocated to every 100 beds. At this time there was still debate as to the value of general hospitals, principally because of their administrative inefficiency and their higher mortality. This was generally due to overcrowding and the cross-infection that inevitably followed.

Those who were designated ward orderlies were drawn from the men who were generally considered to be incapable of undertaking any other tasks in the service. Most were so ill disciplined that they should never have been retained in the service.

From early in 1809, the government and the Medical Board decided that British officers should be seconded to the Portuguese army and to their Medical Service, in the expectation that this would improve the efficiency of these services. General Beresford was transferred to the Portuguese army, to act as its commanding officer with the rank of Field Marshal, and deputy inspector William Fergusson was transferred to the Portuguese Medical Service to act as its inspector general of hospitals.[84] Initially 12 and later 20 medical officers were transferred to him, all with the rank of staff surgeon. The task before Fergusson was a considerable one, as the hospital arrangements within the Portuguese medical system were both antiquated and inefficient. The status of their few medical officers was extremely low, and all were engaged in almost full-time private practice to supplement their derisory army salary.

Initially the Portuguese military hospitals were reorganized along regimental lines, as Fergusson particularly favored this system. Attempts to improve their hygienic arrangements were, however, only very slowly achieved. Fergusson acted in this capacity for three years before returning to his earlier post, but over this period he not only improved the conditions within the hospitals but also dramatically improved the lot of their medical officers.

As the war progressed, many young, ill-prepared regimental and hospital mates were sent out to assist in the treatment of the enormous numbers of sick and wounded, particularly in the general hospitals. A few well-qualified men also arrived, but these tended to be the exception rather than the rule. Some of those sent by the Medical Board had until relatively recently been apothecaries' assistants with often only a few months of clinical training, and were particularly dangerous when expected to perform emergency surgical procedures in the absence of any detailed knowledge of anatomy. Most had had no previous exposure to military discipline or training. On arrival at their posting, no appropriate accommodation was provided for them, nor were they allowed a military servant to assist them in acclimatizing to the conditions to which they were exposed. They were expected to fend for themselves, with no knowledge of the local language or customs. Not surprisingly, many suffered as a consequence.

The illogicality of the hierarchical system in the Army Medical Department particularly distressed Fergusson, who stated in his *Notes and Recollections*:

> Taking the medical staff of regiments, where all act as army physicians, prescribing for diseases whether medical or surgical, and performing operations as the first circle of duties, it might be supposed that all would continue to walk in the same line through the different grades of military service. But no. Promote the operator among the regimental surgeons to the rank of physician, and the knife is forthwith taken out of his hands; he is never to touch it again. Make him a staff-surgeon, with superior rank, but the same pay,

he may indeed preserve the amputation-knife, but he is deprived of his home with the regiment, the accommodations of his mess and his servant, and made to shift for himself as he best can. Still more,—promote him to the highest ranks of Deputy-Inspector, or Inspector-General of Hospitals, and he ceases to be a medical man altogether, whether physician or surgeon. He is from henceforth to be a man of office entirely, an officer of administration alone: the book of physic, including surgery, is shut in his face, never to be opened unless by the less experienced juniors. Many, it must be owned, have continued to read and to inquire, but they have done so not in accordance with, but in defiance of, their prescribed duties.[85]

During the first half of 1813, the medical arrangements organized by McGrigor were beginning to bear fruit, in that many lives were saved by not having to be exposed to the rigors of the journey by bullock cart from the regimental to the general hospitals. In the latter, separate wards were created to cater to the surgical patients and for the needs of the patients with the different types of fever then prevalent, in order to reduce the incidence of cross-infection. Separate hospital accommodation was also provided for the officers, although they could still be treated in their own quarters if they so wished.

In the regimental hospitals, the overall organization of the auxiliaries and orderlies was now transferred into the control of the PMOs, rather than retained in the hands of the commanding officers of the regiments. The PMOs' authority was also extended to cover advice on clothing, diet, and messing arrangements for the sick. McGrigor ran into considerable difficulty, for example, when he wished to support the promotion of meritorious medical officers in the Peninsula. Despite Wellington's support, the Medical Board blocked most of his recommendations. They claimed that they had to take into account the expectations of the many equally meritorious medical officers who were on active service in more distant parts of the Empire. Much to McGrigor's and Wellington's annoyance, the Duke of York, the commander-in-chief supported the director-general of the Army Medical Board's view.

As the war progressed, the standard of surgery improved dramatically. During the early part of the war, amputations were very commonly performed, but were only rarely carried out during its later stages. After the battle of Toulouse, in the spring of 1814: "Out of 1,242 capital (major) operations only 48 times were amputations performed, or 4 per cent of the total; and out of 304 wounds of the upper extremity there were 7 amputations or between 2 and 3 percent. The mortality in these 1,242 operations . . . amounted to 146 or 11.7 per cent; in the upper extremity the mortality was 1 per cent; in the lower extremity 4 per cent; but in secondary amputations for compound fractures it was 33 per cent."[86] There was also "not a single case of hospital gangrene." Guthrie believed that amputations were far too commonly performed,[87] and he rarely amputated the upper extremity, performing, where appropriate, the excision of the head of the humerus, or the elbow joint. In most areas of military surgery, great strides were made, and these were soon reflected in civilian practice.

The reputation of the Army Medical Service during the last decade of the 18th century was not good. It has been said that "the mismanagement of hospitals had been exceeded only by the chaos in the Army as a whole, and this in turn by

Government mismanagement, and misappropriation of public funds."[88] During the early years of the Peninsular War, the situation was only slightly better. Lack of funds and government indifference, associated with incompetence on the part of the members of the Medical Board, greatly frustrated all Wellington's efforts and those of his senior medical staff to improve the situation.

Despite the improvements initiated in surgical practice by George Guthrie during the Peninsular campaigns, both hospital administration and the organization of the transport of the wounded and supplies were still often grossly inadequate. Many of the wounded officers and men died before they reached the base hospitals, and even if they did survive to full recovery, they were often reluctant to return to duty. Guthrie recommended to Wellington that the regimental hospitals should be both enlarged and better equipped, and that those being treated in them should be kept in closer contact with their regimental colleagues. This alone had a dramatic effect not only on decreasing the mortality rates, but also in encouraging a high proportion of those who recovered to return to duty. It was only after the appointment of McGrigor as Wellington's inspector of hospitals that improvements gradually began to be made in the efficiency of the Army Medical Department in the Peninsula.

Shortly after his appointment, McGrigor investigated rumors of financial irregularities in the general hospitals in Lisbon and Coimbra that had previously come to his attention. The cause of the latter was due largely to the inexperience of the individuals in the accounts departments of these hospitals, rather than that there was misconduct on the part of specific individuals, and this problem was relatively easily rectified. He then investigated the apparently very large number of convalescent patients in these two hospitals. This was a considerable problem in Lisbon, where officers in particular were happy to prolong their "convalescence" in the company of their wives and ladies, rather than recovering from their supposed ailments. The large number of convalescent patients required a substantial number of doctors at all levels to cater to their needs. By March 1812, after firm words were spoken in certain quarters, many of these troops, as well as their medical attendants, returned to more useful duties elsewhere.

The alleviation of the unacceptable position in Lisbon and to a lesser extent in Coimbra freed many of the beds in these hospitals. McGrigor believed that the majority of both the sick and wounded officers and men should be treated in the regimental hospitals. Only those to be invalided back to England were sent to the general hospital in Lisbon. This change in policy also had the advantage that only those who were soon to leave the service would be exposed to the lengthy overland journey by bullock cart to Lisbon. The harshness of the journey, which could last from one to three weeks, invariably traumatized the most seriously ill patients, very few of whom ever recovered to return to their regiments. In those instances where patients did successfully recover, the duration of their illness was considerably prolonged, compared to those retained in the regimental hospitals. More important, most of the sick preferred to be treated in the regimental hospitals where they found the atmosphere friendly and, moreover, they received treatment from individuals, both doctors and orderlies, who were familiar to them. In the general hospitals, the patients often found that many of the staff appeared to be indifferent to their welfare.

The changes that McGrigor planned to implement were not new, and had the support of the vast majority of the regimental medical officers. This arrangement was implemented with little difficulty during the winter months when relatively few individuals needed to be transported by bullock cart to the general hospitals. As the weather improved, the number of bullocks that would be required to move the regimental hospitals when the army was on campaign was more than could be spared for patient transport. McGrigor's plan had therefore to be temporarily shelved.

The close bond that soon developed between McGrigor and Wellington, as Wellington was in the habit of seeing the heads of his administrative sections on a daily basis, for the first time allowed the medical service advance warning of intended operations. This provided Wellington, for the first time, with insight into the difficulties encountered by the members of the Army Medical Department. This closeness to Wellington also allowed McGrigor to provide him with up-to-date casualty figures. "Being with his Lordship the whole time the business went on I saw everything and heard everything . . . when the account came that our people had been repulsed from the two breaches. . . . Lord Wellington was extremely anxious to know the number of men that came wounded to the different posts."[89] Equally, anything that improved the efficiency of the medical service also increased the manpower available to the commanding officer.

The Events Soon after the Peninsular War

During 1814, Wellington's successes were confined to the southern part of France. Elsewhere, his allies advanced toward Paris and both the Austrian and Prussian armies entered and occupied the city on March 30. Napoleon abdicated and was banished to Elba. During the early part of the year, the British Government had decided to send a small force to the Low Countries to capture Antwerp. This force attacked Bergen op Zoom in March, but was unable to capture it, and lost over 3,000 men out of a total force of 4,600. Half were killed and the other half taken prisoner. Hostilities in Holland continued until the end of April, although Antwerp and Bergen op Zoom were not occupied until May 5. The British then set up their headquarters in Brussels.

In February 1815, the Great powers, known as the "Concert of Europe," met to divide up the territories that formerly belonged to France and her allies. A Victory Ball was held on March 7, in Vienna, but the celebrations were short-lived when news reached them that Napoleon had escaped from Elba. He was in Lyons by March 10, and by the 20th in Fontainebleau. The Allied forces had mobilized, and the British and Prussians were required to defend the Low Countries. The British had earlier established their headquarters in Brussels, and the Duke of Wellington was confirmed as commander-in-chief. His force occupied the territory between Brussels and Ostend. The Prussian army, with a force of 110,000 men under the command of Field Marshal Gebhard von

Blücher, had its headquarters at Namur, and looked after the territory to the southeast of the rivers Sambre and Meuse.

Initially, Wellington had at his disposal only six regiments of cavalry (about 6,000 men) and twentyfive infantry battalions (about 20,000 men). The original nucleus of about 5,000 Peninsular War veterans already in the Netherlands was soon increased to about 71,000, many of them from second battalions consisting of fresh and inadequately trained recruits. Most of the Peninsular War veterans were with the army in America[90] or had been disbanded. To the British contingent was added a variety of foreign corps, including the German Legion, Hanoverian troops, and those from Brunswick and Nassau. There were also Dutch and Belgian troops, the latter of indifferent quality and dubious reliability. These in all increased the strength of the Allied force by about 15,000 cavalry and 70,000 infantry.

THE BATTLE OF WATERLOO

Napoleon planned to capture Brussels, and aimed to destroy individually both the British army (including those of its allies) and the Prussian army. On June 15 he attacked the Prussians at Charleroi, and on June 16 he also engaged them at Ligny. The British were attacked at Quatre Bras and sustained over 600 killed and 2,400 wounded, but managed to hold their position. The Prussians were forced to withdraw to Wavre, about 15 miles from Waterloo. This was where Wellington had previously decided that the principal encounter between Napoleon and his enemies should take place.

While not wishing to discuss Wellington's tactics during the ensuing battle, as others have covered this in great detail,[91] it is appropriate to note here the principal components of the battle as far as this sheds light on the enormous casualties sustained by all the combatants involved. The two sides were drawn up against each other on June 18, the majority of the British on a ridge south of the village of Mont St. Jean, with others in front of them holding the farms of Hougoumont on the right and La Haye Saint in the center.

The French infantry attacked the relatively small Allied force at Hougoumont, which held its position, and shortly afterward the Allied center and left. These were mostly held at bay by sustained musket fire, followed by bayonet charges. French cavalry were then sent in to support their infantry, but were routed by a charge of the Household Brigade, although they were overwhelmed when they encountered the main French lines. It was essential that Napoleon should defeat Wellington's force before the arrival of the Prussians, in order to ensure a victory. The French now employed cavalry unsupported by artillery or infantry against the Allies. Further assaults on the Allied lines severely weakened their center. They now formed into squares, and additional troops were called in from Wellington's left and right wings.

The Allies held until the arrival of the Prussians. After a heavy bombardment, Napoleon sent in his Imperial Guard, and these were directed against Wellington's right center. After numerous volleys of musket fire from the British infantrymen, which killed many and had a dramatic effect on the morale of the rest of the Imperial Guard, the British guardsmen charged, and successfully routed them. Wellington then ordered his counteroffensive. The French force was completely routed, and Wellington claimed a great victory. About a month later, Napoleon abdicated, and on this occasion was exiled to St. Helena, where he died in 1821.[92]

At Waterloo, the medical position was only marginally better than it was in 1809. The Army Medical Service, in 1815, under the direction of Dr. James (later Sir James) Grant (1773–1864),[93] could only muster 52 staff officers,[94] though Grant was able to allocate one surgeon and two assistant surgeons to each regiment, being the minimum number previously requested by Wellington.[95] Each regiment now had a spring wagon to carry the sick and wounded. The medical establishment was grossly inadequate for the task at hand, because it was only intended for an army of about 40,000 men. It also had to serve the needs of five general hospitals, the first at Ostend, and then others at Ghent, Bruges, Brussels, and Antwerp. In addition, many of the junior medical officers had no experience of combat.

The British losses at Waterloo were 1,417 killed and 4,923 wounded; an additional 582 men were reported missing, a proportion of whom were probably also killed, although a considerable number would have gone to the rear with wounded officers and men. Although this practice was strictly forbidden, it commonly occurred, due in particular to the absence of an organized system of stretcher-bearers.

The Immediate Aftermath of the Battle of Waterloo

At the end of the day, within a two-mile area, 40,000 men and 25,000 horses lay dead or wounded, and it took at least four days to extricate the Allied wounded from the battlefield.[96] This figure may be an underestimate; Howard reported that "in the space of about six square miles lay more than 52,000 dead and wounded. About 6,700 were Prussians, 15,000 were from the allied army, and the rest [i.e., over 30,000] were French."[97]

The medical service dealt with about 12,500 Allied sick and wounded and an additional 2,500 sick and wounded French prisoners, so that nearly 15,000 hospital beds had to be provided to cope with these numbers. It took far longer to rescue the French wounded from the battlefield and from the surrounding countryside, and many remained there for more than 10 days before being transported to a hospital. The majority either died where they were wounded or died of their wounds, which had now become gangrenous, after they had reached the hospital. "For the first 24 hours, nothing effectual could be done, for assistant surgeons only carried a small pocket case of instruments, and they were without their amputating knives. But while awaiting their arrival, the doctors were not idle, for with their lancets we bled our fellows all around."[98]

The bodies on the battlefield soon proved a health hazard, and the majority were disposed of in mass graves. During the weeks after the battle, local peasants from miles around were rounded up at bayonet-point by the Prussians to expedite the disposal of the decomposing and putrefying corpses of the men and horses from the battlefield. These had already contaminated most of the local sources of water within three miles of the battlefield.[99]

Many of the Allied wounded were operated on either on the battlefield or in relatively crude field stations, and many limbs were probably sacrificed which could otherwise have been saved. According to Guthrie, "Few, if any, of the medical staff officers had seen a field of battle. I found the assistant surgeons doing everything they should not have done. The greatest efforts were made to obviate this state of things. Amateur surgeons flocked over from London. They rectified these evils as far as they could, but nothing could recall the past or the irretrievable mischief insufficient care had occasioned in the first few days."[100]

Guthrie did not publish his conservative views on the treatment of gunshot fractures of the long bones until many years later,[101] and he may well have taken a different view at the time. His monograph published shortly after the battle advocated immediate rather than delayed amputation for the majority of cases of compound fractures following gunshot wounds of the extremities, before the appearance of "fever, inflammation, suppuration and gangrene."[102] This was the accepted wisdom at that time.[103] Thomson[104] estimated that at Waterloo some 500 amputations were done; one-third of them before the onset of inflammation, and noted that the highest mortality was seen where amputation was for any reason delayed. In cases where the fracture was located above the middle of the femur, the majority died from septicemia or from shock.[105]

Examples are available of the advantages to be gained by less extreme surgical measures, but in the early years of the Peninsular War these seemed to be the exception rather than the rule. Toward the end of this war, far fewer amputations were performed (see section entitled "Medical Arrangements during the Peninsular War"). If amputations had to be performed, Guthrie was in favor of them being undertaken as soon as the patient was able to bear the operation.[106] He was extremely hostile to secondary amputations because of their much poorer prognosis.

Guthrie gave a long interview in 1850 to one of the *Lancet*'s editorial staff in which he detailed some of his more heroic exploits in the Peninsular War. In one of the episodes cited, an example of the conservative approach occasionally employed by Guthrie is given, almost as though this was the accepted practice of the time—which it clearly was not, as many surgeons were still enthusiastic to amputate limbs, rather than excising joints in an attempt to preserve some limb function. When the interview was published Guthrie, curiously, described his activities in the third person:

> At the last battle in France, Toulouse, the late Lord, then Sir Hussey Vivian, commanding the cavalry, had his left arm broken by a musket-ball, and was advised by the surgeons present to have it amputated. This he refused until he saw some persons of more experience, and Mr. Guthrie, then in charge of that part of the army, engaged on the Right Bank of the Garonne, decided that it should not be removed. Many years afterwards, when Lord Vivian presented him to his second wife on her marriage, he did it with the compliment: "I introduce you to Mr. Guthrie, to whom you and I are both indebted for the arm on which you are now leaning." The precepts laid down in his last work on this subject, scarcely admit of an arm being cut off for any injury save by cannon-shot. The

elbow-joint has been cut out, the head of the bone has been sawed off from its connexion with the shoulder, any portion of the middle part removed, but not the arm itself has been excised, not even if its principal artery be injured, unless mortification has taken place.[107]

In 1854, an anonymous article was published in the *Lancet* that provided an abstract of Guthrie's then current views on the emergency treatment of battle casualties.[108] This was in the form of 34 key points that always had to be borne in mind by army surgeons when attending to the wounded. In this pamphlet, many of Guthrie's key points referred to conditions where amputation of a limb would previously have been the favored course of action. Here, amputation was recommended only when so much tissue had been destroyed that the limb, and probably the patient, would inevitably be lost if this procedure were not undertaken. Amputation was only rarely necessary except following the effects of cannon-shot. In most cases of gunshot injury to the upper limb involving a joint, it was nearly always possible to successfully excise the damaged joint, thus leaving the individual with a useful arm. When there was much splintering of bone, the bony fragments had to be removed and the limb then carefully splinted. The hand was never to be amputated unless all or nearly all of its parts were destroyed.

With regard to gunshot wounds involving the lower limb, a similar conservative approach was recommended. Amputation was necessary only when much of the limb was destroyed by cannon-shot or, in thigh injuries, when the removal of the damaged soft tissues of the thigh exposed the femur, so that there was no possibility of limb function. Equally, amputation was necessary when a gunshot wound involved the principal artery to the thigh. In cases of fractures, splinting of the fractured bones was essential. Wounds of the arteries of the thigh required compression to avoid the death (i.e., mortification) of more distal parts of the limb. Ligatures should then be secured above and below the damaged vessel as soon as possible afterward to avoid death by exsanguination.

The British civilian surgeons mostly operated on the French wounded, as the majority of the Allied wounded had already been attended to by the time they reached the hospitals. Ten days after the battle, Grant wrote to Wellington that there were 2,376 British and Hanoverian wounded in the various hospitals in Brussels. He also noted that the evacuation of others to Antwerp was proceeding slowly, but that no transport was available to take the wounded to the hospitals in Bruges, Ghent, or Ostend. Numerous accounts were published of the horrendous conditions that were encountered shortly after the battle.[109]

A contemporary account draws attention to the high regard that the combatants often had for their wounded adversaries as soon as the hostilities had ceased.[110] According to a letter written from Brussels by a wounded British officer from the 92d Regiment, shortly after the battle of Waterloo:

We marched from Brussels at one in the morning, and arrived at three o'clock in the afternoon at the place of action, having marched nine leagues. We were engaged in five minutes after, and continued so till night. I was wounded about half past eight, when I was obliged to walk six miles to the nearest village, where I lay in pain and sleepless till day-light. I was again obliged to walk to Brussels, seven leagues; not being able to bear the motion of a waggon. The exertion has done me no good. I am indeed surprised that I was able to stand it out. The poor fellows who had escaped, bivouacked in the field, without tents or baggage—last night the same—and it has rained incessantly.

Our regiment was again engaged, and suffered severely. There is scarcely one officer left. Never was there sight so touching, so extraordinary, as this town presents—the people in crowds going out to meet the wounded with refreshments, bandages, &c.—all the women employed in the kindest offices. I returned to the house of my former landlord, where I am treated as if I were his own brother. The French prisoners are treated by the populace in the most violent manner; the escort can with difficulty protect them from being attacked.

A note follows from the hand of Viscount Vanderfosse:

The Scotch regiments, who had during the battle of the 18th, given such proofs of intrepidity, offered a most sympathetic example in appearing to forget their wounds, to render services to their wounded Iron Foe, who, but the minute before, had been attempting with all their might to destroy them. . . . Upwards of 500 of the French owe their lives to their generous enemies; "among these respectable warriors, the Scotch deserve to be particularly commemorated; and this honourable mention, is due to their discipline, their mildness, their patience, their humanity, and their bravery without example."

On the 16th and 18th of June 1815, their valour was displayed in a manner the most heroic. Multiplied, constant, and almost unheard of proofs were given, I do not merely say of courage, but of devotion to their country quite extraordinary and sublime—nor must we forget that these men so terrible in the Field of Battle, were mild and tranquil out of it.

Thomson[111] wrote one of the most important accounts of the treatment of the wounded in the hospitals in Brussels, although he did not arrive there until about three weeks after the battle. He produced a considerable series of rough ink sketches of the wounded in Brussels that he presented to Ballingall. These were bound together and relatively recently transferred to Edinburgh University Library.[112] Charles Bell also produced a large series of watercolor sketches of the wounded, and his widow in 1866 presented these and a number of related items to the army.[113] Bell also sketched in other media.[114] Charles Bell mostly attended French casualties as almost all of the Allied wounded had already been attended to a week or more before he arrived in Brussels. The British wounded who survived were mostly sent either to York hospital, Chelsea, under the care of Guthrie, or to Colchester, under the care of James Forbes.

THE LIGHT MOBILE AMBULANCES DESIGNED BY LARREY, AND THE MOBILE AMBULANCE UNITS

The most outstanding contribution by the French military surgeon Baron Dominique Larrey was the concept developed by him and first employed by the French army during the last decade of the 18th century, of the light mobile ambulance wagon (Ambulance Volantes).[115] This could keep up with the troops as they marched into battle, and would also allow surgeons to collect the wounded and transport them from the battlefield to distant field hospitals without suffering additional trauma (see Figure 2.1). These vehicles also allowed the surgeons to undertake emergency and often life-saving procedures while under enemy fire, in reasonable safety. Their presence close to the battlefield was clearly reassuring to their own men, and must have saved countless lives, making the French army the envy of their enemies. A less sophisticated French-designed ambulance, or temporary hospital, had originally been employed at the Battle of Fontenoy, in 1745, having the great advantage that it could be located close to the front lines. Stretcher-bearer parties (Corps de Brancardiers) had also been introduced by Baron Percy.[116]

The French ambulances would have been of little value on their own, had they not been backed up by teams of surgeons, orderlies, and an adequate supply of first-aid equipment. Each ambulance unit worked under the direction of a chief surgeon, and was staffed by about 340 men. The unit was divided into three divisions; each supervised by a surgeon of the first class, assisted by two assistant surgeons of the second class, and twelve assistant surgeons of the third class. The latter were only partially trained, and the units also contained two qualified pharmacists.

Each division had eight two-wheeled wagons, and four four-wheeled wagons each with their drivers and orderlies. Four additional ordinary transport wagons were assigned to each division. The light two-wheeled wagons were well sprung and specifically designed for working in flat country. Each could accommodate two stretchers lying side-by-side, and were drawn by two horses, each with a postilion. The larger four-wheeled wagons could accommodate four men, and were designed for more uneven terrain; they were drawn by four horses, two of which had postilions. In mountainous terrain, mules or packhorses each with panniers to carry the essential medical dressings and equipment accompanied the wagons. These units were also employed to collect and bury the dead. When engaged in this activity, they were accompanied by a mounted military policeman who could utilize local inhabitants to assist with this task.[117]

REMOVAL OF THE CASUALTIES FROM THE BATTLEFIELD—THE BRITISH APPROACH

One of the greatest problems encountered by McGrigor in the Peninsula was the lack of means to evacuate the wounded from the battlefield, and to evacuate these men, and the sick, to the field and regimental hospitals.

The system of field ambulances employed by the French contrasted with the very limited number of poorly sprung, often bullock-drawn, general-purpose wagons that had to be withdrawn from other activities for this purpose. In addition to their other duties, senior medical officers were also responsible for applying to the commissary general for the transport needed to evacuate the sick and wounded to the rear. More particularly, those soldiers who were associated with the transportation of the French wounded and sick were well disciplined and well organized. Those who undertook this function for the Allies tended to

Figure 2.1. French Ambulance Men and Surgeons Attending to a Wounded Soldier on the Battlefield

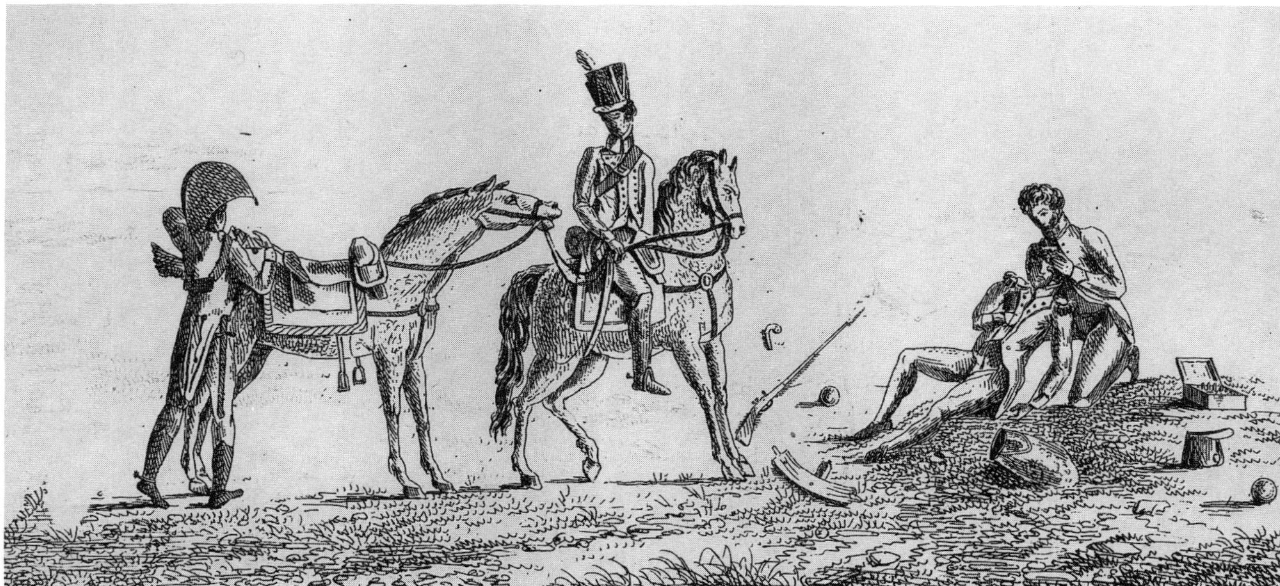

From: D. J. Larrey, 1812-1817. *Mémoires de Chirurgie Militaire, et Campagnes*. 4 Volumes (Paris: J. Smith) [Volume 1, 1812; Plate II].

be drawn from the dregs of the army, those who were generally considered to be unsuitable for any other useful role.

Most British regiments sent out parties of noncombatants, such as the drummers, often in the charge of a medical officer, to collect their own wounded from the battlefield, to bring them to medical attention. This was clearly both inadequate and unsatisfactory. More often, their comrades assisted the casualties to the rear, thus depriving the force of some of its firepower. This was also not infrequently used as an excuse for those who were less keen to be in the midst of the action to retire to the rear. At Waterloo, many of the wounded were not removed from the battlefield for up to four days after the conflict. Descriptions are available of surgeons forcing peasants to assist in this exercise, rather than pillaging the dead.

In the field, the British in India used the *Dooly*. This consisted of a framework to protect the patient against the weather, suspended by a pole or length of bamboo passing through it, and was carried on the shoulders of four men. While adapted to the terrain in India, it was considered unsuitable for general use in Europe. Larrey had designed his camel litter for use when accompanying Napoleon's expedition to Egypt in 1798. Two large boxes were slung, one on either side of the camel, and each could carry a wounded man. This was not a comfortable conveyance, and "Bonaparte is said to have experienced a sensation like sea-sickness, from riding on the back of a camel."[118] The wagons in use in the British army during the Peninsular War and previously were said to be in all respects inferior to those used by the French, poorly designed for the conveyance of the wounded, very cumbrous, and unwieldy.

Ballingall, in Edinburgh, was well aware of the value of mobile ambulances and ambulance units, and had a number of illustrations and models of them in the museum associated with his class of military surgery. The design and discussions of the role of these ambulances also featured in his *Outlines of Military Surgery*,[119] and in less detail in his earlier *Introductory Notes*.[120] Tufnell, in Dublin, had also collected a substantial museum which contained these and similar appliances to illustrate his lecture course on military surgery. His collection was subsequently transferred to the Army Medical College, at Netley, in 1863, after the government withdrew funding to support his Regius Chair in 1860.[121]

THE FORMATION OF A HOSPITAL CORPS TO ASSIST THE MEDICAL OFFICERS IN THEIR DUTIES

In Ballingall's *Outlines of Military Surgery*,[122] in a section entitled "Transportation of the sick and wounded," he not only detailed the various carriages that were used for this purpose, but also discussed what assistance was generally available to the medical staff to collect the wounded from the battlefield and transport them to the hospital.

Ballingall recommended "the formation of a *hospital corps*, placed entirely at the disposal of the medical staff, and consisting of men either enlisted and embodied solely with this view . . . a body of men trained in the particular duties required of them, qualified to attend the sick in the hospitals as well as to succour and bear off the wounded in the field, would preserve the effective forces of regiments; would afford a degree of comfort to the sick and wounded, to which they are too often strangers; and would give an efficiency to the medical staff, which the most zealous devotion to the duties of the service cannot otherwise ensure."[123]

Despite the excellent example displayed by the French, no comparable arrangement was established in the British army despite the well-intentioned but abortive attempt made by Colonel Gilbert Waugh in 1795 in the West Indies campaign which barely survived for six months. The detailed plans proposed by surgeon van Millingen were published in his *Army Medical Officer's Manual.*[124]

Van Millingen suggested that the noncombatants, such as the drummers and pioneers, would remove the casualties from the battlefield and deliver them to the regimental Aid Posts. The Hospital Ambulance Corps, which was commanded by a regimental assistant surgeon, would then transport the wounded, and remove them to the brigade hospital which, critically, was out of musket-ball range. Here the regimental surgeons and assistant surgeons would dress the wounded and undertake all measures necessary to stop the bleeding. The wounded would then be transported by ambulance wagons to the brigade hospital (equivalent to the regimental hospital), which was to be located out of cannon range, where essential lifesaving operations would be performed. In his plan, the noncombatants would be withdrawn when there was no action to serve as hospital orderlies, returning to their battlefield duties in times of action. Untrained personnel requisitioned from the regiments would then take their place on the wards. This plan was terminated with the dramatic manpower cuts that were implemented during the early post-Waterloo era.[125]

Van Millingen's book has, as its frontispiece, an engraving of a private in his imaginary "Hospital Corps," dressed in an appropriate uniform of the period. In his hand he carries a long pike, and on his back a "traverse" (or cross-piece made of wood) with two holes, as well as a length of canvas (see Figure 2.2). Thus, two members of the corps, between them, had the means of making a stretcher, the two pikes being used as stretcher poles. Such a stretcher is shown in use in the background. When necessary, these poles could be used as offensive weapons.

Ballingall and many others clearly saw the need for a Hospital Ambulance Corps associated with a corps of hospital orderlies. No corps along these lines was established in the British army until after the Crimean War, which incorporated the critical elements of (1) an efficient and rapid means of removing casualties from the battlefield by an adequate number of non-combatants, (2) individuals who could attend to their immediate first aid need, (3) the provision of a means of transporting them to the regimental hospitals where essential lifesaving operations could be performed, and (4) providing adequately trained hospital orderlies who could exclusively attend to the needs of the sick and wounded on the wards.

It is likely that one of the principal reasons why the French Medical Corps with its light mobile ambulance units worked so efficiently was because at that

Figure 2.2. Private in Hospital Corps

He is carrying a long pike that could be used as a stretcher pole or, if necessary, as an offensive weapon. He carries on his back a length of canvas and a "traverse" with two holes the other items needed to form a stretcher.

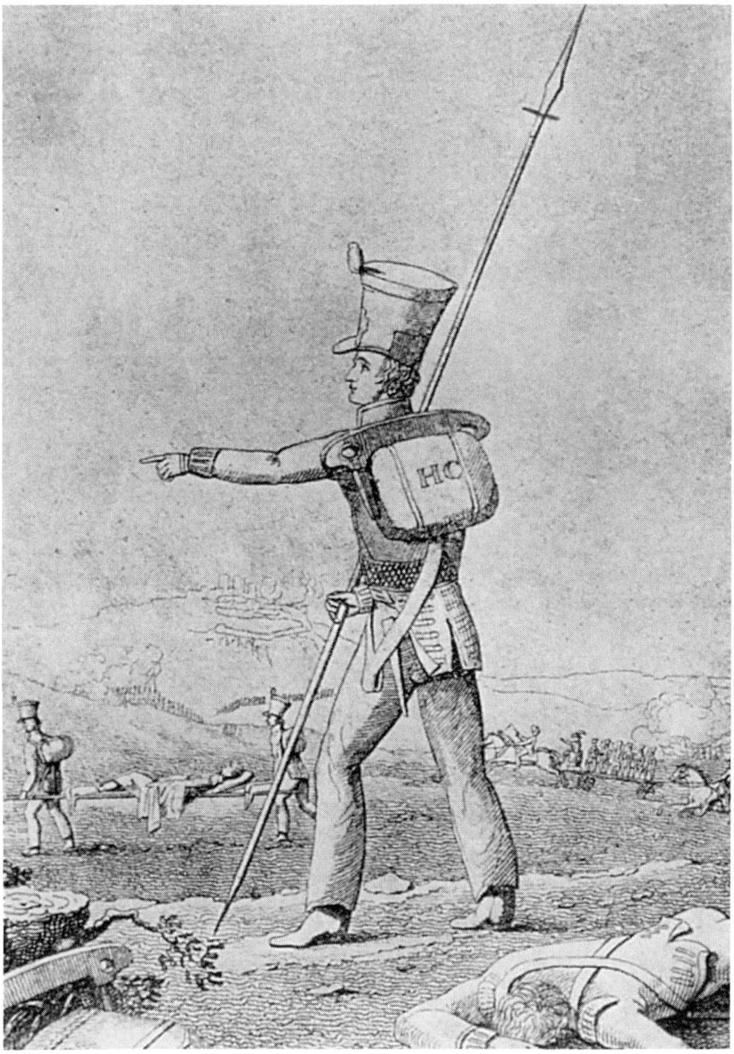

From: J. G. van Millingen, 1819. *The Army Medical Officer's Manual upon Active Service; Precepts for his Guidance in the Various Situations in which he may be placed; with Observations on the Preservation of the Health of Armies upon Foreign Service* (London: Burgess & Hill) [According to F. Smith, 1929, *A short history of the Royal Army Medical Corps* (Aldershot: Gale & Polden Ltd.), this volume was first published in 1805, and reprinted in 1819].

time they had conscription in France, and consequently no significant manpower problem. Each unit had an establishment of 113 officers, noncommissioned officers, and men, including 14 mounted surgeons under the command of a surgeon major, 1st class. All had specific duties to perform, and carried the instruments or dressings they required either in a pouch on their back or, if a surgeon, in a pannier.

The absence of anything comparable in the British army also extended to the poor treatment of their medical officers during this period. Medical officers had no mess, and had to live in civilian lodgings, were looked after by a civilian servant, and fed individually. Had they the opportunity of living in a mess, it is likely that the junior staff would have soon come under the beneficial guidance of their more senior colleagues, and established a corporate spirit, like their colleagues in the executive branch of the service.

NOTES

1. P. J. Haythornthwaite, 1994. *The Armies of Wellington* (London: Arms and Armour Press), p. 22.
2. J. W. Fortescue, 1899–1930. *A History of the British Army*. 13 Volumes (London: Macmillan & Co.), 1906, Volume 4, Part 1, p. 213.
3. Fortescue, *British Army*, Volume 4, Part 1, pp. 94–95.
4. N. Cantlie, 1974. *A History of the Army Medical Department*. 2 Volumes (Edinburgh and London: Churchill Livingstone), Volume 1, pp. 214–215.
5. Haythornthwaite, *Wellington*, p. 14.
6. Fortescue, *British Army*, Volume 4, Part 1, p. 72.
7. He had been appointed a Knight Bachelor in 1782, and inspector general of prisons in Ireland from May 1788. He was later appointed inspector of health for the Land Forces in September 1794, was retired on half-pay in December 1802, and died in 1810; Anon., 1810. *The Gentleman's Magazine: and Historical Chronicle (New Series)* **80**, 187 [brief obituary notice for Sir Jerome Fitzpatrick]; A. Peterkin, and W. Johnston, 1968. *Commissioned Officers in the Medical Services of the British Army 1660–1960*. 2 Volumes. Vol. 1, 1660–1898, 638 pp., Vol. 2, 1898–1960, 452 pp. (London: Wellcome Historical Medical Library) [This volume is sometimes referred to as "Drew, R. (Editor)," with the same details], Volume 1, ref. no. 1303, p. 82.
8. Cantlie, *Army Medical Department*, Volume 1, pp. 223–224.
9. Fortescue, *British Army*, Volume 4, pp. 320–321.
10. Cantlie, *Army Medical Department*, Volume 1, p. 225.
11. J. Hennen, 1818. *Observations on Some important points in the Practice of Military Surgery, and in the Arrangement and Police of Hospitals. Illustrated by Cases and Dissections* (Edinburgh: A. Constable & Co.; London: Longman, Hurst, Rees, Orme & Brown; Dublin: J. Cumming) [dedicated to Sir James McGrigor, Knt. M.D. F.R.S.], pp. 53–54; Anon., 1959–1960. Hennen, John, M.D. (1779–1828). *Dictionary of National Biography* **9** (Oxford: Oxford University Press), 424.
12. Anon., 1908. Jackson, Robert, M.D. (1750–1827). *Dictionary of National Biography* **10** (London: Smith, Elder & Co.), 542–543, p. 542.
13. R. Jackson, 1791. *A Treatise on the Fevers of Jamaica, with some Observations on the Intermitting Fever of America, and an Appendix Containing Some Hints on the Means of Preserving the Health of Soldiers in Hot Climates* (London: J. Murray).

14. An outbreak of an epidemic occurred at Parkhurst, with an increase in sickness and mortality for which Jackson was personally held responsible.

15. J. Fergusson, 1846. *Notes and Recollections of a Professional Life, by the Late William Fergusson, Esq. M.D. Inspector General of Military Hospitals. Edited by his son, James Fergusson* (London: Longman, Brown, Green & Longmans).

16. R. Jackson, 1817. *A Sketch of the History and Cure of Febrile Diseases; More Particularly as they appear in the West-Indies among the Soldiers of the British Army* (Stockton: T. & H. Eeles; London: R. Fenner). [606 pp.].

17. R. Jackson, 1805. *A System of Arrangement and Discipline for the Medical Department of Armies* (London: J. Murray).

18. H.A.L. Howell, 1911. Robert Jackson, M.D., Inspector of Hospitals. *Journal of the Royal Army Medical Corps* **16**, 121–139; Anon., 1908. Jackson, Robert, M.D. (1750–1827). *Dictionary of National Biography* **10** (London: Smith, Elder & Co.), 542–543.

19. Fortescue, *British Army*, Volume 10, p. 195.

20. Cantlie, *Army Medical Department*, Volume 1, p. 228.

21. Fortescue, *British Army*, Volume 4, pp. 323–324.

22. Fortescue, *British Army*, Volume 4, p. 77.

23. Cantlie, *Army Medical Department*, Volume 1, p. 252.

24. D. Monro, 1780. *Observations on the Means of Preserving the Health of Soldiers: and of Conducting Military Hospitals. And on Diseases Incident to Soldiers in the Time of Service, and on the same Diseases as they have appeared in London*. 2 Volumes. Volume 1 and Volume 2 bound together. 2nd Edition. Vol. 1, 374 pp., Vol. 2, 304 pp. (London: J. Murray and G. Robinson).

25. Fergusson, *Recollections*, pp. 62–63.

26. Fergusson, *Recollections*, pp. 206–214.

27. Fortescue, *British Army*, Volume 4, Part 2, pp. 848–870.

28. G. A. Kempthorne, 1930. The Egyptian campaign of 1801. *Journal of the Royal Army Medical Corps* **55**, 217–230, p. 220; Cantlie, *Army Medical Department*, Volume 1, pp. 264–273.

29. Peterkin and Johnston, *Commissioned Officers*, Volume 1, Reference No. 972, p. 56.

30. Kempthorne, *Egyptian Campaign*, p. 223.

31. Anon., 1963–1964. Abercromby, Sir Ralph (1734–1801). *Dictionary of National Biography*. **1** (London: Oxford University Press), 43–46; Cantlie, *Army Medical Department*, Volume 1, p. 268.

32. Kempthorne, *Egyptian Campaign*, pp. 224–225.

33. Kempthorne, *Egyptian Campaign*, p. 229.

34. The causal organism, *Yersinia pestis*, is carried by rat fleas.

35. J. H. Dible, 1970. *Napoleon's Surgeon* (London: William Heinemann Medical Books Ltd.), pp. 26–29.

36. Cantlie, *Army Medical Department*, Volume 1, pp. 273–281.

37. The French method of treating ophthalmia avoided surgical intervention and exposure of the eyes to solutions that were likely to be caustic. The patients were instead bled from the neck veins and treated with leeches and the temples scarified. The eyes were exposed to steam and anodyne lotions made from decoctions of poppy-head, linseed, and oriental saffron. At night the eyes were bathed in a solution of egg white to which was added rose water and a few grains of alum and camphor. As the inflammation diminished, Larrey substituted lotions containing a little lead acetate, oxychloride of mercury, or copper sulphate, and when resolution began a decoction of pomegranite bark or zinc sulphate. See: Dible, *Napoleon's Surgeon*, pp. 28–29.

38. In cases where individuals had gonorrhea, Larrey believed that the ophthalmia observed was more rapid and more serious than that seen in Egyptian ophthalmia, and had additional special features. The redness of the edges of the eyelids was more pronounced, and the pus greenish and very irritant. Such patients particularly suffered during the night. As soon as the local irritation of the conjunctivas was relieved by scarification of the temples and by anodynes, Larrey believed that the best form of treatment in these patients was to reestablish the gonorrhea, for example by local irritation of the urethra either by inoculation or with an alkaline injection. The gonorrhea was then treated with Balm of Gilead or Copaiba balsam in large doses, both of which apparently cured this condition in a matter of days. See: Dible, *Napoleon's Surgeon*, p. 28.

39. Fergusson, *Recollections*, pp. 110–116.

40. G. J. Guthrie, 1815. *On Gun-Shot Wounds of the Extremities, Requiring the Different Operations of Amputation, with their after-treatment: Establishing the Advantages of Amputation on the Field of Battle to the Delay usually recommended, &c. &c. With Four Explanatory Plates* (London: Longman, Hurst, Rees, Orme and Brown); G. J. Guthrie, 1853. *Commentaries on the Surgery of the War in Portugal, Spain, France, and the Netherlands, from the Battle of Roliça, in 1808, to that of Waterloo, in 1815, Showing the Improvements made during and since that period in the great art and science of surgery on all the subjects to which they relate.* 5th Edition (London: Henry Renshaw); Hennen, *Practice of Military Surgery*; Anon., 1850. Biographical Sketch of G. J. Guthrie, esq., F.R.S., Late President of the College of Surgeons. *Lancet* **I**, 726–738.

41. J. McGrigor, 1861. *The Autobiography and Services of Sir James McGrigor, Bart. Late Director-General of the Army Medical Department, with an Appendix of Notes and Original Correspondence* (London: Longman, Green, Longman & Roberts).

42. R. L. Blanco, 1974. *Wellington's Surgeon General: Sir James McGrigor* (Durham, N.C.: Duke University Press); Cantlie, *Army Medical Department*, Volume 1, pp. 292–394; G. A. Kempthorne, 1930. The medical department of Wellington's army, 1809–1814. *Journal of the Royal Army Medical Corps* **54**, 65–72, 131–146, 212–220; J. M. Matheson, 1966. Comments on the medical aspect of the Battle of Waterloo, 1815. *Medical History* **10**, 204–207; M. R. Howard, 1988. British medical services at the Battle of Waterloo. *British Medical Journal* **297**, 1653–1656.

43. W.F.P. Napier, 1828–1840. *History of the War in the Peninsula and in the South of France, from the Year 1807 to the Year 1814* [The complete set consists of 6 Volumes: Volume 1, 1828 (London: John Murray); Volume 2, 1829; Volume 3, 1831; Volume 4, 1834; Volume 5, 1836; Volume 6, 1840 (Volumes 2–6, London: Thomas & William Boone)]; Fortescue, *History of the British Army*, Volumes 1–13; Haythornthwaite, *Wellington*.

44. [John] Gurwood, 1834–1838. *The Dispatches of Field Marshall The Duke of Wellington K.G during his various Campaigns in India, Denmark, Portugal, Spain, The Low Countries, and France. From 1799–1818. Compiled from Official and Authentic Documents.* 12 Volumes, and Supplement to the 1st, 2nd, and 3rd Volumes relating to India 1799–1818 (London: John Murray) [The dates are 1799–1818 in all volumes except Volume 12, where the dates are from 1799–1815; the years of publication are as follows: 1834 (Vol. 1), 1835 (Vols. 2–4), 1836 (Vol. 5 and 6), 1837 (Vols. 8 and 9), 1838 (Vols. 10–12), 1839 (Index to The Dispatches of Field Marshall the Duke of Wellington)].

45. Haythornthwaite, *Wellington*, pp. 233–234.

46. Numerous public meetings were held, and the King was petitioned to hold a public inquiry. As an example of the outrage felt, Byron (quoted by Haythornthwaite, *Wellington*, p. 234) wrote:

Here Folly dash'd to earth the victor's plume,

And Policy regain'd what arms had lost;
For chiefs like ours in vain may laurels bloom!
Woe to the conqu'ring, not the conquer'd host

47. R. Chambers, ed. 1864. Moore, (Sir) John. In: *A Biographical Dictionary of Eminent Scotsmen*. New Edition. Volume 4 (London: Blackie & Son), pp. 50–63.

48. G. Gordon-Taylor and E.W. Walls, 1958. *Sir Charles Bell: His Life and Times* (Edinburgh and London: E. & S. Livingstone); Blanco, *Wellington's Surgeon General*, pp. 89–91.

49. Bell had always regretted letting the opportunity slip of tending the wounded from Trafalgar, and determined on this occasion to proceed at once to the port of arrival, at Haslar, despite the fact that the journey would take him several days by coach from London (Gordon-Taylor and Walls, *Sir Charles Bell*, p. 41).

50. C. Bell, 1814. *A Dissertation on Gunshot Wounds* (London: Longman, Hurst, Rees, Orme & Brown). This book is entirely illustrated by Bell's engravings, many of which are based on a series of sketches in oil displayed in the Playfair Hall of the Royal College of Surgeons of Edinburgh; J. Struthers, 1867. Sir Charles Bell. In: *Historical sketch of the Edinburgh Anatomical School* (Edinburgh: Maclachlan & Stewart), pp. 44–55.

51. Kempthorne, *Wellington's army*, pp. 131–134.

52. Gurwood, *Dispatches*, Volume 5, pp. 11–12:

An exertion ought to be made immediately to clothe them in a national uniform. By the adoption of this measure, the practice which prevails . . . very generally, of throwing away their arms and accoutrements and running away, and pretending to be peasants, would be discontinued. Large bodies could not change their clothing or the distinctive modes of dress in a soldier; and it is probable that as they would not only find no security, but rather increase their danger by throwing away their arms and accoutrements in their flight. . . . Another advantage is . . . that it would be in the power of the general to punish the troops who misbehave before the enemy, in the manner most likely to affect the feelings of Spaniards, viz. by disgrace. . . . Whole corps, officers and men, all run off upon the first appearance of danger.

53. Fortescue, *British Army*, Volume 7, pp. 226–261; Cantlie, *Army Medical Department*, Volume 1, pp. 313–314.

54. Cantlie, *Army Medical Department*, Volume 1, pp. 313–319.

55. Cantlie, *Army Medical Department*, Volume 1, p. 318; Haythornthwaite, *Wellington*, p. 238.

56. Anon., *Sketch of G. J. Guthrie*, p. 729.

57. Cantlie, *Army Medical Department*, Volume 1, p. 317; Hennen, *Practice of Military Surgery*, pp. 53–54.

58. Napier, *War in the Peninsula*, Volume 1, p. 496.

59. Kempthorne, *Wellington's army*, pp. 134–138.

60. Fergusson, *Recollections*, pp. 67–68.

61. Gurwood, *Dispatches*, Volume 5, p. 276.

62. Gurwood, *Dispatches*, Volume 5, p. 282.

63. Gurwood, *Dispatches*, Volume 5, pp. 299–300.

64. Cantlie, *Army Medical Department*, Volume 1, p. 320.

65. Fortescue, *British Army*, Volume 7, p. 472.

66. Kempthorne, *Wellington's army*, p. 140.

67. Napier, *War in the Peninsula*, Volume 3, pp. 534–558; Fortescue, *British Army*, Volume 8, pp. 184–215.

68. Kempthorne, *Wellington's army*, p. 146.

69. Fortescue, *British Army*, Volume 7, pp. 606–629.

70. The Java Medal is inscribed "Java conquered 28th August 1811," and, for some reason, omits the final defeat and capitulation of the force under Janssens that occurred during mid-September. One hundred and thirty-three gold medals were issued, and 5,761 natives and 750 Europeans received silver medals. Only individuals in the service of the HEIC were allowed to wear their medal.

71. Kempthorne, *Wellington's army*, p. 212.

72. Cantlie, *Army Medical Department*, Volume 1, pp. 342–343.

73. McGrigor, *Autobiography of Sir James McGrigor*, p. 278: "Nothing could more gratify those officers, nothing could be a greater incentive to their exertions on future occasions, than his noticing them in his public despatches." Wellington asked, "Is that usual?" McGrigor's reply was "It would be of the most essential service," and "really their extraordinary exertions gave them in justice a claim to this."

74. Gurwood, *Dispatches*, Volume 9, p. 50:

Camp at Badajoz, 8th April, 1812.
It gives me great pleasure to inform your Lordship that our numerous wounded officers and soldiers are doing well. I have had great reason to be satisfied with the attention paid to them by Mr. McGrigor, the Inspector General of Hospitals, and the medical gentlemen under his direction, and I trust that the loss to the service, upon this occasion, will not eventually be great.

75. McGrigor, *Autobiography of Sir James McGrigor*, p. 278.

76. Guthrie related the following cautionary tale concerning an episode that occurred during the siege of Salamanca. "Everybody of all ranks passed along the road . . . within range of the guns without the slightest molestation, until . . . a handsome captain of the Welsh Fusiliers . . . put on a new road coat, with a pair of large gold epaulettes, and mounted himself on a white horse to attract the attention of the . . . ladies of Salamanca. Mr. Guthrie rode by his side . . . when a round shot dropped under Mr. Guthrie's horse's nose on the road, throwing the dirt in his face. Both gentlemen rode off . . . Mr. Guthrie protesting he would never again ride by the side of a white horse, the ordinary attribute of [a] marshal of France, or general commanding, and for which his friend was . . . presumed taken. Chance was soon afterwards more successful . . . the captain fell from a grape shot, which entered his abdomen on one side, carrying out with it, on the other, several feet of his bowels, which were lying on the ground when Mr. Guthrie reached him." (Anon., *Sketch of G. J. Guthrie*, p. 730).

77. Napier, *War in the Peninsula*, Volume 5, pp. 248–250.

78. Cantlie, *Army Medical Department*, Volume 1, p. 353.

79. Cantlie, *Army Medical Department*, Volume 1, p. 352.

80. Haythornthwaite, *Wellington*, pp. 169–170; Gurwood, *Dispatches*, Volume 10, p. 617. "The best of the story is, that all parties ran away. Maurice Mathieu ran away; Sir John Murray ran away; and so did Suchet." (Wellington to Colonel Torrens, Lesaca, August 8, 1813.)

81. Kempthorne, *Wellington's army*, pp. 215–216. The spelling of the name of this city is variable; in some texts it is spelled "Vitoria," e.g., Cantlie, *Army Medical Department*, elsewhere "Vittoria."

82. Kempthorne, *Wellington's army*, pp. 65–69.

83. Kempthorne, *Wellington's army*, p. 69.

84. Kempthorne, *Wellington's army*, pp. 131–133.

85. Fergusson, *Recollections*, p. 65.

86. Cantlie, *Army Medical Department*, Volume 1, pp. 374–375.

87. The figures presented here do not include those amputations carried out shortly after Waterloo, a considerable proportion of which would later be considered as unnecessary.

88. Matheson, *Battle of Waterloo*, p. 204.

89. Cantlie, *Army Medical Department*, Volume 1, p. 342.

90. For observations on this campaign, which lasted from July 1812 until January 1815, see Cantlie, *Army Medical Department*, Volume 1, pp. 407–410.

91. Cantlie, *Army Medical Department*, Volume 1, pp. 382–394.

92. Cantlie, *Army Medical Department*, Volume 1, pp. 392–393.

93. Anon., 1864. Sir James Robert Grant, M.D., C.B., K.H., K.S.A. *Lancet* **I**, 112–113; his sister married, in 1810, Dr. James (later Sir James) McGrigor, and his brother, Colquhoun Grant, was Wellington's intelligence officer.

94. This was only one less than the number requested for an army of 40,000, namely, an inspector of hospitals, 3 deputy inspectors, 3 physicians, 13 staff surgeons, 22 hospital assistants, a purveyor, 3 deputy purveyors, 3 apothecaries, and 4 dispensers (G. A. Kempthorne, 1933. The Waterloo campaign. *Journal of the Royal Army Medical Corps* **60**, 52–58, p. 52). The figures provided here do not appear to be in exact agreement with the total on the list provided by G. Jones, 1817. *The Battle of Waterloo, also of Ligny, and Quatre Bras, Described by the Series of Accounts Published by Authority, with Circumstantial Details. By a Near Observer. Also Important Particulars, Communicated by Staff, and Regimental Officers, Serving in Different Parts of the Field, with every Connected Official Document; Forming an Historical Record of the Campaign in the Netherlands, 1815; from the Testimony of Eye-Witnesses, and of those who had the Honour to Share in its Operations. To which is added a Register of the Names of the Officers Employed, with their Respective Ranks, and the Several Casualties, Arranged in Regimental Order, and Alphabetically.* Tenth Edition, Enlarged and Corrected (London: John Booth, and T. Egerton) [This is in 2 Volumes, bound together. The second volume has a similar title to that of Volume 1, except that its full title is: *Additional Particulars to the Battle of Waterloo.* The title pages of these two volumes indicate that they are "Illustrated with the Portraits of Field Marshals Wellington and Blucher, Maps and Enlarged Plans, View of the Field of Waterloo, and Thirty-four etchings Descriptive of the Positions of the British Lines, and of regimental and Individual Acts of Heroism, Gallantry, and Incidents Arising During the Operations, from Sketches"], Volume 2, *A List of Officers in the Netherlands, 1815. Commissariat, Medical Staff, and Chaplains*, columns 60 and 61). This contains the names of 58 medical staff officers who served in the Netherlands in 1815, all of whom were at Waterloo. It does not include McGrigor's name or the names of medical staff officers who served in the hospitals in Brussels, but who were not present at Waterloo, such as Robert Knox and Theodore Gordon; Kempthorne, *Waterloo campaign*, pp. 57–58.

95. Kempthorne, *Waterloo campaign*, p. 52.

96. Kempthorne, *Waterloo campaign*, p. 55.

97. Howard, *British medical services*, p. 1653.

98. Cantlie, *Army Medical Department*, Volume 1, p. 389.

99. Jones, *Battle of Waterloo*.

100. cited by Kempthorne, *Waterloo campaign*, p. 56, though he was of the view that Guthrie "was never one to understate his case").

101. G. J. Guthrie, 1838. *Clinical Lectures on Compound Fractures of the Extremities, on Excision of the Head of the Thigh-Bone, the Arm-Bone, and the Elbow-Joint: On the Diseases of the Peninsula, and on Several Miscellaneous Subjects. Delivered at the*

Westminster Hospital (London: John Churchill) [The copy in Edinburgh University Library is a presentation copy from the author to Sir George Ballingall].

102. This approach was clearly contrary to that previously advocated by Hunter, who recommended that amputation "should not be performed until after suppuration had been established, a period probably of six weeks, which, even if the patient survived, was often found to be too late to be serviceable. . . . From the failure of this practice, the contrary one of immediate amputation became more general during the [Peninsular] war." See: G. J. Guthrie, 1827. *A Treatise on Gun-Shot Wounds, on Inflammation, Erisipelas, and Mortification, on Injuries of Nerves, and on Wounds of the Extremities Requiring the Different Operations of Amputation; in which The Various Methods of Performing these Operations are Shown, Together with their After-Treatment; and containing an account of the author's successful Case of Amputation at the Hip-Joint. Being a Record of the Opinions and Practice of the Surgical Department of the British Army, at the Termination of the Wars in Spain, Portugal, France, and the Netherlands, in 1814 and 1815*. The Third Edition (London: Burgess & Hill), pp. vi–vii.

103. Bell, *Gunshot Wounds*, p. 60: "If the knife could follow the shot directly, it would be the more effectual in preventing the accession of those symptoms which have been described as consequent to the commotion of the limb." In the second edition of Guthrie's *Treatise on Gun-Shot Wounds* (1827, pp. 505–507), he is extremely critical of Charles Bell's early teaching on the treatment of gunshot wounds.

104. J. Thomson, 1816. *Report of observations made in the British Military Hospitals in Belgium, after the Battle of Waterloo; with some remarks upon amputation* (Edinburgh: W. Blackwood; London: T. Cadell & W. Davies), p. 228; for general observations on amputations, pp. 159–279.

105. Thomson, *British Military Hospitals*, p. 256. Thomson cites Guthrie, who stated "that those whose thigh-bone has been fractured in its upper part by a musket-bullet, generally die with great suffering before the end of the sixth or eighth week; and that few even of those escape in whom that bone has been fractured in its middle part." The estimate for total number of amputations performed after Waterloo is quite variable. According to Gordon-Taylor and Walls, *Sir Charles Bell*, the figure was closer to 371.

106. "When the surgeon is satisfied there is no chance of saving the limb by prudent delay, the operation [of amputation] is to be performed as soon after the receipt of the injury as the state of the patient will permit; the only point to be considered is, if the patient has so far recovered the shock of the injury as to be able to bear the additional one of the operation." See: Guthrie, *Gun-Shot Wounds* (1827), p. 231. "The general result . . . which is decidedly in favour of allowing the first *moments* of agitation to pass over before any thing be done; a period extending from that, to one, six, or eight hours, according to the difference of constitution and the different injuries that have been sustained. But from one to three hours will in most cases be found sufficient." See: Guthrie, *Gun-Shot Wounds* (1827), p. 234.

107. Anon., *Sketch of G. J. Guthrie*, pp. 729–730. This story is first recounted in Guthrie's *Treatise on Gun-Shot Wounds.*

108. Guthrie's advice had previously been published in a *Pamphlet on the Hospital Brigade.* See: Anon., 1854. Mr. Guthrie's directions to army Surgeons (Extracted from his pamphlet on the Hospital Brigade). *Lancet* **II**, 155–157.

109. Jones, *Battle of Waterloo*; Napier, *War in the Peninsula*; H. P. Elkington, 1911. Some episodes in the life of James Goodall Elkington, an army surgeon in the Peninsular days, together with extracts from his journal. *Journal of the Royal Army Medical Corps* **16**, 79–104; Kempthorne, *The Waterloo campaign*; Matheson, *Battle of Waterloo*; Cantlie, *Army Medical Department*, Volume 1, pp. 292–394; Howard, *British medical services.*

110. Jones, *Battle of Waterloo*, Volume 1, pp. 80–81.

111. Thomson, *British Military Hospitals*.

112. Edinburgh University Library Reference Number: Gen.594. Each drawing is associated with the name of the soldier, and has a brief description of his injuries.

113. The series of 17 watercolor drawings of injuries sustained at the battle of Waterloo, executed by Sir Charles Bell, were illustrations of cases treated by him in Brussels in 1815. This collection was donated to the army by Sir Charles' widow, Lady Bell, in 1866, and is presently housed in the RAMC Muniment Collection in the Library of the Wellcome Institute for the History of Medicine. For details of the items presented, see: T. Longmore, (undated). *Army Medical School Museum. Description of a series of watercolour drawings, executed by the late Sir Charles Bell, illustrative of wounds received at the Battle of Waterloo, presented by his widow to the Army Medical School, together with a Sketch-book, book of manuscript notes, and some original letters* [12 pp.] [No publisher's name cited]. These life-size paintings were prepared in 1836 when he was professor of surgery in the University of Edinburgh, and used as illustrations for his lectures. They had been selected and enlarged from the drawings in his sketch-book which were generally outline sketches in black lead, highlighted by the addition of red chalk.

114. Bell's series of sketches in oil of the wounded after the retreat to Corunna are all displayed in the Museum of the Royal College of Surgeons of Edinburgh, and formed the basis for many of the engravings that were used to illustrate his *Dissertation on Gunshot Wounds*, published in 1814. He was an extremely accomplished artist, and his drawings formed the basis for the etchings and engravings, many of which he prepared, that were used to illustrate his books, as he encountered great difficulty in persuading engravers to incorporate the details and emphasis he required. Despite the fact that he was "the greatest artistic anatomist of the day, but he failed twice, if not thrice, in his application for the Professorship of Anatomy to the Royal Academy in London." See: H. Lonsdale, 1870. *A Sketch of the Life and Writings of Robert Knox the Anatomist. By his Pupil and Colleague* (London: Macmillan & Co.), p. 221. For additional observations on Bell's suitability for this post, see: Struthers, *Sir Charles Bell*, p. 54; Gordon-Taylor and Walls, *Sir Charles Bell*, pp. 25–26.

115. D. J. Larrey, 1812–1817. *Mémoires de Chirurgie Militaire, et Campagnes*. 4 Volumes (Paris: J. Smith), Volume 1, Plates III–VIII.

116. Dible, *Napoleon's Surgeon*, p. 16.

117. Dible, *Napoleon's Surgeon*, p. 17.

118. G. Ballingall, 1844. *Outlines of Military Surgery*. Third Edition (Edinburgh: Adam & Charles Black; London: Longman, Brown, Green & Longmans), p. 97.

119. G. Ballingall, 1833. *Outlines of the Course of Lectures on Military Surgery, delivered in the University of Edinburgh* (Edinburgh: Adam Black; London: Longman, Rees, Orme, Brown & Green) [This is the 1st Edition of Ballingall's *Outlines of Military Surgery*; 589 pp.], pp. 94–108.

120. G. Ballingall, 1830, *Introductory Lectures to a Course of Military Surgery, Delivered in the University of Edinburgh* (Edinburgh: Adam Black; London: Longman, Rees, Orme, Brown & Green), pp. 189–226.

121. Anon., 1963–64. Tufnell, Thomas Joliffe (1819–1885). *Dictionary of National Biography* **19** (Oxford: Oxford University Press), 1220–1221.

122. Ballingall, *Military Surgery*, pp. 94–108.

123. Ballingall, *Military Surgery*, pp. 94–95.

124. J. G. van Millingen, 1819. *The Army Medical Officer's Manual upon Active Service; Precepts for his Guidance in the Various Situations in which he may be placed; with Observations on the Preservation of the Health of Armies upon Foreign Service*

(London: Burgess & Hill) [According to F. Smith, 1929, *A short history of the Royal Army Medical Corps* (Aldershot: Gale & Polden Ltd.), this volume was first published in 1805, and reprinted in 1819].

125. Cantlie, *Army Medical Department*, Volume 1, pp. 447–448.

3

THE REGIUS CHAIR OF MILITARY SURGERY AT THE UNIVERSITY OF EDINBURGH, 1806–1856, AND THE REGIUS CHAIR OF MILITARY SURGERY AT THE ROYAL COLLEGE OF SURGEONS OF IRELAND, DUBLIN, 1855–1860

BACKGROUND

The most important recent authoritative account of the Army Medical Department makes little mention of the contribution of the Regius Chair of Military Surgery in the University of Edinburgh to the training of army and navy surgeons during the first half of the 19th century.[1] This chair functioned from 1806 until the government early in 1856, shortly after the death of Sir George Ballingall,[2] withdrew funding for it. Ballingall had been appointed in 1822 to succeed John Thomson,[3] the first holder of this commission. In Dublin, Tufnell had lectured privately on military hygiene since 1846, but was only formally appointed to the Regius Chair of Military Surgery in 1855. He held this post until the government also withdrew the funding for it with the establishment of the Army Medical School at Fort Pitt, Chatham in 1860.[4] Additional lectures on military surgery were given by George Guthrie in London during the period between the end of the Peninsular War and the early part of the Crimean War,[5] but despite repeated pleas from various sources, no chair of military surgery was established in London during this period.[6]

While an account of the Edinburgh Chair of Military Surgery was published in 1918,[7] this was in the context of the various chairs of surgery that existed in Edinburgh before the time of Lister. While it considered the personalities of the two individuals who filled this chair, it did not take into account its two principal roles, in introducing large numbers of medical students to all aspects of military medicine and surgery, and in providing postgraduate teaching facilities gratis for medical officers in the armed services. The students that attended this course were provided with both lectures and practical sessions where they were exposed to a wide range of topics not taught elsewhere in the Edinburgh medical curriculum and that were relevant to a career in one of the services.[8] The medical officers were not only updated on recent advances in the field, but also given the opportunity of passing an examination that qualified them for promotion to a higher grade in the service.[9] Moreover, attendance at the course was strongly recommended by the heads of both the Army and Navy Medical Departments as well as by the senior medical authorities of the Honourable East India Company.[10]

FACTORS LEADING TO THE ESTABLISHMENT OF THE REGIUS CHAIR OF MILITARY SURGERY IN EDINBURGH

The stimulus for the teaching of military medicine and surgery in Edinburgh came from John Bell, who was a leading teacher of anatomy and surgery within the extramural school associated with Surgeons' Hall during the last decade of the 19th century.[11] He was one of the civilian surgeons who volunteered to attend the British wounded after the Battle of Camperdown.[12] Bell was not impressed with the skills of the naval surgeons with whom he worked when they attended the large number of casualties that were brought ashore at Yarmouth after the battle. While it is clear that some of the naval surgeons behaved heroically during the conflict,[13] Bell was aware that many of the surgeons with whom he had worked had neither adequate training nor the surgical expertise to treat the conditions that they encountered. He believed that this lack of training was not exclusively a naval problem, but was also encountered among the majority of military surgeons. More important, he believed that it would be possible to make up for this deficiency if they were provided with an adequate period of appropriate instruction. He was aware that there were schools of military and naval medicine established on the Continent that had been functioning for almost a century. Indeed, there had been a strong tradition of training in military medicine and military surgery in Prussia, Russia (in the military academies at St. Petersburg and in Moscow), Holland, and France. In Paris, the Val-de-Grâce Military Hospital and Medical School had been established since the Revolution, and had rapidly acquired an international reputation for excellence.[14] There was also a particularly strong tradition of naval medicine in France, with academies at Rochefort, Nice, Brest, and Toulon, all of which dated from the 1720s and 1730s. All of these military and naval academies were associated with large teaching hospitals.[15]

Bell prepared a detailed Memoir while he was at the naval hospital at Yarmouth, which he submitted privately to Earl Spencer, the First Lord of the Admiralty in the then Whig administration.[16] Bell proposed the establishment of "one great School of Military Surgery." This was to be a national school for the training of medical officers for the army and navy. He detailed the subjects that he thought should be covered in its curriculum. He particularly emphasized that they should be suitable for those that planned a career in one of the services, and that they were different from the subjects normally covered in the curriculum leading toward the M.D. degree. Bell envisaged that it was essential that the students have a solid grounding in military medicine as well as in military surgery. They would also be taught military geography—the manner of conducting soldiers on a foreign expedition, the general care of their health, the choice of encampments, and how to convert buildings into occasional hospitals. He also discussed the number of staff that he envisaged would be required in such an institution, as well as the backup facilities it would require, such as a library, lecture room, practical classes, and other necessary facilities. Similar views were also expressed by Jackson in his book *The Medical Department of Armies*, published in 1805,[17] and by Turnbull in *The Naval Surgeon*, published in 1806.[18]

While Bell did not indicate where such a school might be located, he emphasized that it should have an academic environment, and would probably be best associated with a university and a teaching hospital. When his Memoir was written, medical faculties of an adequate size were available only in Scottish universities. While Oxford and Cambridge may have had the appropriate academic environment, neither had a teaching hospital, nor the facilities nor probably the interest to accommodate large numbers of medical students or military and naval postgraduates. While Bell may not have mentioned Edinburgh as an appropriate location, he must have considered this as a likely possibility, with himself as an eminently suitable candidate for heading such an institution. It was also relevant that the Royal Infirmary of Edinburgh, established in 1729, had been rebuilt in 1742, and could accommodate about 200 patients.[19] Shortly after 1745, nearly all of its patients had been military, while during the second half of the century, a significant proportion of its patients consisted of sick soldiers and sailors who were looked after in its military wards. From about 1770 to 1800, the payment received to accommodate and treat the soldiers accounted for almost 10% of the total income of the infirmary over this period. During the period between 1795 and 1800, the fees paid by the government for the seamen alone accounted for almost 16% of the infirmary's total income.[20]

As his privately prepared Memoir produced no obvious response from Earl Spencer, Bell decided that the issue was too important to be ignored. He therefore revised and substantially enlarged his pamphlet, and then published it. While his Memoir was only 21 pages long, the "Memorial" now contained 41 pages of text. This document was submitted to Earl Spencer, and while its receipt may have been acknowledged, it again appears to have been filed away for possible future reference. Soon afterward, the Whig government was ousted from office and replaced by a Tory administration, and Bell's proposal was not pursued. Bell had other matters on his mind in Edinburgh as, following Professor Gregory's suggestion, the managers of the infirmary decided that it would be better for continuity of patient care to appoint six surgeons to the permanent staff of the infirmary, rather than allowing all fellows of the College of Surgeons to attend the infirmary on a monthly rotation.[21] Bell was not selected to be on the surgical staff of the Royal Infirmary. Following this great personal disappointment, he decided to devote his time to teaching and writing, as well as pursuing his private surgical practice. Over the years and with the assistance of his younger brother Charles he had established an anatomical museum. The majority of its contents moved to London in 1804 with Charles, who was then aged 30 and planned to become a teacher of anatomy in the metropolis, as he saw little prospect of advancement as an independent teacher of anatomy in Edinburgh.[22]

THE FIRST HOLDER OF THE EDINBURGH CHAIR: JOHN THOMSON

One of those who were selected to be a member of the surgical staff of the infirmary in 1800 was John Thomson.[23] He had initially been a medical student in Glasgow during 1788–1789, and had then transferred to Edinburgh to continue his medical studies there, commencing in 1789–1790. He appears to have had ambitions toward both an academic and a medical career, and in 1791–1792 was elected junior president of the Royal Medical Society. He took up a junior post in the infirmary, but resigned this in 1792. He went to London, where he studied at John Hunter's extramural medical school at Leicester Square. He initially considered teaching anatomy, but soon abandoned this plan partly because of the capital costs involved, and partly because of the high opinion he had formed of Mr. John Bell's expertise in this area.[24] He then decided to pursue a career in surgery, and gained the fellowship examination of the Royal College of Surgeons of Edinburgh in 1793.[25] While in London, as well as in Edinburgh, Thomson entered a political circle with strong Whig affiliations. He must have been a reasonably competent surgeon, and at the age of 39 was one of the youngest of those selected to be on the surgical staff of the infirmary,[26] despite the fact that in all respects he was an inferior candidate to John Bell. It is possible that the pamphlet he produced entitled *Regulation of the Surgical Department of the Infirmary*[27] may have been a crucial factor in the managers' decision in selecting him rather than Bell. From 1801, Thomson taught surgery at the extra-academical school of medicine and surgery. More important in the present context, during the winter of 1803–04, Thomson gave a series of lectures on the nature and treatment of those injuries and diseases that might reasonably be expected to come under the care of the military surgeon.[28] This course of lectures was well received, and was repeated during the following summer. These added to his reputation as a scholar as well as a competent clinician.

In the winter session of 1804–1805, a memorial was presented to the College of Surgeons, signed by a number of the fellows all previously solicited by Thomson, recommending that the College establish either a lectureship or professorship in surgery.[29] Most fellows were unhappy with the way that surgery had been taught in the University of Edinburgh, largely as an adjunct of anatomy, by the Monros secundus and tertius.[30] Thomson was unanimously elected to the College's Chair of Surgery, and a public announcement was made to this effect on October 5, 1804.[31] It was predicted that this appointment would not be well received by Monro, by the town council or by the senatus of the university, as all considered it to be an infringement on their authority.[32] The university sought legal opinion but was advised not to pursue the matter through the courts.[33] Thomson's lectures on surgery delivered at Surgeons' Hall were delivered in two series. The first half was given at almost daily intervals between November and February, and consisted of 61 lectures on the principles of surgery. The second half of the course consisted of a series of practical lectures, some of which were illustrated with anatomical specimens.[34]

Less than two years later, with the re-election of a Whig administration under Mr. Charles James Fox, Lord Lauderdale encouraged Mr. Thomson to apply to His Majesty's Government for a commission to be professor of military surgery in the University of Edinburgh.[35] Earl Spencer, now Secretary of State for the Home Department, declared that after a brief interview he was satisfied with Thomson's academic and political credentials, and recommended him for the appointment.[36] Because of the tense situation with France, this was clearly an opportune time to establish such an appointment. As only a Regius Chair was contemplated, it also involved the expenditure of far less funds than had Bell's original plan been implemented in its entirety. The chair was not associated with clinical responsibilities for military or naval patients who were housed in the military wards in the infirmary, although the staff of the infirmary were allowed to use these patients for their clinical teaching.[37] While resident in the military wards, the men were technically always under the care of their own medical officers, although they were encouraged to consult with their clinical colleagues in cases of particular difficulty.[38] It is clear that individuals in the military wards were cared for by the physicians-in-ordinary during the 18th century.[39] Reference to the *Royal Infirmary Minute Book* for 1821 indicates that in later years, members of the infirmary staff were paid to attend patients in the military wards. The Treasury informed the managers that they wished to discontinue this practice,[40] possibly because the number of soldiers and seamen resident in the infirmary was now so small.

In 1810, Thomson resigned from his surgeoncy in the infirmary, following an acrimonious argument with John Bell over his surgical competence,[41] although Thomson continued to lecture on surgery to his extramural class.[42] His reason for resigning was that the managers had refused to hold an inquiry into the affair, which he believed had damaged his reputation. There was initially no overlap between Thomson's surgery lectures and his teaching course in military surgery, but in later years it is difficult to establish whether he gave a single combined course which covered both series of lectures. In 1815 he visited the Continent to observe the medical and surgical condition of the men who had been wounded at Waterloo.[43] He offered advice to his clinical colleagues, and this exercise, but particularly the report he subsequently published on his observations, greatly enhanced his reputation.[44] Shortly after his return from Belgium he wrote to H.R.H. the Duke of York requesting a formal military association, and although he had no military experience he was duly appointed "Surgeon to the Forces,"[45] which then allowed him access to the military hospitals in and around Edinburgh.

According to Thomson, in the winter session of 1815–1816, and for a number of years after Waterloo, he gave his lectures to the students of surgery without fee, and nearly 200 had attended.[46] Because of the large number of senior army and navy surgeons who attended gratis, there were probably close to 250–280 in the audience.[47] His military surgery lectures covered a wide range of topics, including: gunshot wounds; dressing of wounds; contused wounds; penetration wounds; tetanus; injuries of the head; fractures; concussion; wounds of the brain, eyes, cheeks, chest, thorax, intestines, and the extremities,[48] and were highly regarded. From 1816 he was put in clinical charge of the depot hospital in Edinburgh, under the authority of the director general of the Army Medical Department. The medical officers who attended his course were also allowed access to the hospital of the 92nd Regiment at Edinburgh Castle. These patients supplemented those in the military wards in the infirmary, and were used by Thomson to conduct clinical trials into the treatment of syphilis without mercury.[49]

Thomson resigned from the College of Surgeons' Chair of Surgery in April 1821, having held this office for seventeen years[50] in order to become a candidate for the Chair of Physic. This was vacant since the death of Dr. James Gregory. While his strong Whig sympathies allowed him to obtain his Crown commission in 1806, the Tories that dominated the Edinburgh town council and the senatus were not equally sympathetic, and his application for the Chair of Physic was unsuccessful. Thomson had for some time decided to pursue a career as a physician, and in 1815 had become a licentiate of the Royal College of Physicians of Edinburgh, and by the 1820s was acting both as a consulting physician and as a consulting surgeon.[51] During the post-Waterloo period, Thomson became an active teacher of medicine, with a considerable interest in medical education. During 1822, he lectured in the extramural school on the practice of physic, in active rivalry to Home.[52] He was also keenly interested in pathology,[53] and had made a collection of about 2,400 illustrations of morbid pathology, many of which were painted in watercolor.[54] At some stage during the summer of 1822, Thomson resigned from his Regius Chair of Military Surgery.[55] The exact reasons are unclear, but it is likely that it allowed him more time to pursue his many other interests. It should not be surprising therefore that, with the return of a Whig administration, he was considered a suitable candidate for the Regius Chair of General Pathology when the Crown established this post in 1831.[56] It was at about this time that the first volume of his *Life of Cullen* appeared,[57] and this is still regarded as the definitive work on him.[58] He resigned from this appointment in 1842 due to ill health. Dr. Robert Knox had referred to him as "The Old Chair-maker" as well as the "Medical Commissioner of the Whigs,"[59] as he had held three chairs in Edinburgh, and because of his well-known political affiliations. He also established a professorial dynasty. His elder son William held the Practice of Physic Chair in Glasgow University,[60] while his younger son, Allen, successively held the Chairs of Anatomy in Aberdeen, Institutes of Medicine (Physiology) in Edinburgh, and finally Anatomy in Glasgow University.[61]

THE SECOND HOLDER OF THE EDINBURGH CHAIR: GEORGE BALLINGALL

Thomson offered his resignation from his Regius Chair to the senatus of the university on November 13, 1822,[62] and only 8 days later Dr. George Ballingall (see Figure 3.1) received his commission from the Crown.[63] Exactly why the time interval between these two dates is so short is unclear. The only reasonable explanation must be that Thomson indicated his plans to resign to Robert Peel, the Home Secretary, some considerable time before he submitted his formal letter of resignation to the senatus. An "unofficial" appointments committee must have been established in Edinburgh to investigate possible candidates, and they suggested to Peel the names of Ballingall and Dr. David Maclagan as individuals who were in their view worthy of serious consideration.[64] Peel then wrote to Lord Melville on October 26, 1822, seeking his advice regarding these two candidates, indicating that of the two applicants, the best-qualified man, "irrespective of any other considerations," must get the chair.[65]

In many respects the two candidates were very similar, both having served for almost the same number of years in the Army Medical Department. Ballingall had matriculated at the University of Edinburgh during the sessions 1803–1806, entering the University at the age of 17.[66] He also studied at the extramural school associated with Surgeons' Hall, and obtained his diploma from the Royal College of Surgeons of Edinburgh in December 1805.[67] He entered the army in May 1806 as a hospital mate, being promoted to assistant surgeon to the 2nd Battalion of the Royal Scots in July 1806, with whom he went to Madras. His colonel was the Duke of Kent. In 1811 he voluntarily transferred to the 22nd Dragoons and accompanied them on their expedition against Java, and was present at the capture of that island. He then returned to India. While a student he had attended Dr. Barclay's extramural anatomy classes,[68] acting for a time as one of his assistants and, it must be assumed, as no correspondence between them survives, maintained a close relationship through his correspondence with him during his period abroad in the army.[69] Shortly after Barclay's death, Ballingall prepared a brief but fulsome memoir of him, and this is the only contemporary account of his life and work.[70] In 1815, Ballingall was stationed with the army of occupation in Paris, and three years later, in September 1818, now a surgeon with the 10th Regiment, he was retired from the Army Medical Department on half-pay and engaged in private practice in Edinburgh.

Ballingall matriculated for a second time in the university during the 1816–1817 session, attending the chemistry class, which he had failed to attend when

Figure 3.1. Sir George Ballingall

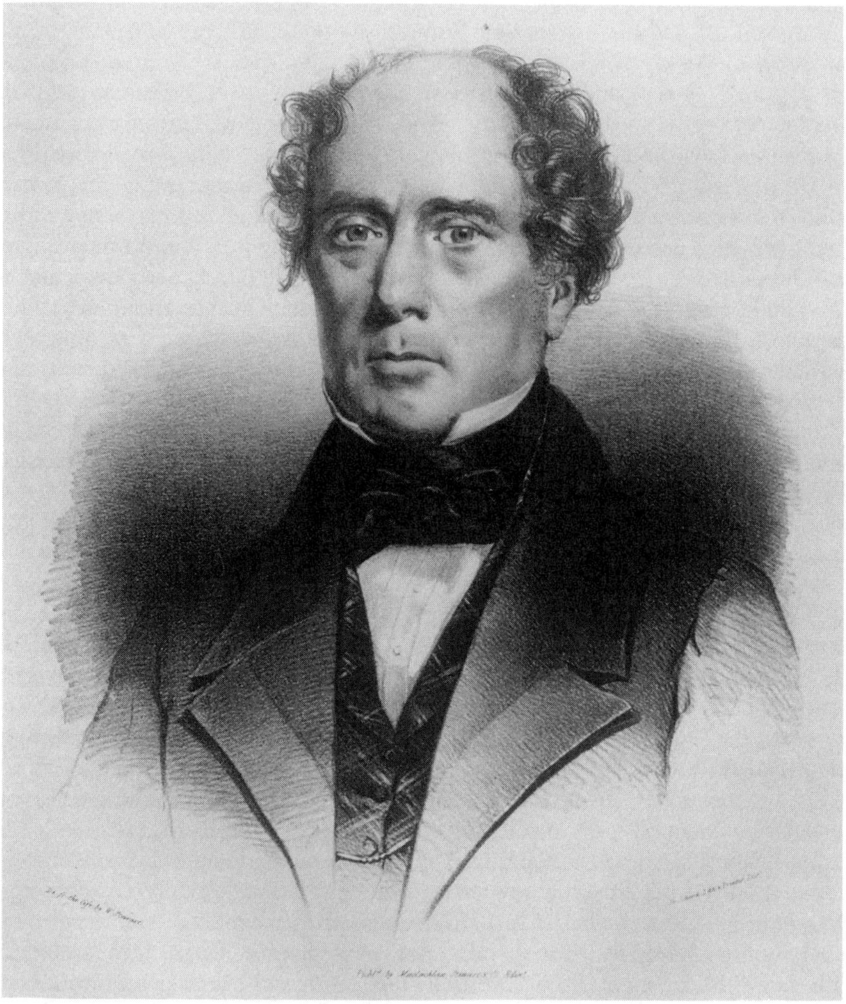

Drawn from life by W. Stewart, published by Maclachlan, Stewart & Co., date unknown.

he was first a student at the University, and which was obligatory in order to allow him to submit his M.D. thesis.[71] He also attended Thomson's lectures on military surgery. He was awarded his M.D. degree in 1819,[72] and shortly afterward he submitted a second thesis, on this occasion in English, being his probationary (fellowship) essay to the Royal College of Surgeons of Edinburgh.[73] Ballingall was also elected to the Royal Society of Edinburgh in June 1820. He had been proposed by Sir George Mackenzie, the mineralogist, on behalf of its physical class, although after his election he played no part in the Society's activities.[74] Ballingall had also gathered together a substantial collection of testimonials, principally dating from August and September 1821, presumably to use when the appropriate opportunity arose.[75]

Ballingall's principal rival for the chair, Dr. David Maclagan, had also studied in Edinburgh, graduating with the M.D. degree in 1805.[76] Maclagan then gained the membership of the Royal College of Surgeons of England in 1807. His first military appointment was with the 91st Regiment, and he went with them to Walcheren where a considerable proportion of the men either died of malaria or needed to be invalided out of the regiment. In November 1811, he sailed to Lisbon to join Wellington there. He was seconded as a staff surgeon to the 9th Portuguese Brigade, while still attached to the Fourth Division in which he served until September 1814. He was present at many of the major battles, and was awarded the Peninsular Medal with six clasps. He was then promoted to physician to the forces, and was retained at the specific request of Sir Benjamin d'Urban, quartermaster general of the Portuguese army, to superintend the hospital arrangements of the Portuguese army. He was retired on half-pay in 1816 and settled in Edinburgh. With his particularly distinguished record of military service in the Peninsular War, it is difficult to see why he was not the chair committee's first choice. The fact that he was not the successful candidate did not appear to have any detrimental effect on his subsequent clinical career, as he was elected President of the Royal College of Surgeons of Edinburgh in 1826, and President of the Royal College of Physicians of Edinburgh in 1856.[77] Ballingall's commission of appointment was signed on behalf of the King by Robert Peel. It was dated November 20, 1822, and he was aged 36 at the time of his appointment. As he had been elected to a Regius Chair, directly after his commission had been read before the senatus, there was, by tradition, a formal protest made by the College Baillie.[78] As Ballingall's salary consisted of £100 per annum from the Crown, his only other sources of funding were from his half-pay from the army[79] and whatever fees he would receive from students who might wish to attend his lecture course[80] and so he desperately needed to supplement his income. This was clearly the situation whether he was successful in this appointment or otherwise. Some time before the announcement of the name of the successful candidate had been made, Ballingall wrote to the managers of the Royal Infirmary in order to be considered for one of their junior surgeoncy posts. In the *Minute Book of the Managers of the Royal Infirmary* dated December 24, 1822, it was announced that he had been appointed one of the assistant surgeons to the infirmary.[81] Ballingall accepted this post, but it is difficult to know how time-consuming this appointment would have been. In

1824, he was promoted to senior assistant surgeon, and in 1825 promoted to acting surgeon. Several years later, though the exact date is unclear, he was appointed consulting surgeon to the infirmary.[82] In 1833, after he had received his knighthood following the accession of William IV in 1830,[83] he was appointed extraordinary surgeon to the Royal Infirmary.[84]

It took some time for Ballingall to establish his teaching course in military surgery. His first *Prospectus*[85] was published in November 1824, and the *Introductory Lectures* he published[86] formed the basis for his successful *Outlines of Military Surgery*, the first edition of which appeared in 1833.[87] This went to five editions by the time of his death in 1855.[88] In his *Prospectus* he indicated that his lectures were to be given on Monday, Wednesday, and Friday each week at 2 P.M. during the winter session, and that surgical operations would be demonstrated on cadavers when appropriate. He also continued the tradition established by his predecessor in office of allowing serving medical officers admission to his lecture course gratis.

All of his teaching was undertaken in the Old College of the University of Edinburgh. As the space available in the Old College was so limited,[89] it is likely that he would have had to use the Anatomical Lecture Theatre for his lectures, for which an arrangement would have had to be made with Professor Monro tertius. The exact number of lectures given in each series differed slightly. During the periods between 1837–1838 and 1841–1842, for which figures are available, the number varied between 25 and 31, and the winter session ran from early December until the beginning of April.[90] In addition to establishing a library for the use of the students that attended his course, Ballingall also collected a considerable number of artifacts to illustrate his lectures (see Figure 3.2). These formed the basis for his museum, which was substantially enlarged when he obtained £150 from the Reid Fund to purchase the specimens collected by Dr. Rutherford Alcock when Alcock was deputy inspector general of hospitals with the British Auxiliary Legion in Spain during 1835–1837.[91]

It is difficult to know where Ballingall stored and displayed his museum collection, although it is possible that after the acquisition of the material from Alcock, some or possibly all of it may have had to be displayed in an appropriate section of the anatomical museum. The *Printed Catalogue* associated with the collection,[92] which was based on an earlier manuscript catalog,[93] indicates that it was divided into Pathological and Miscellaneous sections. While the Pathological section consisted principally of "osteological specimens," most of which had been obtained from Alcock,[94] there were also examples of "exfoliations, bony fragments and exostoses." This section also contained a substantial number of potted "soft-tissue" specimens. The items in the Miscellaneous section had mostly come from Ballingall's own collection, and consisted of (i) plaster of Paris casts, (ii) models, instruments, and apparatus, (iii) balls, missiles etcetera, and (iv) drawings, plans, etcetera. A considerable proportion of the osteological specimens from this collection is still available for inspection and analysis.[95]

Figure 3.2. Sabre Injury to the Right Lower Occipital Region

This wound shows the characteristic features of an edged weapon injury—a clearly defined edge, and a flat smooth surface—in association with the lateral border of the lesion. A lack of evidence of healing suggests that the wound proved fatal.

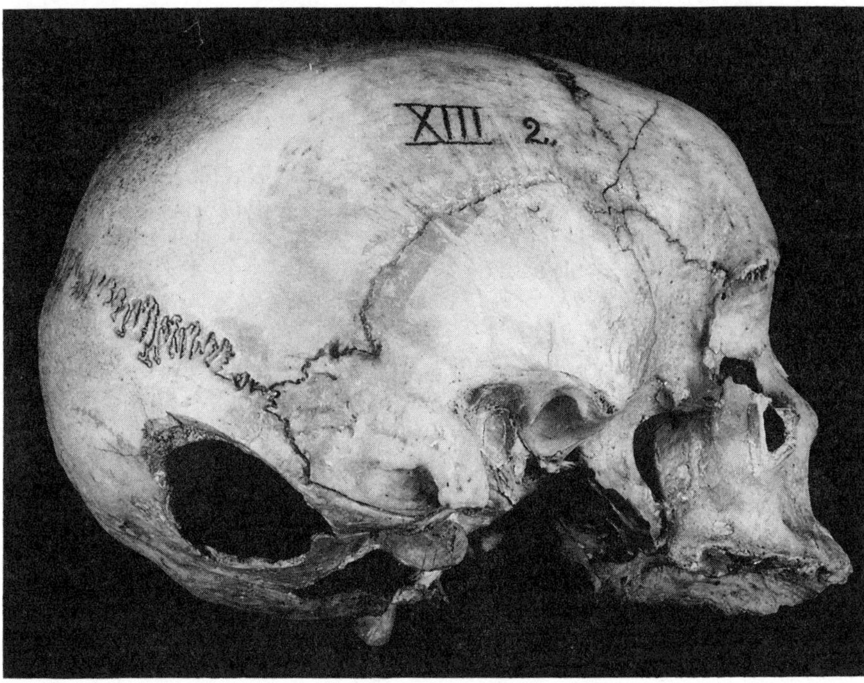

From: M.H. Kaufman, D. Whitaker and J. McTavish, 1997. Differential diagnosis of holes in the calvarium: application of modern clinical data to palaeopathology. *Journal of Archaeological Science* **24**, 193–218 [Figure 23]. Used with permission.

EFFECTIVENESS OF THOMSON'S AND BALLINGALL'S TEACHING

While no exact figures are available for the size of Thomson's classes, beyond the information indicated previously, reasonably exact figures are available for those that attended Ballingall's classes. These figures come from a number of different sources,[96] and Rosner[97] in particular has stressed that the variation observed is largely due to the fact that matriculation lists only provide information on the number of students who paid the fees to the professor. In reality, many more students may have attended lectures than those noted on these lists. Attendance figures for medical students and medical officers who attended Ballingall's lecture courses on military surgery between 1839 and 1846 are available,[98] and while the figures vary a little among the various sources indicated above, they provide a reasonable indication of his class sizes during this period (Table 3.1). It is assumed that the figures provided for medical officers in the public service included commissioned officers in the army and navy as well as in the service of the Honourable East India Company.

Table 3.1
Numbers Attending Ballingall's Lecture Course between 1839 and 1846

Session	Medical officers in the public service	Medical students	Total
1839–1840	17	63	80
1840–1841	15	60	75
1841–1842	13	39	52
1842–1843	9	23	32
1843–1844	13	23	36
1844–1845	13	32	45
1846 (Summer)	7	25	32
Totals:	87	265	352
Numbers previous to 1839–40	434	443	877
Annual average of audience for the period between 1823 and 1846			53

It is relevant to note that both Thomson's and Ballingall's courses were strongly supported by Sir James McGrigor, on behalf of the Army Medical Department, and Dr. William Burnett, medical commissioner of the navy, on behalf of his service. Both of these gentlemen provided glowing testimonials in which they indicated their approval of the overall standard of the Edinburgh medical graduates which they had encountered over the years. In part of the evidence presented to the Royal Commissioners by Professor Alison, dean of the faculty of medicine, on October 23, 1826, he noted:

Sir James McGregor [*sic*] . . . mentions . . . that about one-third of the medical officers in the army, and certainly the best informed part of them, have been educated here [i.e. in the University of Edinburgh]. . . . Dr. Burnet says, "For several years past it has been my duty, in connexion with my colleague Dr. Weir, to examine candidates for admission into the medical Department of the Navy, and, though they are all young men of superior medical education, I can with the utmost truth declare, that those young gentlemen who have obtained the Degree of M.D. at the University of Edinburgh are by far the best informed in their profession of any I have met with, and whom, without any other recommendation, we have immediately admitted into the service." Many of the medical officers of the Navy, independently of those lately admitted, have, since the return of peace, obtained Degrees from the same University; and it is but justice to add, that, when employed...they have invariably distinguished themselves by their superior acquirements and Knowledge.[99]

Letters indicating their approval of Ballingall's course, and recommending it to potential candidates and those who were already serving in the medical branches of these two services were published as "Notices" and appeared before the Preface section of his *Outlines of a Course of Lectures on Military Surgery*.[100] It is only possible to gain an indirect indication of the effectiveness of Thomson's and Ballingall's lecture courses based on the number of students who entered one of the public services. It is, however, possible to gain a reasonably accurate estimate of the number of individuals who entered the Army Medical Department during the period between 1806 and 23 when Thomson held the Regius Chair in Edinburgh, and between 1823 and 1855 when Ballingall held the Regius Chair. This information is provided in Tables 3.2 and 3.3. Because of the dramatic reduction in the number of medical officers that entered the service after Waterloo, the figures in Table 3.2 are divided into those who entered between 1806 and 1815, and those between 1816 and 1823.[101] The post-Waterloo admission rate was only about 5% of the pre-Waterloo figure.

Table 3.2

Academic Origin of Medical Officers in Army Based on University Medical Degree or Fellowship Diploma (if No University Medical Degree Held); 1806–1815 and 1816–1823

Year	Nil	Edinb.	Glasg.	Aberd.	St. Andr.	Dublin	Other	FRCS	Total
Totals:	1,095	168*	39	16	15	13	41		1,392
1806–1815	*(78.7)*	(57.5)	(13.4)	(5.5)	(5.1)	(4.5)	(14.0)		
Totals:	48	8**	2	1	1	3			65
1816–1823	*(73.8)*	(53.3)	(13.3)	(6.7)	(6.7)	(20.0)			

* Edinburgh University: 16.8 graduates per year; *Scottish Universities 81.5% of medical graduates*

**Edinburgh University: 1 graduate per year; *Scottish Universities 80.0% of medical graduates*

Table 3.3
Academic Origin of Medical Officers in Army Based on University Medical Degree or Fellowship Diploma (if No University Medical Degree Held); 1823–1856

Year	Nil	Edinb.	Glasg.	Aberd.	St. Andr.	Dublin	Other	FRCS	Total
Totals:	834	247*	102	52	46	49	37	15	1,382
1823–1856	*(60.3)*	(46.3)	(19.1)	(9.8)	(8.6)	(9.2)	(6.9)		

*Edinburgh University: 7.7 graduates per year; *Scottish Universities 83.9% of medical graduates*

Key for Tables 3.2 and 3.3: Nil, Number of medical officers who did not possess an M.D. degree; Edinb., Edinburgh University; Glasg., Glasgow University; Aberd., Aberdeen University; St. Andr., St. Andrews University; Dublin, Dublin University; Other, Non-Scottish universities; FRCS, Those with fellowship diplomas of either the Royal College of Surgeons of England, Edinburgh, Glasgow or Ireland.

What emerges from the information provided in Tables 3.2 and 3.3 is that during the period between 1806 and 1823 when Thomson was in the chair, between 74 and 79% of those who entered the Army Medical Department did not possess a medical degree. These candidates all possessed the lesser medical qualification of a diploma from one of the colleges of surgeons. More interestingly, of those who were medical graduates, between 1806–23, about 80% were graduates of a Scottish university, and of these 53–58% were graduates from the University of Edinburgh. During the period between 1823 and 1856, while those who had a medical degree now accounted for 40% of the entry, 84% were graduates of a Scottish university, and of these 46% were graduates of the University of Edinburgh. Furthermore, the figures indicate that during the two periods when there was a reasonable medical intake, 1806–1815 and 1823–1856, the Army Medical Department received respectively an average of 16.8 and 7.7 graduates per year from the University of Edinburgh. Considering that the annual intake during these two periods fell dramatically from about 155 to 33 per year, respectively, the proportion of the candidates who were graduates of the University of Edinburgh had increased considerably to take this overall reduction in the intake into the service into account. These figures do not take into account the substantial proportion of medical students who attended the military surgery lectures but decided against taking the M.D. degree. They qualified in medicine, as had Ballingall in 1805, by passing the diploma examination of the Royal College of Surgeons of Edinburgh. Since it is highly likely that a number of these students also entered the Army Medical Department, this strongly suggests that the Edinburgh students were not only enthused by their lecturer, but also decided to pursue a medical career within one of the public services. Unfortunately, Peterkin and Johnston's book[102] does not usually supply information on the education of those candidates who did not graduate with the M.D. degree.

While the intake into the Naval Medical Department during the period between 1806 and 1856 is not readily available, figures for the overall intake into the navy are available for selected years during the period between 1813 and 1900 (Table 3.4).[103] These figures clearly reflect the great reduction in the navy that took place during the early post-Waterloo era, as well as the reduction that occurred during the post–Crimean War period. What figures are available indicate that the medical intake was also dramatically cut back due to the financial constraints imposed by the government during these periods. Many naval medical officers were put on half-pay or on the retired list after Waterloo due to government cutbacks. Information for those on full-pay in the years 1814, 1835, and 1838 are presented in Table 3.5.[104]

Table 3.4
The Size of the Navy at Selected Dates during the 19th Century

Year	No. of men
1813	130,127
1835	21,141
1846	36,181
1855	61,246
1875	33,902
1900	114,880

Table 3.5
A Comparison between Numbers on Full-Pay in Various Grades of the Naval Medical Service in 1814, 1835 and 1838

Rank	1814	1835	1838
Physician	15	11	3
Surgeon	840	560	186
Assistant surgeon	600	280	261
Dispenser	19	11	–
Hospital mate	18	3	2

BALLINGALL'S EVIDENCE PRESENTED BEFORE THE ROYAL COMMISSIONERS IN 1826 REGARDING THE TEACHING OF MILITARY SURGERY AND OTHER TOPICS

In 1826, Ballingall presented a memorial to the Royal Commissioners who were visiting the Scottish universities. His presentation was principally concerned with the value of military surgery as an independent discipline within the context of surgery. He also indicated that he was well aware that there were many even within the Edinburgh faculty of medicine, particularly among his surgical colleagues, who felt that military surgery should not be separated from surgery.[105] He indicated his views to the commissioners in the following terms:

> With regard to military surgery . . . I have been repeatedly told, that military surgery differs in no respect from common surgery; and I have even been pressed . . . to model my course, so as to render my tickets admissible at Surgeons' Hall, as equivalent to a full course of surgery: This I have hitherto declined, and still decline, doing . . . it is my duty to embrace, in my course, an extensive range of Surgical subjects . . . to dwell upon those Surgical diseases and accidents to which soldiers and seamen are more particularly exposed; and to point out those peculiarities of practice which military and naval surgeons are often compelled to adopt, from the singular and unforeseen circumstances in which they are placed . . . I do not therefore urge any claim in favour of the chair which I now have the honour to fill; and however unpleasant it may be for me to be the only medical Member of the Senatus whose class it is not considered necessary for graduates to attend.[106]

He was given a sympathetic hearing by the commissioners, who stated in their report with regard to the teaching of military surgery:

> It is not to be expected that the course of study for Physicians generally should include the whole extent of peculiar qualifications required by the Medical Boards of the Army and Navy. But, at the same time, there are certain requisites established by these Boards, which ought to be kept in view in framing the Regulations for the Course of Study at the Universities. It may also safely be inferred, that such Regulations as have been found by the Army and Navy Medical Boards to be quite practicable as to the class of person offering themselves as surgeons for either service, may, without the risk of much inconvenience, be required from Candidates for the medical Degree at the Universities. We apply this observation particularly to the Regulations of the Army Board respecting Practical Chemistry, a separate class of surgery, the Practice and Theory of medicine separately, a competent knowledge of the Greek Language, and even of an acquaintance with Mathematics and Natural Philosophy.[107]

While Ballingall was probably a meticulous but fairly dull surgeon, and certainly not in the same league as Liston or Syme,[108] it is clear that he took an active interest in all aspects of the medical curriculum. He believed that the academic standard of the majority of the medical graduates was less than he would have wished, and it was for this reason that he suggested that all individuals who wished to take the M.D. degree should previously have obtained an arts degree.[109] In this regard, his views were probably closer to those of the profession in general than those of his colleagues in the faculty of medicine. The fact that he was prepared to express an opinion contrary to those of his colleagues was guaranteed to increase their hostility toward him. It is also clear that some of his detractors were against the post that he held, and the undemocratic way that the university was forced to accept his crown appointment. It was almost as though the holder of this post were irrelevant.

Many were prepared to go to almost any lengths to deprive Ballingall of his professorship. These detractors persistently dogged him in an attempt to wear him down and force him to resign from his chair. Throughout his academic career, numerous scurrilous articles were published about him, criticizing all aspects of his professional activities. Most of these articles were either anonymous[110] or signed "Scotus," although these mostly appeared during the late 1820s,[111] and it appears likely that a considerable proportion of these came from the pen of Professor James Syme. Wakley, its proprietor and editor, published numerous extremely critical editorials in the *Lancet*, and these were especially associated with critical reviews of Ballingall's lecture courses and his books.[112] He was, for example, referred to as "The Military Blusterer,"[113] appointed to a "sham" professorship, and not fit to succeed Thomson.[114] For reasons that are not entirely clear, the critical editorials in the *Lancet* ceased during the 1840s, as did the anonymous articles and those signed by "Scotus."

BALLINGALL'S OTHER ACTIVITIES

In addition to his various university duties, Ballingall wrote numerous letters to journals and Ministers in support of military surgery topics, including his view that the government should establish separate chairs of military surgery in London and in Dublin,[115] the too-early enlistment of recruits particularly for service abroad,[116] that serving medical officers should be eligible for awards for gallantry and other military honors, [117] and the poor pay and conditions of medical officers in the various services.[118]

Ballingall had applied for the Regius Professorship of Surgery, in 1831, but was unsuccessful, and J. W. Turner, who already held the College of Surgeons' Chair of Surgery as successor to John Thomson,[119] was appointed to the Regius Chair. Ballingall indicated that he had wanted a chair of surgery separate from that of military surgery, and separate from the chair of anatomy. He was well aware that there were many on the faculty who were hostile to the existence of his chair of military surgery, and he had informed the commissioners in 1826 that he had been approached with the proposal that his chair should be converted into a chair of general surgery, but that at that time he had vigorously resisted this suggestion. He indicated in his letter of application for this appointment that he still believed that the chair of military surgery should not be sacrificed to form a chair of general surgery.[120] It is possible that the reason why he applied for this chair was that it held out the prospects of a significantly increased income from private practice, which was clearly not forthcoming through his present appointments. He was also particularly distressed because his half-pay from the army ceased in 1831, and had a dramatic effect on his income.[121]

From about 1850 until his death in 1855, Ballingall maintained a close correspondence with Guthrie,[122] and they both actively campaigned in support of military medical educational reform. Both also maintained an active correspondence with the editor of the *Lancet*, and a number of their letters appeared in the columns of this influential journal. More importantly, the unsolicited editorials that commonly appeared in the *Lancet* were now entirely supportive of the causes they espoused, including the suggestion that the government should establish chairs of military surgery in London and elsewhere. Even Ballingall's *Outlines of Military Surg*ery was very favorably reviewed.[123] He was even referred to as "that veteran military teacher."[124] Ballingall became increasingly unwell during the 1850s, and during the latter period was no longer able to deliver his lecture course during the winter months. For several years, he was forced to deliver an abbreviated version of his course during the summer months.[125]

WITHDRAWAL OF GOVERNMENT FUNDING FOR THE REGIUS CHAIR OF MILITARY SURGERY IN EDINBURGH IN 1856, AND FROM THE REGIUS CHAIR OF MILITARY SURGERY IN DUBLIN IN 1860

With Ballingall's death in December 1855, Syme immediately wrote to Lord Panmure to suggest that the time was now opportune to withdraw the funding for the Regius Chair of Military Surgery in Edinburgh by the Crown. No mention was made of the animosity that existed between Syme and Ballingall over the years, and the impression was given that any decision to withdraw funding for the chair would be in the best interest of the Edinburgh medical school. According to Syme: "The circumstances under which the chair was established by the Crown in 1806 were so entirely different from those now existing [with the establishment of the chair of systematic surgery in 1831] . . . in offering this suggestion [to withdraw funding for the chair], my only objects are to free the school [i.e., Edinburgh] of a useless incumbrance."[126]

It appears to be clear that the government was happy to accept Syme's advice in this matter, and indeed requested advice from him several years later with regard to some of the appointments to the Army Medical School at Fort Pitt.[127]

During these last few years of his life, Ballingall seriously considered who might be his possible successor. Several names came to mind, the most likely being his assistant, Dr. Richard James Mackenzie. Because of his lack of military experience, Mackenzie volunteered to serve in the Crimea, but unfortunately died of cholera.[128] Ballingall acknowledged his indebtedness to him in the Preface to the 5th Edition of his *Outlines of Military Surgery* in the following terms: "that if I had been aware that my work was so nearly out of print, its revision would have been a very agreeable occupation to me during a tedious winter in the country; and had my late lamented friend and colleague, Dr. Mackenzie, whose surgical talent was so generally acknowledged at the battle of the Alma, been spared to return, and to give me his assistance in the revisal of this volume, which I at one time ventured to hope for, I should have been enabled to make the work more worthy of the patronage it has met with."[129]

Another serious candidate was Dr. Patrick Heron Watson. He also served in the Crimea, but was not considered for the post.[130] After a brief delay, the name of Ballingall's successor was published in a brief article in the Medical News section of the *Edinburgh Medical Journal*. Dr. Thomas Patrick Matthew, a distinguished Crimean veteran, was named as Ballingall's successor, but within a short time of the announcement the government withdrew the offer. According to this article: "Chair of Military Surgery.—This professorship, vacant by the death of Sir George Ballingall, has at length been filled up by Government, by the appointment of Dr. Matthews [sic], a staff-surgeon of great experience. Dr. Matthews served in the Crimea, and is reputed in the profession to be in every respect well qualified to perform the duties of the chair. Though comparatively unknown in Edinburgh, Dr. Matthews may rely on a cordial reception."[131]

The only reason that was given at the time was that the government planned to redirect the funds that would have been used to support this chair toward the establishment of an army medical school. According to his obituary notice: "Mr. Matthew was selected to fill the chair of the Regius Professorship of Military Surgery in Edinburgh; but the new Army Medical School altered the proposed plans and upset his appointment."[132]

In Dublin, a retired military surgeon, Mr. Thomas Joliffe Tufnell had lectured on military hygiene from 1846, and in 1855 was formally appointed to the Regius Chair of Military Surgery in the Royal College of Surgeons of Ireland, in Dublin. Despite running an extremely successful course, Tufnell's funding was also withdrawn in 1860, with the establishment of the Army Medical School. The extensive museum that he had gathered together, which contained an impressive collection of models of ambulance appliances and other artifacts relevant to his teaching course, was donated to the army medical college.

NOTES

1. N. Cantlie, 1974. *A History of the Army Medical Department*. 2 Volumes (Edinburgh and London: Churchill Livingstone).

2. Anon., 1963–1964. Ballingall, Sir George, M.D. (1780–1855). *Dictionary of National Biography* **1** (London: Oxford University Press), 1008.

3. J. Thomson, 1859. *An Account of the Life, Lectures, and Writings of William Cullen, M.D., Professor of the Practice of Physic in the University of Edinburgh. 2 Volumes. Volume 1. First Published in 1832. Now re-issued along with the second volume, and having pre-fixed to it a biographical notice of the author* (Edinburgh and London: W. Blackwood & Sons) [For biographical notice of Dr. John Thomson, see pp. 5–84].

4. Anon., 1963–1964. Tufnell, Thomas Joliffe (1819–1885). *Dictionary of National Biography* **19** (London: Oxford University Press), 1220–1221; A. Peterkin and W. Johnston, 1968. *Commissioned Officers in the Medical Services of the British Army 1660–1960.* 2 Volumes. Vol. 1, 1660–1898, 638 pp., Vol. 2, 1898–1960, 452 pp. (London: Wellcome Historical Medical Library). Volume 1, Reference Number 4649, p. 315. Both of these sources indicate that he was appointed to his Regius Chair in 1851. Tufnell received a letter from Peel, written on behalf of Lord Panmure and dated August

19, 1855, formally notifying him of his appointment to the Regius Chair of Military Surgeons in Dublin. See letter in Special Collections Section Edinburgh University Library from the War Office. Manuscript Reference Number M.S. 3082.3 Fol. 7.

5. G. J. Guthrie, 1855. Military Surgery in the Crimea. A Lecture delivered at the Royal College of Surgeons of England, on Saturday, April 14, 1855. *Lancet* **I**, 413–417; G. J. Guthrie, 1855. Surgical Practice in the Crimea. *Lancet* **I**, 544 [A brief letter]; G. J. Guthrie, 1856. Cases in Military Surgery Occurring in the Crimea. Communicated by G. J. Guthrie, Esq., F.R.S. *Lancet* **I**, 65–67; G. J. Guthrie, 1856. The Crimean Army. Wounds of the Head. Communicated by G.J. Guthrie, Esq., F.R.S. *Lancet* **I**, 257–260; G. J. Guthrie, 1856. The Crimean Army. Wounds of the Head. Communicated by G. J. Guthrie, Esq., F.R.S. *Lancet* **I**, 310–312.

6. A chair of military surgery was to be established for Dr. Rutherford Alcock, deputy inspector general of hospitals with the British Auxiliary Legion in Spain, in King's College, London, on his return from the Carlist War in 1838. As a consequence of an illness contracted in Spain which left his thumbs paralyzed, Alcock was unable to return to a career in surgery. As no others were considered for this post, no chair in this discipline was established. Alcock subsequently became a successful diplomat in China and Japan, and was awarded the K.C.B. (Knight Commander of the Order of the Bath) in 1862. See: A. Michie, 1900. *The Englishman in China During the Victorian Era: As Illustrated in the Career of Sir Rutherford Alcock, K.C.B., D.C.L. Many Years Consul and Minister in China and Japan.* 2 Volumes (Edinburgh and London: William Blackwood & Sons).

7. A. Miles, 1918. The Chair of Military Surgery. In: *The Edinburgh School of Surgery before Lister* (London: A. & C. Black Ltd.), pp. 108–120.

8. Universities of Scotland, Report (1831). *Report Made to His Majesty by a Royal Commission of Inquiry into the State of the Universities of Scotland* (London: The House of Commons) [Ordered to be Printed, October 7, 1831], pp. 56–59.

9. Anon., 1817. Medical Department of the Army. *Edinburgh Medical and Surgical Journal* **13**, 124–125.

10. Medical officers in the service of the Honourable East India Company regularly attended Ballingall's course of lectures in military surgery from 1825–1826.

11. J. Struthers, 1867. John Bell. In: *Historical sketch of the Edinburgh Anatomical School* (Edinburgh: Maclachlan & Stewart), pp. 37–44.

12. The British fleet under Admiral Adam Duncan had engaged a Dutch fleet under the command of Admiral de Winter on October 11, 1797. While the British lost only 203 killed and 620 wounded, and the Dutch losses were far greater, the battle was an important tactical victory, because in this one action the French lost their greatest ally. It was also the end of Dutch aspirations to being a great naval power.

13. C. Lloyd and J.L.S. Coulter, 1961. *Medicine and the Navy 1200–1900. Volume 3: 1714–1815* (Edinburgh and London: E. & S. Livingstone Ltd.), pp. 365–366; L. Haire, 1786. Remarks on Mr. Lucas's practical observations on amputation. *London Medical Journal* **7**, 377–390; E. Home, 1786. An account of Mr. Hunter's method of performing the operation for the popliteal aneurism. *London Medical Journal* **7**, 391–406.

14. J. H. Dible, 1970. *Napoleon's Surgeon* (London: William Heinemann Medical Books Ltd.).

15. J. Bell, 1800. *Memorial Concerning the Present State of Military and Naval Surgery. Addressed Several Years ago to the Right Honourable Earl Spencer, First Lord of the Admiralty; and now Submitted to the Public* (Edinburgh: Longman & Rees; London: Cadell & Davies).

16. J. Bell, 1798. *Memoir on the Present State of Naval and Military Surgery. Addressed to the Right Honourable Earl Spenser [sic], First Lord of the Admiralty* [21 pp. Yarmouth, January 20, 1798].

17. R. Jackson, 1805. *A System of Arrangement and Discipline for the Medical Department of Armies* (London: J. Murray).

18. "One advantage, however, attends the regular commencement of study at a university, namely, that the student is there taught to entertain enlarged and scientific views of his subjects, which, in the more confined situation of an inferior seminary, he has neither the opportunities to do, nor is he so apt to imbibe them. It is for this reason that the University of Edinburgh has been so deservedly distinguished for the scientific acquirements of its medical pupils; and though in the metropolis a great display of abilities prevails among the teachers, still the course of study is seldom so beneficial to the student, from the want of that connexion among the different professional branches, which a university so happily possesses." See: W. Turnbull, 1806. *The Naval Surgeon; Comprising the Entire Duties of Professional Men at Sea. To which are Subjoined, a System of Naval Surgery, and a Compendious Pharmacopoeia. The Whole Illustrated by Plates* (London: Richard Phillips & B. McMillan).

19. A. L. Turner, 1937. *Story of a Great Hospital: The Royal Infirmary of Edinburgh, 1729–1929* (Edinburgh: Oliver & Boyd).

20. G. B. Risse, 1986. *Hospital Life in Enlightenment Scotland: Care and Teaching at the Royal Infirmary of Edinburgh* (Cambridge: Cambridge University Press), p. 36.

21. J. Gregory, 1800. *Memorial to the Managers of the Royal Infirmary* (Edinburgh: Murray & Cochrane) [p. 260. Section IX, "Proposal for a more rational system of the attendance of the surgeons in the Royal Infirmary, on the pure principle of what would be best for the patients."]

22. J. Struthers, 1867. Sir Charles Bell. In: *Historical Sketch of the Edinburgh Anatomical School* (Edinburgh: Maclachlan & Stewart), pp. 44–55; G. Gordon-Taylor and E. W. Walls, 1958. *Sir Charles Bell: His Life and Times* (Edinburgh and London: E. & S. Livingstone), pp. 15–31, for observations on his early London days.

23. Anon., 1963–1964. Thomson, John (1765–1846). *Dictionary of National Biography* **19** (London: Oxford University Press), 740–742.

24. L. S. Jacyna, 1994. *Philosophic Whigs: Medicine, Science and Citizenship in Edinburgh, 1789–1848* (London: Routledge), p. 87.

25. J. Thomson, 1793. Probationary essay FRCSEd, topic believed to be 'Catarrhus' [Not located in Royal College of Surgeons Library or Edinburgh University Library].

26. Thomson, *Life of Cullen*, p. 19.

27. J. Thomson, 1800. *Outline of a Plan for the Regulation of the Surgical Department of the Royal Infirmary. Submitted to the Consideration of the Managers of that Institution* (Edinburgh: C. Stewart & Co.) [14 pp.].

28. These lectures were given on the recommendation of Dr. Thomas (later General Sir Thomas) Maitland, because of the renewal of hostilities with France and the fear of an imminent invasion from the Continent.

29. Jacyna, *Philosophic Whigs*, p. 89.

30. R. E. Wright-St. Clair, 1964. *Doctors Monro: A Medical Saga* (London: Wellcome Historical Medical Library), pp. 86–87.

31. The only other chair of surgery in Edinburgh at that time, apart from that associated with the chair of anatomy, was the Regius Chair of Clinical Surgery to which James Russell had been appointed by the Crown in 1803, but in order not to infringe the rights of Professor Monro tertius he had agreed not to give courses of lectures on systematic surgery. See: J. D. Comrie, 1932. *A History of Scottish Medicine*. 2nd Edition. 2 Volumes (London: Baillière, Tindall & Cox), Volume 2, p. 503.

32. Wright-St. Clair, *Doctors Monro*, p. 86.

33. For details, see: D. C. Simpson, 1977. The Chairs of Surgery at Edinburgh. *Journal of the Royal College of Surgeons of Edinburgh* **22**, 91–102.

34. Several sets of notes taken down by students who attended Thomson's lectures are available. See: Royal College of Surgeons of Edinburgh Manuscript Reference Number B.S. 03, Ref. No. 2685; the first lecture in this series was delivered on February 12, 1810; Edinburgh University Library Reference Number Dc.7.122.

35. Jacyna, *Philosophic Whigs*, pp. 92–97.

36. It was particularly important to the Whig administration that whoever was appointed to this post was politically sound, and represented a safe pair of hands within the Tory town council-dominated university senatus.

37. Risse, *Hospital Life*, pp. 92–97.

38. Risse, *Hospital Life*, p. 93.

39. Risse, *Hospital Life*, pp. 96–97.

40. "The Paymaster of Contingent Accounts [was directed] to discontinue the allowance of 5/- per diem granted to Drs. Hamilton and Spens for attending the military wards in the Royal Infirmary after the 24th ulto." See: *Minute Book, Managers, Royal Infirmary of Edinburgh*, Volume 9, pp. 254–255. This relates to a meeting of the managers held on October 22, 1821.

41. Thomson, *Life of Cullen*, pp. 32–34.

42. Thomson bought No. 9 Surgeons' Square, the premises previously occupied from 1808–1818 by Dr. John Gordon, and taught surgery here for a number of years. In this house, Dr. Sharpey, afterward professor of physiology in University College, London, taught anatomy here until 1836, during which period Thomson's son Allen, who also lectured on physiology, assisted him. This house was later acquired by the Royal Infirmary from Thomson's family, and used as a fever hospital. It was pulled down in 1850 to make room for the new surgical hospital. See: C. W. Cathcart, 1882. Some of the older schools of anatomy connected with the Royal College of Surgeons, Edinburgh. *Edinburgh Medical Journal* **27**, 769–781, pp. 777–778.

43. This visit to the Continent was undertaken with the blessing of the director-general, Sir James McGrigor, and he was accompanied by Dr. Somerville, a principal inspector in the Army Medical Department.

44. J. Thomson, 1816. *Report of observations made in the British military hospitals in Belgium, after the Battle of Waterloo; with some remarks upon amputation* (Edinburgh: W. Blackwood; London: T. Cadell & W. Davies). He also donated "an extensive series of sketches of the wounded at Waterloo, made, on the spot, by himself and Dr. Somerville" to the University of Edinburgh [Edinburgh University Library Reference Number: MS. Gen.594 B] and these are first noted in these terms. See: G. Ballingall, 1844. *Outlines of Military Surgery*. 3rd Edition (Edinburgh: Adam & Charles Black; London: Longman, Brown, Green & Longmans), p. viii.

45. This caused considerable distress within military medical circles in Edinburgh at that time, as many serving medical officers were retired on half-pay. Numerous anonymous letters were sent to the Secretary-at-War requesting that his commission should be withdrawn. He received a full salary from the Army Medical Department, and was retired on half-pay in March 1821 and was paid this until he died in October 1846. See: A. Peterkin & W. Johnston 1968. *Commissioned Officers in the medical Services of the British Army 1660–1960*. 2 Volumes (London: Wellcome Historical Medical Library), Volume 1, p. 264, John Thomson, Reference Number 3961.

46. Thomson, *Life of Cullen*, p. 34.

47. Thomson, *Life of Cullen*, pp. 47–48.

48. See: Royal College of Surgeons of Edinburgh Manuscript Reference Number B.S. 03, Ref. No. 2685; the first lecture in this series was delivered on February 12, 1810; Edinburgh University Library Reference Number Dc.7.122.

49. J. Thomson, 1817. Extracts from a letter from a physician in London. 3. Syphilis cured without mercury. *Edinburgh Medical and Surgical Journal* **13**, 250–251 [An anonymous item, said to have been written by Thomson, who claimed that it had been sent privately to Dr. Andrew Ducan junior, but that he had submitted it to the journal for publication; see: Thomson, *Life of Cullen*, p. 49]. Thomson "invariably followed the same modes of treatment in private practice, and was led from his experience, to place the most entire confidence in the non-mercurial treatment of every form of the disease, whether primary or secondary." See: Thomson, *Life of Cullen*, p. 48.

50. Thomson's successor in office was Mr. J. W. Turner, who since about 1811 had assisted him in his class of military surgery, and from 1819 had also assisted him in demonstrating the operations of surgery during the practical component of his College lecture course on surgery. Ten years later, in 1831, Thomson was appointed to the newly established Regius Chair of Pathology, and Turner was appointed to the newly established Chair of Surgery. On Turner's sudden death from pneumonia in 1836, his chair was offered to Sir Charles Bell, who retained it until his death in 1842. See: Comrie, *Scottish Medicine*, Volume 2, p. 507. Turner's Fellowship dissertation was dedicated to Dr. Thomson. See: J. W. Turner, 1812. *A probationary surgical essay on dislocation of the shoulder joint; submitted, by authority of the President and his Council, to the examination of the Royal College of Surgeons of Edinburgh, when candidate for admission into their corporation, in conformity to their regulations respecting the admission of ordinary members* (Edinburgh: James Ballantyne & Co.).

51. He "became a licentiate of the Royal College of Physicians, Edinburgh, a measure though not necessary, yet expedient to one who was now acting as consultant surgeon, and occasionally as consulting physician." See: Thomson, *Life of Cullen*, p. 44.

52. Between 1828 and 1830, these lectures were given in conjunction with his son William, who later became professor of the practice of physic in the University of Glasgow.

53. In 1813, he published his *Lectures on Inflammation*, which discussed the pathological basis of inflammation. It was well received, and clearly demonstrated his early interest in pathology. See: J. Thomson, 1813. *Lectures on Inflammation, exhibiting a view of the General Doctrines, Pathological and Practical, of Medical Surgery* (Edinburgh: W. Blackwood; London: T. Cadell).

54. These were initially used to illustrate his extramural lectures on the practice of physic, but were later used to illustrate his university lectures on general pathology.

55. His extremely brief letter of resignation that was read before the senatus of the university was dated November 13, 1822. No reasons for this decision were provided in this letter

56. This followed his memorial addressed to Lord Melbourne, then Secretary of State for the Home Department.

57. Thomson, *Life of Cullen*; J. Thomson, 1859. *An Account of the Life, Lectures, and Writings of William Cullen, M.D., Professor of the Practice of Physic in the University of Edinburgh. 2 Volumes. Volume. 2. Commenced by Dr. John Thomson and Dr. William Thomson, and concluded by David Craigie, M.D., F.R.C.P.E., F.R.S.E., &c. &c.* (Edinburgh and London: W. Blackwood & Sons)..

58. M. Barfoot, 1997. Introduction. In: *Lives of the Literati. An Account of the Life, Lectures, and Writings of William Cullen. Volume 1. John Thomson* (Bristol: Thoennes Press), pp. v–xvii.

59. H. Lonsdale, 1870. *A Sketch of the Life and Writings of Robert Knox the Anatomist. By his Pupil and Colleague* (London: Macmillan & Co.), p. 201.

60. Thomson, *Life of Cullen* [For biographical notice of Dr. William Thomson, see pp. 85–92].

61. Comrie, *Scottish Medicine*, Volume 2, pp. 521–522; 555–556; 607–608.

62. Thomson's letter of resignation from his Regius Chair appointment had been sent to the Minister for the Home Department. See: *Senatus Minutes* (i.e., College Minutes Book), 1812–1824, pp. 323–324.

63. Ballingall was informed in a letter from the Prime Minister, Sir Robert Peel, dated November 20, 1822, of his appointment. This letter is addressed from Whitehall, and reads as follows: "I have the satisfaction of acquainting you that after considering the several applications which have been made for the appointment of Professor of Military Surgery, I have recommended your name to His Majesty for that Office, and His Majesty has been graciously pleased to give directions for your appointment." See: Special Collections Manuscript Reference Number MS 3082.2. Fols. 371–372. A copy of his commission of appointment dated November 21, 1822 was entered into the *College Minutes Book 1812–1824*. See: Quarterly Meeting, Senate Room, January 18, 1823, pp. 336–338. According to p. 336: "The King's Commission to Dr. Ballingall was read & ordered to be recorded—as was also the usual protest by the Town Council for preservation of their rights as Patrons—likewise a Certificate of Dr. Ballingall having signed the Formula ordained by Act of Assembly—Dr. Ballingall was then admitted in the usual form and took his seat accordingly."

64. Dr. Borthwick's name had also been proposed as a candidate by one of the town council whose brother-in-law he was. As he was not a fellow of the College of Surgeons, his candidature did not have their support.

65. In Peel's letter to Lord Melville, he asked him: "Which would be the best appointment in the interests of surgery which have the first claim to be consulted in this case. If Ballingall be equally well qualified in regard to science with Dr. Maclagan there can be no reason why he should not be preferred. If he be his inferior in the qualifications of a professor I think he ought not to owe his appointment to the politics of his rival." See: R. Peel, 1822. *Peel papers*. Letter from Peel to the second Lord Melville, dated October 26, 1822 [BM Add MS 40317, fo. 5]. As Ballingall's political sympathies were somewhere between neutral and conservative, it is likely that this would have been acceptable to the Tory government.

66. He matriculated in all the classes in the university necessary to obtain the M.D. degree with the exception of chemistry, possibly because he had no intention of graduating with this degree. If he planned at this stage to enter the Army Medical Department, he would only have needed the lesser qualification of a diploma from the Royal College of Surgeons, which he obtained in December 1805.

67. He was elected president of the Royal College of Surgeons of Edinburgh during the 1836–1838 Session.

68. J. Struthers, 1867. Barclay. In: *Historical Sketch of the Edinburgh Anatomical School* (Edinburgh: Maclachlan & Stewart), pp. 56–70.

69. In April 1813, Ballingall purchased an elephant that had formerly been employed by the East India Company for transporting camp equipment and stores. It had been removed from service because of a progressive lung disease. Ballingall dispatched the elephant and with assistance from a number of natives cleaned and prepared its skeleton. The disarticulated skeleton was subsequently sent to Barclay, and the skeleton reassembled when Ballingall returned to Edinburgh in 1814. The skeleton was initially displayed in Barclay's rooms at 10 Surgeons' Square, and later formed the centerpiece of Barclay's Comparative Anatomy Collection displayed in the main hall of the Royal

College of Surgeons of Edinburgh. See: G. Ballingall, 1820. *Memoir of the skeleton of an Elephant dissected at Bangalore in 1813, and now deposited in Dr. Barclay's Museum* (Edinburgh: George Ramsay & Company); M. H. Kaufman, 1996. Observations on Barclay's elephant. *Journal of the Royal College of Surgeons of Edinburgh* **41**, 75–81.

70. G. Ballingall, 1827. *The life of Dr. Bar*clay, pp. i–xix [Prefixed to *Introductory lectures to a course of anatomy by John Barclay* (Edinburgh: Maclachlan & Stewart)].

71. Universities of Scotland, Report, 1831, pp. 58–63; L. Rosner, 1991. *Medical Education in the Age of Improvement: Edinburgh Students and Apprentices 1760–1826* (Edinburgh: University Press), pp. 62–85.

72. G. Ballingall, 1819. *Dissertatio medica inauguralis de apoplexia sanguinea* (Edinburgh: P. Neill) [M.D. Thesis, Edinburgh University, 24 pp.].

73. G. Ballingall, 1820. *An essay on syphilis submitted, by authority of the President and his Council, to the examination of the Royal College of Surgeons of Edinburgh, when candidate for admission into their corporation* (Edinburgh: Balfour & Clarke) [30 pp.] [Fellowship of the Royal College of Surgeons of Edinburgh probationary essay].

74. It is possible that he was elected to the Royal Society of Edinburgh either because of the influence of Barclay or Thomson, elected in 1807 and in 1812, respectively, on the basis of his publications, or more likely "on the promise of things to come." He had published only a small monograph, and several reports based on clinical cases he had seen while on military service in India. See: G. Ballingall, 1818. *Practical observations on fever, dysentery and liver complaints, as they occur amongst the European troops in India; with introductory remarks on the disadvantages of selecting boys for Indian military service* (Edinburgh: David Brown, & A Constable & Co.); G. Ballingall, 1818. Case of hydrophobia, which occurred in the Regimental hospital of His Majesty's 1st Foot, or Royal Scots. *Edinburgh Medical and Surgical Journal* **11**, 74–77; G. Ballingall, 1818. Two cases of dislocation of the thumb. *Edinburgh Medical and Surgical Journal* **11**, 188–192; G. Ballingall, 1820. Case of hydrophobia originating without any obvious cause. *Edinburgh Medical and Surgical Journal* **16**, 209–212.

75. A copy of the original set of printed testimonials that was submitted with his application for the professorship is available in Edinburgh University Library Special Collections Reference Number MS 3082.10. These testimonials were obtained from ten individuals and were accompanied by extract of the reviews of his two books that had recently been published.

76. D. Maclagan, 1805. *De sanitate tuenda* (Edinburgh: Adam Neill & Son).

77. His eldest son, Andrew Douglas (later Sir Douglas) Maclagan, professor of Medical Jurisprudence in the University of Edinburgh, is the only other individual who has been elected President of both the College of Surgeons and College of Physicians of Edinburgh. Another son became the Archbishop of York, while others distinguished themselves in the public service. See: Anon., 1865. Dr. Maclagan. *Edinburgh Medical Journal* **11**, 94.

78. Such a hollow gesture of defiance was always made after the announcement of an appointment to a Regius Chair, to indicate that the appointment had been awarded at the whim of the government. It was not technically a university appointment, as it had not been made at the discretion of the town council or of the senatus of the university.

79. This probably amounted to about £125 per annum in 1820. It is difficult to assess exactly how much Ballingall received each year that he was on half-pay between 1818 and 1831. The half-pay for a surgeon in the Ordnance Medical Department for the year 1820 was £127-15-0. See: Parliamentary Papers (1821). *Estimates and Accounts, Volume 1, Army; Navy; Ordnance; Chelsea Hospital; Ophthalmia; Commissariat; etc. Session 23 January to 11 July 1821*. Volume **XV** [Ordered to be printed by the House of Commons]. In 1858, a surgeon on full-pay received £273-15-0 per annum gradually rising after 25

years to £456-5-0 per annum, as a result of the Medical Warrant of 1858. See: W. Rivington, 1879. *The Medical Profession: being the Essay to which was awarded the First Carmichael Prize of £200 by the Council of the Royal College of Surgeons, Ireland, 1879* (Dublin: Fannin & Co.; London: Longmans & Co.; Baillière, Tindall, & Cox; Edinburgh: Maclachlan & Stewart), pp. 211–212.

80. Each student that matriculated to attend his course paid him a fee of 3 guineas per session. See: Universities of Scotland, Abstract (1836). *An Abstract of the General Report of the Royal Commissioners Appointed to Visit the Universities of Scotland. With Notes and Tabular States Relating to the State of These Institutions in 1826* (Edinburgh: Adam & Charles Black; Glasgow: James Brash & Co.; Aberdeen: Alex. Brown & Co.; St. Andrews: M. Fletcher), Table, pp. 8–9.

81. *Minute Book, Royal Infirmary of Edinburgh*, Volume 9, p. 327. "Dr. George Ballingall to be one of the Assistant Surgeons."

82. During this period, he also accepted an invitation from Syme to act as a consulting surgeon in what is believed to be his surgical hospital in Minto House, although this was not formally opened until 1829. Syme had established this hospital in 1827–1828, in rivalry to the Royal Infirmary, because the managers there had decided that only Liston should be allowed to continue practicing there. See: Comrie, *Scottish Medicine*, Volume 2, p. 594.

83. Anon., 1830. *London Gazette*, Volume 2, p. 1689.

84. *Minute Book, Royal Infirmary of Edinburgh*, Volume 11, p. 107.

85. G. Ballingall, 1824. *Prospectus of the Course of Lectures on Military Surgery. University of Edinburgh, 10th November 1824.*

86. G. Ballingall, 1830. *Introductory Lectures to a Course of military Surgery, Delivered in the University of Edinburgh* (Edinburgh: Adam Black; London: Longman, Rees, Orme, Brown & Green), [246 pp.].

87. G. Ballingall, 1833. *Outlines of the Course of Lectures on military Surgery, delivered in the University of Edinburgh* (Edinburgh: Adam Black; London: Longman, Rees, Orme, Brown & Green) [This is the 1st Edition of Ballingall's *Outlines of Military Surgery*; 589 pp.].

88. G. Ballingall, 1855. *Outlines of Military Surgery*. 5th Edition (Edinburgh: Adam & Charles Black; London: Longman & Co.).

89. The college commissioners stressed that professors had only certain rights, that is "to be furnished with sufficient accommodation for his teaching," rather than having rights of occupancy, although the Medical Faculty at that time occupied a disproportionate amount of the available space in the Old College. See: A. G. Fraser, 1989. *The Building of Old College: Adam, Playfair & The University of Edinburgh* (Edinburgh: Edinburgh University Press), p. 190.

90. The information presented here comes from the analysis of the various class lists and attendance books for Ballingall's course available in Edinburgh University archives.

91. The receipt of Alcock's collection was first publicly acknowledged in 1843. See: G. Ballingall, 1843. Instruction for medical officers of the army and navy. *Lancet* **I**, 268–270, p. 269.

92. G. Ballingall, 1855. *Catalogue of the Museum attached to the Class of Military Surgery in the University of Edinburgh* (Edinburgh: R. & R. Clark).

93. The *Printed Catalogue* was largely based on a manuscript catalogue prepared during the 1843–1844 session by two students as a joint prize essay, and was updated at intervals as additional items were added to the collection.

94. R. Alcock, 1838. *Notes on the Medical History and Statistics of the British Legion of Spain; Comprising the Results of Gun-Shot Wounds in Relation to Important Questions in Surgery* (London: J. Churchill).

95. For publications on some of the items in this collection, see: M. H. Kaufman, B. N. Purdue, and A. L Carswell, 1996. Old wounds and distant battles; the Alcock-Ballingall collection of military surgery at the University of Edinburgh. *Journal of the Royal College of Surgeons of Edinburgh* **41**, 339–350; M. H. Kaufman, J. McTavish, and R. Mitchell, 1997. The gunner with the silver mask: observations on the management of severe maxillo-facial lesions over the last 160 years. *Journal of the Royal College of Surgeons of Edinburgh* **42**, 367–375; M. H. Kaufman, 2000. Howison, The Cramond Murderer, and last person to be hanged and dissected. *Scottish Medical Journal* **45**, 28-30; M. H. Kaufman and M. T. Royds, 2000. Excision of a remarkable tumour of the upper jaw in 1834 by Robert Liston. *Scottish Medical Journal* **45**, 58-60; M. H. Kaufman and M. T. Royds, 2000. The Penman case: a re-evaluation. *Journal of the Royal College of Surgeons of Edinburgh* **45**, 51–55.

96. Edinburgh University Library Manuscript Reference Number MS 3082.6, Fols. 2–7. Between sessions 1823–1824 and 1840–1841, the names of all of the students who attended the military surgery course are listed. From 1841–1842 until 1853–1854, only the totals attending are provided. The information available includes matriculation lists and the professor's class returns lists.

97. L. Rosner, 1991. *Medical Education in the Age of Improvement: Edinburgh Students and Apprentices 1760–1826* (Edinburgh: University Press), pp. 109–205.

98. Source of information. See: Edinburgh University Library, Manuscript Reference Gen. 1733/28.

99. Universities of Scotland, Evidence (1837). *Evidence, Oral and Documentary, Taken and Received By The Commissioners Appointed by His Majesty George IV. July 23d, 1826; And Re-appointed by His Majesty William IV., October 12th 1830; For Visiting The Universities of Scotland. Volume 1. University of Edinburgh. Presented to both Houses of Parliament by Command of His Majesty* (London: W. Clowes & Sons), p. 192.

100. Ballingall, *Outlines of Military Surgery*, 1833.

101. The figures presented here have been abstracted from Peterkin and Johnston. *Commissioned Officers*, Volume 1. It is now accepted that these figures may not be completely accurate. They are, however, the only figures available covering this period, and are therefore useful for showing important trends.

102. Peterkin and Johnston, *Commissioned Officers*, Volume 1.

103. C. Lloyd and J.L.S. Coulter, 1963. *Medicine and the Navy 1200–1900*. In 4 Volumes (Edinburgh and London: E. & S. Livingstone Ltd.), Volume 4, p. 11.

104. Lloyd and Coulter, *Medicine and the Navy*, Volume 4, pp. 1, 3.

105. Universities of Scotland, Report (1831), pp. 56–59; Universities of Scotland, Abstract (1836); Universities of Scotland, Evidence (1837), p. 192. For the manuscript copy of his memorial, in the hand of an amanuensis, see: Edinburgh University Library Manuscript Reference MS 3082.7, Fols. 1–7.

106. Universities of Scotland, Evidence (1837), p. 301.

107. Universities of Scotland, Report (1831), p. 61.

108. For Liston, see: Comrie, *Scottish Medicine*, Volume 2, pp. 496–497; D. J. Coltart, 1972. Surgery between Hunter and Lister as exemplified by the life and works of Robert Liston (1794–1847). *Proceedings of the Royal Society of Medicine* **65**, 556–560; For Syme: see: R. Paterson, 1874. *Memorials of the Life of James Syme* (Edinburgh: Edmonston & Douglas).

109. Universities of Scotland, Evidence (1837), pp. 300–303.

110. See, for example: Anon., 1843. *Lancet* **I**, 270 [Editorial—untitled, as a follow-up to Ballingall's article entitled "Instruction for Medical Officers of the Army and Navy." *Lancet*, 1843, **I**, 268–270]; Anon., 1844. Remarks on Schools of Instruction for Military

and Naval Surgeons, in a letter to the Right Hon. Sir Robert Peel, Bart. By Sir George Ballingall, M.D., Regius Professor of Military Surgery in the University of Edinburgh. *Medico-Chirurgical Review. New Series* **40**, 355–361 [This represents another article critical of Ballingall's letter to Sir Robert Peel, previously published in the *Lancet*, 1843, **I**, 268–270].

111. See, for example: Scotus, 1827. Review of some of the surgical cases which have lately occurred in the Royal Infirmary of Edinburgh—A clinical lecture delivered to the students of surgery in that institution, on the evening of Monday 26 February, 1827. By George Ballingall (Edinburgh: A. Balfour & Co.). *Lancet* **II**, 774–778; Scotus, 1827. A new method of performing the operation for the radical cure of hydrocele. By Dr. Ballingall. *Lancet* **II**, 444–445; Scotus, 1828. Dr. Ballingall's clinical lecture. *Lancet* **I**, 89–90; Scotus, 1828. Letters from the Army, Navy and East India Medical Boards, to Dr. Ballingall. *Lancet* **I**, 258–260.

112. These principally appeared between 1827 and 1844. For example, see: Anon., 1843. *Lancet* **I**, 270 [Editorial—untitled, as a follow-up to Ballingall's article entitled "Instruction for Medical Officers of the Army and Navy." *Lancet*, 1843, **I**, 268–270].

113. Anon., 1828. Review of some of the surgical cases which have lately occurred in the Royal Infirmary of Edinburgh—A clinical lecture delivered to the students of surgery in that institution, on the evening of Monday, 28th July, 1828. By George Ballingall. *Lancet* **II**, 757–759.

114. "It would appear never to have occurred to the founders of sham professorships of this kind. . . . The succession to the "Chair," after so illustrious a predecessor as Dr. Thomson. . . . It would, we think, speak more for Dr. Ballingal's [sic] sagacity and integrity had he interpreted Dr. Thomson's resignation in another way, and imitated his conduct." See: Anon., 1830. Dr. Ballingal's [sic] Introductory Lectures. *Lancet* **II**, 130–132.

115. G. Ballingall, 1843. Instruction for medical officers of the army and navy. *Lancet* **I**, 268–270. After numerous letters from Ballingall to successive Secretaries of State for War, the government eventually included in the army estimates for 1854 the sum of £400 to endow additional professorships of military surgery in London and Dublin. While a chair was funded in Dublin for five years, no funds were directed toward establishing a similar chair in London.

116. G. Ballingall, 1823. *Practical observations on fever, dysentery, and liver complaints, as they occur amongst the European troops in India; illustrated by numerous tables and cases. To which is annexed an essay on syphilis.* 2nd Edition (Edinburgh: Adam Black; London: T & G Underwood; Dublin: Hodges & McArthur); G. Ballingall, 1855. On the too early enlistment of recruits. *Lancet* **I**, 78–79.

117. G. Ballingall, 1844. Letter addressed by Sir George Ballingall, M.D. to Sir De Lacy Evans on the subject of the right of military surgeons to military honours. *Lancet* **II**, 215–216; Anon., 1851. Abstract of the Introductory Lecture to the Course of Military Surgery. Delivered in the University of Edinburgh, May 1, 1851. By Sir George Ballingall. *Lancet* **I**, 566–568.

118. Anon., 1855. Sir George Ballingall and the War Department. *Lancet* **I**, 53; Anon., 1855. Sir George Ballingall's letter to the Secretary-at-War. *Lancet* **I**, 74–75.

119. Turner, since 1819, had assisted Thomson while he was College professor of surgery in conducting the operative part of his course, as Thomson found this part distasteful.

120. Edinburgh University Library Special Collection Manuscripts Reference QP.386/14.

121. He had been given an ultimatum by the War Office, that either he return to the Army Medical Department on full-pay or continue to hold his university post and be put

on the retired list. He decided on the latter course of action, and as a consequence his salary dropped dramatically.

122. Possibly as a result of the publication of an interview with him that was published in the *Lancet* which drew attention to his numerous heroic exploits in the Peninsular War, his reputation was much enhanced, and his opinions on military surgical topics were greatly respected. On three separate occasions he was elected president of the Royal College of Surgeons of England, in 1833, 1841, and 1854. See: Anon., 1850. Biographical Sketch of G. J. Guthrie, esq., F.R.S., Late President of the College of Surgeons. *Lancet* **I**, 726–738; Z. Cope, 1959. *The Royal College of Surgeons of England. A History* (London: A. Blond).

123. Anon., 1855. Reviews and Notices of Books. *Outlines of Military Surgery*. By Sir George Ballingall, M.D., F.R.S.E., &c. &c. Fifth Edition (Edinburgh: A. & C. Black. 1855, 634 pp.) *Lancet* **II**, 226–227.

124. Anon., *Ballingall's letter*.

125. For example, Ballingall wrote on March 5, 1853 to Dr. Andrew Smith to inquire whether his six-month winter course could be replaced with a three-month summer course. See: Edinburgh University Library Reference Number MS 3082.2, Fols. 1–492.

126. Paterson, *James Syme*, pp. 129–130.

127. Paterson, *James Syme*, pp. 127–129.

128. Anon., 1855. Brief Memorial of the life and writings of the late Richard James Mackenzie, M.D., F.R.C.S. *Edinburgh Medical and Surgical Journal* **82**, 281–316; J. A. Shepherd, 1989. Richard Mackenzie – a forgotten hero. *Journal of the Royal College of Surgeons of Edinburgh* **34**, 185–188.

129. Ballingall, *Outlines of Military Surgery*, 5th Edition, p. xiii.

130. He had a distinguished clinical career, and was President of the Royal College of Surgeons of Edinburgh on two occasions, and was also knighted. See: Comrie, *Scottish Medicine*, Volume 2, p. 675.

131. Anon., 1857. Medical News. Chair of Military Surgery. *Edinburgh Medical Journal* **2**, 1131.

132. Anon., 1865. Surgeon-Major Matthew. *Lancet* **II**, 54–55, p. 54.

4

THE CRIMEAN WAR

POLITICAL CONDITIONS THAT LED TO HOSTILITIES IN THE CRIMEA

As a result of Russia's imperialist ambitions to expand its territory and influence into those parts of the Balkans then under Turkish control, the Russians, under Tsar Nicholas I, established a large army on the frontiers of the Turkish provinces in the Balkans. A large Black Sea fleet based at Sebastopol backed this up. In October 1853, the Russians declared war and invaded the Turkish provinces of Moldavia and Wallachia, on either bank of the Danube, under the pretext of protecting the Greek Orthodox Christians there, and in the holy places in Palestine, then under Turkish control. On November 30, 1853, a modern Russian fleet outgunned and totally destroyed an antiquated Turkish fleet at anchor in the harbor of Sinope, with great loss of life. Under cover of fog, the Russian navy, under the command of Admiral Nachimoff, entered the harbor and opened fire with the new high-explosive shells on the Turkish ships, destroying them all. According to a contemporary source, "Five thousand sailors perished; the whole squadron was blown into one mass of broken and burning timber, and blasted and bleeding human flesh. Yet amidst the floating timbers, blackened and blood-stained, the Russian ships fired grape and canister, lest any of the wrecked should swim ashore; and such as did make the harbor were shelled, and aim even directed upon the wounded. It was not war—it was massacre."[1]

A strong anti-Russian feeling was stimulated in Britain in support of the policies of Lord Palmerston, and a warship was dispatched to provide medical assistance to the survivors. The warship arrived seven days after the battle, but relatively few survivors were received from the shore. The British were particularly incensed when they heard that Nachimoff and his men received a hero's welcome from the Tsar.

The Russian army advanced to the Danube, but were resisted by the Turkish army. It was believed that Russia planned to seize the whole of the Ottoman Empire and upset the balance of power in Europe. When the Russians refused to withdraw Britain and France declared war, the French nominally to protect the Roman Catholic community in the Holy Land. A 10,000-strong "Army of Observation" had previously been sent from Britain to Malta before the declaration of war on March 27, 1854, but under the changed circumstances, progressed to the Dardanelles, landing there in April 1854. Shortly before, a larger French force had already been sent to Turkey, in readiness for war. It was generally believed that Britain and its allies planned to destroy the Russian naval base at Sebastopol. An additional British force of 40,000 men was therefore dispatched early in April to the Crimea.

In June, the Turks recaptured a number of key positions on the Danube, although they were supported by the presence of a large Austrian army as well as the various Allied armies. The Russians retreated toward their own border, on the River Pruth. While a peace settlement might have been arranged at this time, no effort was made in that direction, and an all-out war was then inevitable. The Danube delta was marshy and a notorious malarial area, and this was the first large campaign when the British army extensively used quinine as a prophylactic agent against this disease. This was despite the fact that the both the vector and causative agent were at that time unknown. Quinine undoubtedly played a critical prophylactic role in preserving the health of the British force.[2]

While malaria did not prove to be a problem, the British force was nearly destroyed by cholera, even before the onset of hostilities. This involved both the army in Gallipoli and all parts of the fleet in July. The French force was exposed to cholera in Marseilles and Toulon, and the disease was brought with them to the Crimea and rapidly spread throughout the British fleet. During the next few months, more than 1,000 of the French troops died from cholera, and the disease debilitated many more. The mortality on board some of the British ships was particularly high, with an overall mortality rate from cholera of over 64%, with 640 of the 992 men admitted to the hospital during July and August dying from it. Of the 29 orderlies who were sent to assist in the wards, 86% died of cholera.

Despite earlier suggestions that this disease spread through contaminated water, and contemporary *Returns from the Registrar-General's Department* published in the *Lancet*[3] which indicated that the incidence of cholera in different parts of London varied according to the source of water, it was still generally held that this condition was due to poor ventilation on board ship. Those who were exposed to this condition in the East but drank wine and avoided water usually survived without catching cholera.

While the Russian and Turkish armies consisted of nearly three-quarters and just over half a million men, respectively, the French army was also quite substantial. The total British army, by contrast, was far smaller and relatively poorly equipped, having been subjected to both severe neglect and financial constraint by Parliament since the time of the Peninsular War. The chief deficiencies involved the administrative services, the Commissariat and the Medical Department, both of which were civil departments. Equally, there was no transport corps or ordnance corps, the tradition since Peninsular days being to requisition transport from the country in which the army fought. During times of peace, financial savings compelled elimination of the medically qualified purveyors and apothecaries. After a lengthy interval, the first apothecary was appointed toward the end of October 1854 by royal warrant. These officers, with the equivalent rank of lieutenant, were to be put in charge of medical stores in general hospitals and oversee the activities of the dispensers who were to hold the rank of ensign. While the British rifle regiments were equipped with the modern Minié rifle, which had a substantially faster rate of fire and three times the range of the Brown Bess musket, typical of the Peninsular War period, the majority of the troops still used the Brown Bess. The artillery also still used smoothbore weapons.

Since Waterloo, the British army had had little exposure to war, apart from the minor colonial skirmishes against largely untrained and poorly armed native forces in Asia and Africa between 1824 and 1853.[4] The quality of its leadership was also highly suspect; the majority of the senior generals were elderly, and expected to fight a relatively short and Peninsular-style campaign. The situation was particularly complicated because the military infrastructure required to defend the far corners of the British Empire was quite different from that required to fight a modern European war. This dilemma was neither fully appreciated during the interwar period nor reconciled by the time of the Crimean War.[5] Difficulties were also encountered between the British and French high commands.

Twenty-five thousand British troops under the command of Lord Raglan, major-general of the ordnance,[6] joined a French force of 30,000 men, under the command of Marshal Saint-Arnaud, at Varna on the Black Sea, the main forces arriving in September 1854. It was jointly decided that the Russian naval base at Sebastopol had to be attacked and the fleet there destroyed. The joint force crossed the Black Sea, landing at Kalamatia (or Kalamita) Bay, just to the north of Sebastopol, and on the west coast of the Crimea, without any opposition from the Russian forces. Due to a lack of forward planning, minimal facilities were available to transport the food and equipment to the troops. All that was available were primitive country carts that had to be requisitioned from the villagers and their farms in the vicinity. Of the 350 that were obtained from this source, only 24 were allocated for the use of the medical staff. In addition, only two ambulance wagons had arrived to carry the sick and wounded. Unfortunately, there were no horses to draw them. Lord Raglan had deliberately instructed that no regimental hospital equipment nor field ambulance units would be allowed to accompany the expedition.

The Russians were in a strong defensive position overlooking the river Alma. After a bloody frontal attack on September 20, 1854, with over 2,200 Allied casualties (see Figure 4.1), and 5,700 Russian dead left on the battlefield, the position was taken. No means were available to the director-general of the Army Medical Department, Dr. Andrew Smith, and his local senior medical officer, inspector-general Hall, to evacuate the wounded the three miles from the battlefield to the ships anchored off the beaches. Suitable wagons had to be

Figure 4.1. Field Hospital after the Battle of the Alma (Crimean War)

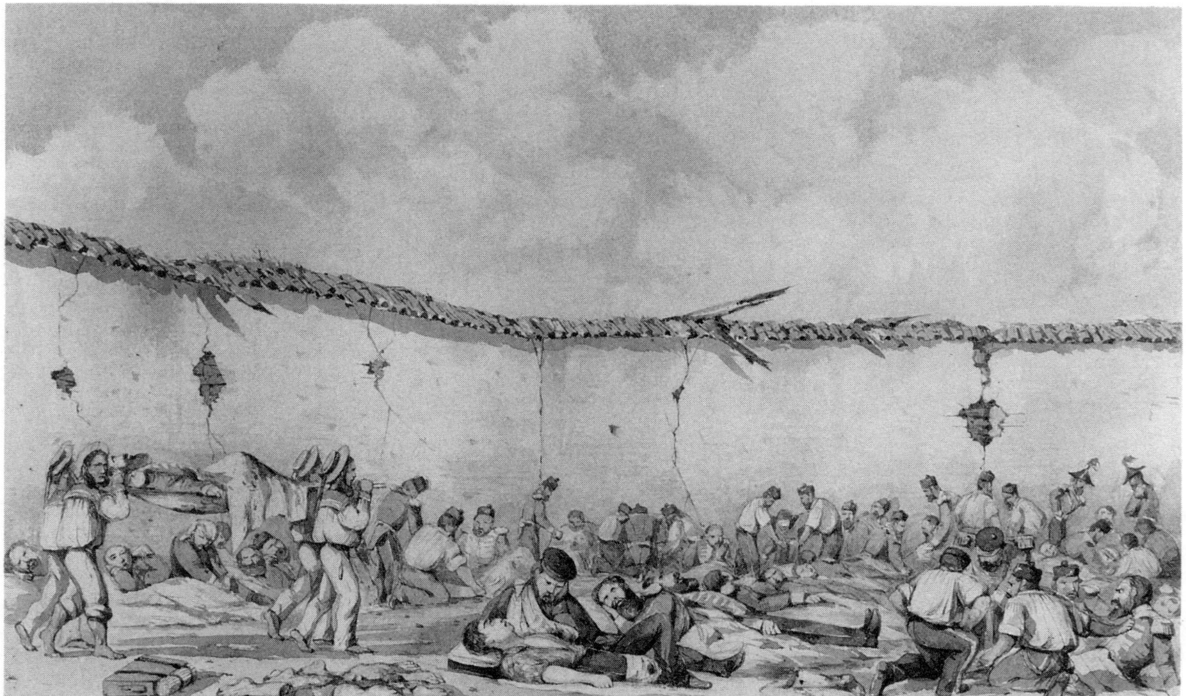

Watercolor painting (artist unknown), in Scottish United Services Museum. Courtesy of the Trustees, National Museums of Scotland.

borrowed from other units for this purpose. Equally, great difficulties were encountered in obtaining enough doctors to accompany the wounded on the transports. The navy came to Hall's assistance, and provided 1,000 seamen with hammocks slung on poles to carry the wounded, as well as medical officers to assist their army colleagues. Assistance was also obtained from the French, who were well equipped with mobile ambulances and mules. Large numbers of the men were taken on board the ships with severe cholera, were often too ill to be accommodated in hammocks, and lay on the decks wrapped in their own blankets. Many were too weak to crawl to the night stools, and died covered in their own excrement. In some of the transports, no orderlies were available to look after the needs of the sick and dying. Very high losses were encountered due to the disgraceful conditions on board these ships.

No attempt was made to pursue the enemy, and any momentum gained was soon lost. The Allies withdrew from the region close to Sebastopol, because it was too exposed to land adequate supplies there. The Allies bombarded Sebastopol on October 17 with their 126 guns, but the Russians replied with counterfire from their 341 guns, which soon silenced the French, and thereafter all thoughts of an early success had to be abandoned. The British then sailed to Balaklava, and the French withdrew to two small ports to the west of the city. The Russians counterattacked, resulting in the Battle of Balaklava, fought on October 25, 1854.

The Russians launched a heavy frontal cavalry attack on the defensive perimeter of the Allied garrison at Balaklava, and quickly overcame the Turkish positions guarding the Allies' supply route. Despite the fact that the Russians outnumbered the British force by about 10:1, their main attack was repulsed by the "thin red line." This consisted of only two rows containing about 550 men of the 93rd Highlanders on the heights, under the command of General Sir Colin Campbell, supported by a small force of marines for the immediate defense of the harbor. The Russian losses were slight, but many of their cavalry were wounded. Once the enemy had a chance to regroup, they organized a second Russian cavalry charge. This was spotted, and the Heavy Brigade, under General Sir James Scarlett, with about 600 cavalrymen, was ordered to charge them.

The 4th Dragoon Guards attacked the Russian flank, while the rest of the regiment went in to support the Heavy Brigade. The Russian force fled in disarray. Lord Cardigan's Light Brigade was held back in reserve, and the infantry sent in to follow up the success of the Heavy Brigade, but were too slow to be effective. The cavalry, under Lord Lucan, was moved over Causeway Heights, and then received orders to charge the enemy to prevent them from carrying away the Turkish guns that had been abandoned on Causeway Heights that had formerly been guarding the approaches to Balaklava.

There was some confusion regarding the exact meaning of Lord Raglan's order.[7] Lucan asked for clarification, because from his position, he could not see any Russians moving guns. Captain Louis Nolan apparently pointed to the Russian artillery at the far end of the North Valley. It is believed that he misinformed Lord Lucan that these were the guns that needed to be rescued. The Light Brigade, with Lord Cardigan at their head, was ordered to advance, and charged directly into the concentrated fire of the Russian guns. The Russian artillery was indeed lined up at the far end of the North Valley, but there was a battery on each flank, which Cardigan was not aware of, and behind these, the Russian army was lined up. The artillery pieces referred to by Lord Raglan in his order were located elsewhere. When Raglan and his staff realized what was happening from their vantagepoint on the Sapoune Heights, efforts were made to countermand the order, but it was too late.

The cavalry that reached the guns had no means of disabling them, so they regrouped in order to return to the Allied lines. On their return, Cossacks and crossfire from the Russian army harried them. Of the 673 men who took part in the cavalry charge, 113 were killed, many more were wounded, and a few were captured by the enemy; only 195 mounted officers and men survived relatively unscathed. Instead of riding to support Cardigan, seeing the outcome of the charge, Lucan withdrew the Heavy Brigade out of the range of the Russian guns. The French Chasseurs d'Afrique bravely charged the Russian positions, and relieved the pressure on Cardigan and those that remained of the Light Brigade. Raglan blamed Lucan for the debacle.[8]

A Russian force of about 40,000 men attacked the Allies' right flank early in the morning on November 5, under cover of a thick mist. The British force was taken by surprise, and only barely escaped destruction at the Battle of Inkerman. The Allies were unable to reach Sebastopol, and were forced to dig in where they stood. The British losses amounted to 2,600 killed or wounded, of whom over 1,900 had to be rescued from the battlefield by the Ambulance Corps assisted by regimental stretcher-bearers.[9]

All 12 available ambulance wagons were fully occupied the whole of that day; the task would clearly have been far easier had Hall received the 40 that had been requested earlier. A considerable number of regimental surgeons had occasion to use their swords or other weapons to defend themselves and their charges to force the enemy to retreat. The wounded tended also to be severely exhausted and, with very few exceptions, the surgery they required was carried out under chloroform anesthesia. The situation was not helped by the loss of 23 store-ships that were destroyed in a severe storm on December 22. At Sebastopol, the Russian garrison was also cut off from its supplies.

As winter set in, the gross inadequacies of the British administration became clear; the poorly-provisioned and poorly-clad British troops lacked winter clothing, transportation was almost nonexistent, they were short on fuel, and the men had only tents to protect themselves against the harshness of the conditions. Large numbers of troops went down with cholera, and many died as a consequence of the poor hygiene and grossly inadequate hospital facilities.

As a result of the daily uncensored accounts that appeared in the *Times* newspaper from as early as April 1854, the British public were soon made aware of the dreadful conditions under which their troops were suffering, and the government was eventually forced into activity. John Roebuck M.P. gave notice of a motion to set up a Committee of Enquiry into the Running of the War, which constituted a vote of no confidence in the then government of Lord

Aberdeen. Aberdeen promptly resigned, and the Queen then invited Lord Palmerston to form a new administration.

The Roebuck Committee's remit was a wide one, and in the spring of 1855, they investigated all aspects of the organization of the army in the Crimea, including the state of the medical services.[10] Other Commissions of Enquiry were also established at that time, including the Sanitary Commission,[11] Supplies Commission,[12] and Pathology Commission.[13] Sidney Herbert's resignation as Secretary-at-War was a particular loss to Dr. Andrew Smith, as he was particularly supportive and understanding of the problems encountered by the medical department. Lord Panmure succeeded him as Secretary-at-War.

Raglan had been severely criticized by the Roebuck Committee,[14] but strongly refuted their assertions. Now a field marshal, he was also severely affected by repeated bouts of dysentery, and his physique destroyed; he died on June 28, 1855, 10 days after the failure of the attack on the Redan and the Malakhoff.

STATE OF MEDICAL SERVICES FOR A CAMPAIGN IN THE EAST—PROBLEMS ENCOUNTERED BY DR. ANDREW SMITH, DIRECTOR-GENERAL OF THE ARMY MEDICAL DEPARTMENT

The director-general of the Army Medical Department at the time of the Crimean War was Dr. Andrew (later Sir Andrew) Smith (1797–1872).[15] He had entered the army as a hospital mate, in 1815, after gaining his license from the Royal College of Surgeons of Edinburgh.[16] He was stationed shortly afterward in Edinburgh, under John Hennen (1779–1828),[17] and while there he completed his medical studies and graduated with the Edinburgh M.D. degree in 1819. He was initially sent to Canada, but was then posted to South Africa. He had been retired on half-pay in July 1837, but was in constant demand as an expert on the fauna, geography, and peoples of South Africa. He returned to full-pay two months later, was then promoted to staff surgeon (first class), and shortly afterward to principal medical officer at Fort Pitt, where most of his time was spent in the selection and training of new recruits for the medical service.

In 1845, he was promoted to deputy director-general of the Army Medical Department, and on McGrigor's retirement, in 1851, Smith succeeded him as inspector-general and superintendent of the Army Medical Department. In 1853, he was appointed director-general of the Army and Ordnance Medical Departments, though he was officially styled superintendent general, with a salary of £1,200 per annum, only slightly more than half that received by his predecessor.[18] His pay was not increased until 1859, when it was increased to £1,500 per annum.

With the death of the Duke of Wellington, in 1852, representatives of all regiments in the army followed the funeral procession. Some of these were regimental surgeons, but no representative of the Army Medical Department was invited to attend, because the civil departments of the army were not officially regarded as worthy participants.[19]

On his appointment, Smith controlled 667 medical officers divided between the staff and the regimental establishments. He had absolute control over the medical staff officers, but only limited control over the medical officers of the regimental establishment as they held commissions in their respective regiments, and they were under the orders of their commanding officers. There were 185 medical staff officers and 482 regimental surgeons and assistant surgeons in the United Kingdom, the Colonies, and India. In India, there were 80 regimental medical officers and a few other medical officers, all paid for by the HEIC, and over which Smith had no authority.

Smith's first significant official task in February 1854 was organizing and revitalizing the Medical Department and equipping it for the inevitable war that was looming in the East. He had no colleagues on his staff who had had any experience of the potential problems associated with the large numbers of sick and wounded likely to be encountered in a major European-scale conflict. Literature from the Peninsular War was studied, but he found little that was either relevant or of value in the official records, and he was forced to depend entirely on his own judgment.[20] Once the orders were received, he moved rapidly, and provided the War Office with a report listing all of the stores, medicines, and equipment likely to be needed to support an army of 10,000 men on active service abroad for a period of six months. This arrangement would have been satisfactory had there not been a severe outbreak of cholera in July 1854 which continued intermittently throughout the rest of the time that the troops were in the Crimea. The force also turned out to be far greater than he had anticipated, and for much of the time, many of the men were also exhausted by severe bouts of diarrhea.

The administrative red tape Smith encountered at all levels in the War Office, although the norm for the time, greatly impeded the implementation of his plans. He was subordinate to five different departments, but on all-important matters he had to approach the military secretary to the commander-in-chief and the Secretary for War, while all matters concerning the artillery had to be referred to the master general of the ordnance. As the Medical Department was a civil department, it possessed less influence with the headquarters' staff; Smith's recommendations carried less weight and received less consideration. Only later during the war was he able to deal directly with the Secretary for War.

One of Smith's greatest causes for concern was the lack of suitable arrangements for rescuing and transporting the wounded from the battlefield, and transporting the sick to appropriate hospital accommodation. The most seriously wounded casualties and men that were only fit enough to be invalided out of the service were repatriated to Britain. Despite repeated pleas for mobile ambulances with a backup force of an appropriately trained ambulance corps, along the lines pioneered by Larrey and employed by the French during the Peninsular War,[21] neither the equipment nor the trained staff were either available or immediately forthcoming.

In mid-February 1854, the military secretary to the commander-in-chief asked Smith about his proposed arrangements for the transportation of the sick and wounded. This had not been seen as a priority over the years when the funding available from government had been so limited. Instructions for the building of appropriate two-wheeled wagons, clearly based on Larrey's earlier successful model, and a larger, but inevitably less manageable, four-wheeled model, were submitted to the War Office in March 1854. These reached the Crimea in relatively small numbers, and rather late in the campaign. The mobile ambulance units were a failure, principally because the War Office had insisted that the lightweight wheels stipulated by Smith be replaced by the far heavier artillery wheels. This made the wagons unstable, and due to their increased weight they tended to get bogged down in the wet and muddy terrain. Because of the bad roads, they caused great discomfort, and many of the wounded men were reticent to be transported in them and preferred to walk. Even when the relatively few ambulances did arrive, their drivers were unsuitable for the task at hand, principally because of their age, infirmity, and, frequently, incompetence.

Because whatever wagons that were available were not under the control of the Army Medical Department, complaints had been received by Smith "that transport for general officers' baggage had invariably been provided before that for the sick. . . . The commanding officer of the regiment must not on any account have anything whatever to do with the same, the whole being in charge of the surgeon, who would be responsible to the divisional medical officer."[22]

Another problem that was encountered was that the local horses were too small for the task at hand; the wagons that should have been drawn by four horses with two drivers required six of the small Bulgarian horses to pull them. More drivers were required than were available, and hospital orderlies had to be removed from their other duties to undertake a task for which they were patently unqualified. The harnesses supplied would not fit, and no specialist staff was available to maintain the wagons or look after the horses.

In April 1854, Smith had formally requested from the War Office the establishment of a hospital corps, with 600 appropriately trained drivers, stretcher-bearers, and hospital orderlies. Only 370 volunteers were recruited from the pensioners who were recalled to the colors. The orderlies contained 10 sergeants and 250 privates, while an additional 10 sergeants supervized the 100 privates who were engaged as ambulance wagon drivers. Smith's suggestion that a further 800 able-bodied men (Armenians) might be recruited locally in Turkey was not acceptable to the general staff, and this force, which was to be termed the Armenian Bearer Corps, failed to materialize. The small ambulance corps that was organized by the War Office arrived in the Crimea in July 1854. While the drivers tended to be of good character, many of the hospital orderlies quickly succumbed to the effects of cholera or drink, and Smith's attempt to produce an efficient ambulance corps ended as a miserable failure. Another request, in October 1854, to raise a hospital corps of 400 volunteers from the depots of the regiments serving in India also failed to materialize.[23]

STAFFING WITHIN THE MEDICAL DEPARTMENT

Because of the great reduction in the medical service over the previous 30–40 years, all of the medical officers with firsthand experience of the conditions in the Peninsular War were too old to be of any assistance. Those with some regimental experience from the intervening colonial wars had no experience that was relevant to the special problems likely to be encountered in the present conflict. Many other medical officers were on half-pay, but few were keen to rejoin the service on a full-time basis.

A total of 174 medical staff were eventually appointed, spanning all ranks, allocating one doctor to every 144 men, sufficient, at least in theory, for a force of about 25,000 men. It soon became apparent that as the force rapidly increased, the medical backup, even allowing for the reengagement of most of the surgeons on half-pay, was going to be grossly inadequate to cope with the medical needs of the British force assembling in the Crimea.

Smith immediately sent out to the Crimea three of his senior staff to investigate firsthand the climatic conditions and features of the terrain, and he received comprehensive reports back from them toward the end of April. Because large areas were subject to considerable climatic variation, it was suggested that changes of uniform suitable for fighting in either hot or cold climates should be provided, rather than a single uniform that was probably inappropriate for all conditions that the troops were likely to encounter. The War Office argued that it was not practicable for the men to carry nonessential items of kit.[24] While the recommendations regarding the adaptation of uniform to suit the local climatic conditions seemed entirely sensible to Smith, this was not viewed to be the case by the War Office, and the suggestions in this regard were generally viewed as impracticable. Most of the senior military staff in the Crimea were extremely conservative and loath to change any traditional item of uniform or equipment, whatever the climate that the troops might encounter. With the arrival of the first signs of winter, the inflexibility of the high command in this regard was seen to be nothing short of stupidity.

The substantial risk of malaria was also appreciated, and the recommendation made that large amounts of quinine be available to cope with this eventuality. During the three months that the army spent in Bulgaria, over one seventh of the force was debilitated by fever, and an additional 20% suffered from diarrhea, though dysentery was less common. Quinine was liberally used to treat a wide range of conditions, and not surprisingly was found to be not particularly useful. The risk of dysentery was also appreciated. While little could be done to treat this condition, it was hoped that the maintenance of the highest standards of hygiene in the camps, associated with the filtration of all water supplies, might reduce these potential health problems to manageable proportions.

The *Lancet*'s special correspondent in the Crimea drew their readers' attention to the recent order from the War Office in London for "Wearing the moustache."[25] The moustache at that time was thought to be of value in malarial country. Deaths from cholera were also said to be causing havoc in the French camp, and the *Lancet*'s special correspondent also reported some British deaths from this condition.

With regard to the transport of the wounded from the base hospitals to intermediate staging posts in the Mediterranean, or directly back to Britain, Smith envisaged an arrangement whereby ships carrying stores and other essential items to the Crimea would act as hospital transports. As these ships were ill-equipped to act as transports, this led to a great deal of unnecessary suffering on the part of the wounded, and the situation was undoubtedly worsened by the lack of coordination between the army and the navy. Spacious steamers, high between decks, with ample means of ventilation and fitted with fixed berths, were not forthcoming, and the sick and wounded men that were transported to Scutari and elsewhere suffered accordingly.

Numerous items were published in the influential medical press, particularly during the period leading up to the war, emphasizing the lack of preparedness of the military medical services. Guthrie,[26] in particular, stressed the shortage of experienced medical officers at Waterloo and during the more recent Indian campaigns and the urgent need for well-equipped mobile ambulances.

COMPETENCE OF THE MEDICAL OFFICERS TO DEAL WITH THE MEDICAL AND SURGICAL SITUATIONS THEY WOULD ENCOUNTER IN THE CRIMEA

None of the medical officers who were recruited by Smith to serve in the Crimea, either from those on full-pay or those on half-pay but who were willing to return to the service, had experience of a European-style war. A considerable number had spent many years in India, or in other similar foreign stations, where their principal concern was the management of tropical diseases. During the various outbreaks of cholera in Britain during the 1830s and later, doctors with military experience were often called upon to advise the civilian medical authorities on the containment of the disease and on other urgent public health measures. Relatively few had any experience of military surgery, as major casualties were only rarely encountered during the colonial wars.[27]

Smith and his senior colleagues gave advice to those who were about to embark for the East concerning the range of medical problems that they were likely to encounter. Little of value regarding the management of surgical emergencies was provided beyond the recommendation that they should rely on the advice that they would find in Guthrie's *Commentaries on Surgery*.[28] The extract from Guthrie's *Pamphlet on the Hospital Brigade* published in the *Lancet*[29] indicated that this volume was provided gratis as a standard item of kit for medical officers in the field. The extract states that "A copy of the *Commentaries* is placed in box No. 7, in Store-wagons A, B, C." Even though the fifth edition of this classic text had only very recently been published, in 1853, few advances in surgical treatment had occurred since the days of the Peninsular War.

The uncertainty that existed in the diagnosis of the various fevers encountered in clinical practice lasted until well after the Crimean War, and applied equally to the wide range of intestinal disorders in most of which diarrhea was a principal feature. In any case, very few specific forms of treatment were available at that time, though improvements in public hygiene undoubtedly assisted in the prevention of the spread of epidemics.

The single greatest advance in the management of surgical cases was the introduction of general anesthesia, ether in 1846, and chloroform in 1847. While such agents rapidly became popular in civilian clinical practice, they were either ignored completely or only very occasionally used by a few military mavericks before the onset of the Crimean War. Guthrie, for example, only barely mentions the use of these agents even in the fifth edition of his *Commentaries on Surgery*,[30] although the value of chloroform is discussed in considerable detail in the sixth edition of this book.[31] In Ballingall's section on Amputation in the 4th edition of his *Outlines of Military Surgery*, no mention is made of the value of general anesthetics in undertaking these capital operations, and chloroform receives only a single mention in relation to the detection of fictitious illnesses.[32] This would seem, on reflection, to be a curious omission, particularly since Robert Liston's successful amputation at the thigh performed at University College Hospital, London, in December 1846 under ether anesthesia had been widely reported in both the medical and lay press.[33]

As an indication of the wide usage of general anesthesia in civilian practice, in the volume of the *Lancet* covering the first half of 1847, there are no less than 32 reports of various types of amputations carried out under ether anesthesia (arm [1]; ankle joint [1]; finger [5]; fore-arm [1]; hand [1]; leg [9]; at inferior third [1]; through the hip-joint [11]; toe [1]). Liston was in a particularly good position to appreciate its value, having previously published extensively on amputation. His *Observations on Amputation*, for example, appeared in the *Edinburgh Medical and Surgical Journal*.[34] This article complements the two previous items by Syme,[35] the first of which describes a successful amputation through the hip joint carried out without the benefit of an anesthetic.

While chloroform had been introduced in 1847[36] and was quickly shown to be both safe for the patient and easy for the surgeon to administer, it is very difficult to understand why its obvious advantages in the field of military surgery could fail to be appreciated by more than a few isolated individuals. Inspector-general Hall, who had previously been PMO, Bombay Presidency, sent a memorandum to his medical officers with a copy to the director-general. Hall cautioned officers against using chloroform in patients with severe shock from gunshot wounds, as he was of the view that few of such cases would survive its use. The advice Hall offered to the men fairly closely followed that of Guthrie, published in his *Pamphlet on the Hospital Brigade*, an extract of which was published in the *Lancet* during the early part of the war.[37] This component of Hall's directive caused much hostility among the younger medical officers, though most ignored him, and chloroform was used extensively throughout the campaign.

Guthrie was considerably more expansive regarding the value of chloroform in 1855.[38] He also provided detailed advice as to how this agent should be administered. He recommended, "in cases of approaching death from the use of chloroform, that the tongue should be drawn forwards by means of a pair of artery forceps, by which it is presumed the epiglottis is raised, and a greater facility afforded for the admission of atmospheric air; the inconvenience resulting from two small holes in the tip of the tongue being amply compensated by the preservation of life."

In the 6th edition of his *Commentaries on Surgery*,[39] Guthrie was able to discuss the use of chloroform in considerable detail, as he had been provided with up-to-date information by a number of senior military surgeons on its extensive use in the Crimea.

"During the whole of the campaign . . . both after the battles of the Alma and Inkermann, as well as throughout the whole siege operations before Sebastopol . . . no operations whatever of any consequence . . . have been performed in the Light Division, without first placing under the influence of chloroform, and in no single instance have either the medical officers of the division or myself seen any bad results follow, or had to reject its use, but quite the contrary . . ."[40]

In 1848, Wakley,[41] editor of the *Lancet*, had published the results of his extensive experimental findings in which he had compared ether with chloroform. A wide variety of animals and birds had been anesthetized to compare the safety of these two agents, and to determine the dosage of each agent required to achieve safe anesthesia.

Because war was viewed as a great adventure, many recently qualified doctors volunteered for service in the Army Medical Department to see service in the East. Only those from the Universities of Edinburgh and Dublin who had attended the lecture courses on military medicine and surgery of Ballingall and Tufnell, respectively, had any knowledge, albeit of an entirely theoretical nature, of what they were likely to encounter before they accepted their commission. Some, at least, who had enlisted before the outbreak of war had the opportunity to spend a period of up to nine months at Fort Pitt, while others who enlisted only shortly before their embarkation had little or no time for such luxuries.

Because of the considerable shortage of the more senior members of the medical profession in the Crimea, there was an urgent need for experienced civilian volunteers, both physicians and surgeons, to support their military colleagues in the running of the base hospitals. Even at some distance from the front lines, these individuals were often at considerable risk due to exposure to the frequent outbreaks of life-threatening contagious diseases, and many were permanently incapacitated or died as a consequence.

PROBLEMS ENCOUNTERED BY THE MEDICAL STAFF IN THE CRIMEA

Reports from medical staff at Gallipoli, later at Scutari, and subsequently at Varna and elsewhere, soon indicated that all was not well. While supplies and other necessities may have been dispatched from Britain, many items seemed not to reach their appropriate destination. The first hospital supplies did not arrive in the East until May 8, and between then and May 27, three ships arrived with medical supplies, including beds, medications, and dressings. Only later did another ship arrive with the regimental panniers, cases of surgical instruments, and splints, as well as more bandages and lint, and the lack of tents led to severe overcrowding. Inflexibility regarding uniforms also caused problems because of the extremes of temperature to which the men were exposed, even in the months of May and June. By July, the incidence of fevers rose dramatically, and the beds in the base hospitals began to fill.

Smith was also encountering difficulties with regard to his senior staff. The first to resign was William Burrell, who had only shortly before been promoted to deputy inspector-general on his elevation to the post of Smith's PMO. Burrell had until then been serving in a similar capacity in Malta. As the size of the expeditionary force rapidly trebled in size, Smith thought it wise to appoint a more experienced medical officer. He recalled inspector-general John Hall, who at that time was serving in Bombay, to take charge of all of the medical services in Turkey. Believing that he had been passed over, Burrell resigned on June 17.

One of the problems encountered by the medical officers in the Crimea was that, as a consequence of their belonging to a civil rather than a combatant department of the army, they were not entitled to a soldier servant. Consequently, medical officers not only had to draw their own rations and cook their own food, but also had to attend to the needs of their horses. In addition, their rate of pay was low; on joining as an assistant surgeon they were entitled to 7s6d per day, and this was raised to only 10s6d per day in February 1855 when the number of those volunteering for active service fell to unacceptably low levels. Equally, pensions paid to doctors' widows were less than that paid to the widows of combatant officers of equivalent rank.

Hall's first task was to complete the planning of the base hospitals at Scutari. It had been estimated that there would be a requirement for bed occupancy of about 5,000, based on a sick-rate of about 20%. This figure was not acceptable to those in the War Office in London, and a maximum of 2,800 beds was eventually conceded. This total did not include the beds in the regimental hospitals, from where the most serious cases would need to be transferred to the base hospitals to receive more specialized treatment.

The overall direction of these hospitals was to be under Dr. Menzies, and he found that almost all of his ward staff were ignorant of all of the basic principles of nursing care. Difficulties were particularly encountered with the recruiting of ancillary staff, at all levels from ward-masters, ward orderlies, stewards, storekeepers, and cooks. These were all obtained from regimental details left behind at Scutari, and with few exceptions were those who had been discarded from their regiments due to their bad character. Those who became orderlies were often the dregs of the army, and dishonesty was rife among them. Miss Terrot, one of the Anglican nurses, stated that "one patient took 2s6d out of his purse to reward an orderly for his services. The orderly, seeing gold in the purse, killed him with one blow on the head. He was seized, tried and hung."[42]

THE BASE HOSPITALS

The largest of the military hospitals was sited at Scutari, at the southern end of the Bosporus. The General Hospital was established in the Turkish military hospital. This was a fine two-story building, three sides of which were composed of wards. The fourth side housed the officers' quarters, operation room, dispensary, and various stores and offices. The wards were large and well ventilated, and could accommodate about 25 patients in the larger rooms and 10–12 in the smaller rooms. With full occupancy of the wards and corridors, the hospital could accommodate 1,086 patients. The wards were heated by stoves in the winter, but the latrines were primitive and drained directly into open cesspits without water seals, so that the odor from them pervaded the wards. The air in the wards was also contaminated by the odors from the local burial ground located close to the southern boundary of the hospital. As many of the dead were only partially buried, and none in coffins, the smell of decomposing bodies was extremely offensive and the ward atmosphere consequently particularly oppressive and not conducive to the well-being of the patients.

The Barrack Hospital was located about three-quarters of a mile from the General Hospital in the Sultan Selive Barracks, and was about 200 yards from the sea. It was a large rectangular building built around a central courtyard that was used as a parade ground. It was not ready for occupancy until September. When fully repaired and appropriately refurbished, it could accommodate about 1,065 patients, 616 in the wards and a further 419 in the corridors. After the Battle of Inkerman, this hospital was full to overflowing, with 1,958 patients, and as a consequence the backup facilities were fully stretched. In addition, over 1,200 men were accommodated in the convalescent hulks. A steamer had to be dispatched from Varna with bedding and stores, and over a thousand palliasses were additionally requested from the stores in the *John Masterman*. These items arrived some three months after they had been requested, and were not landed until early December.

As the Barrack Hospital was intended only to receive the sick, it had no operating room. All essential operations had to be performed in the wards in full view of the other patients. Screens were provided only after the arrival of Miss Nightingale. Because of the overcrowding, outbreaks of hospital gangrene occurred, were highly contagious, and rapidly spread to the other patients.

Only three sites were available in the whole hospital from which water could be drawn, and the state of the sanitation was similar to that in the General Hospital. Because of the nature of the installations, it was never possible to improve the basic sanitary arrangements. For much of the time, it served as both a hospital and a barracks, as a garrison for the reinforcements. Soldiers' wives, whose husbands had been sent to the front, lived in some of the rooms, and it was difficult to keep them and the soldiers from the barracks out of the wards. The single canteen in the hospital was frequently full of drunken soldiers. The total number of medical staff in the Barrack Hospital was considerable, 74 in all, including eight 1st class staff surgeons, and about 20 clinical medical students or "dressers" who assisted the nurses in the wards. The staff was also supplemented with a considerable number of dispensers.

Toward the end of January 1855, there were over 4,500 sick men hospitalized at Scutari, and over 1,000 waiting to disembark from the transports. Of nearly 1,400 admitted with dysentery, the mortality rate was over 60%, and with the high mortality among the fever cases, the losses during this period amounted to about 45 men per day.[43]

As it was generally believed that many of these deaths could be ascribed to the polluted atmosphere in the hospitals at Scutari, arrangements were made to establish hospitals elsewhere, for example, on one of the Aegean islands. It was also mooted that some of the men should be repatriated home. This second proposal was the less favored, because those that recovered their health would have to be returned to the Crimea. Nevertheless, many of the invalids were returned to Plymouth, where they were accommodated in a number of army and naval hospitals. Generous offers of help from a number of civilian hospitals were declined because of possible administrative difficulties. The ragged appearance of the men created a sensation, and the War Office promptly sent out large amounts of clothing and equipment to Scutari, making up for earlier deficiencies for which the Army Medical Department had previously been blamed.

One of the principal concerns raised by the local medical officers, and noted by all of the visitors, was the significant difference between the fabric of the French hospitals and those available to the British. The French had arrived at Scutari first, and took the opportunity of selecting the most suitable buildings, particularly those in the best state of repair. Many of those that remained had previously been used as barracks for the Turkish soldiers. They were generally in a poor state of repair, full of rotten timber, verminous, and in most respects almost impossible to convert into hygienic premises that would be suitable for the recuperation of the sick and wounded. The French hospitals also gave the impression of being better organized than their British counterparts.

The situation regarding stores for the hospitals was extremely difficult, and dealt with by the Purveyor's Department. They were theoretically under the control of the director-general, except that he was only rarely informed of their activities. Bedding and other essential items that had been dispatched during September were delivered three months later to the hospitals at Scutari. Some were unloaded at Varna or Balaklava, and only months later located and returned to Scutari. Conditions in the General Hospital were generally satisfactory, but those in the Barrack Hospital were often extremely poor, principally because of the impossibility of converting the barracks into a satisfactory hospital. Due to gross deficiencies in the cooking facilities, most patients were fortunate if they received one hot meal a day.

NEWSPAPER COVERAGE OF THE CRIMEAN WAR

One of the principal consequences of the daily feedback of information to the British public concerning the dreadful conditions in the Crimea was that there was constant agitation that the conditions in the hospitals in the Crimea were far inferior to those in supposedly comparable civilian hospitals in Britain. Staffing levels in the Crimea were far lower, the number of patients with fevers mostly of unidentifiable origin was far higher, and the general standard of hygiene and cleanliness far poorer, for reasons that were beyond the power of those in the hospitals.

The poor conditions in the front lines were also highlighted in the newspapers in the usually accurate articles from the front that were sent home by their various war correspondents, and in the generally anonymous letters from doctors at the front that were regularly published in the medical press. The deficiencies were so glaring that they could not be hidden. In the end, the government was forced to act. While many of these non-medically-qualified individuals were genuine in their concern to improve the conditions of the men, others were simply troublemakers. The press was also keen to report the problems encountered with attaining adequate levels of medical staffing in all areas, with particular concern being expressed regarding what was perceived to be the poor provision of experienced surgeons near to the front lines.

Russell, the *Times* correspondent, for example, wrote numerous extravagant, and often incorrect, accounts in which the suffering of the men was detailed. It was often claimed that there were insufficient medical staff, dressers, and ward orderlies, and inadequate equipment available to allow the simplest of operations to be performed. Consequently, the men were dying because no staff were available to attend to their wounds. These reports were largely untrue. In the hospitals there were adequate medical staff and supplies for all that needed to be attended. In the field, the situation was often quite different, and the press coverage was usually fairly accurate, due to the deficiencies of ambulance wagons, and the fact that the panniers that were carried by the horses had only a limited capacity.[44] While the War Office or the high commands of the army or navy were usually responsible for these deficiencies, the newspapers held the Army Medical Department responsible, naming the director-general as the principal culprit. Smith was quite unprepared for these attacks, as Hall had passed across little information to him regarding the difficulties he was encountering in the Crimea.

PROBLEMS WITH THE TRANSPORT OF THE SICK AND WOUNDED TO THE BASE HOSPITALS AT SCUTARI

Problems were encountered with the transports for the sick and wounded from Balaklava to Scutari, a distance of about 300 miles. While such a journey, usually undertaken by steamship, could take as little as two days, it often took considerably longer, principally due to poor weather conditions. Many of the vessels were requisitioned and were often in a poor state of repair, were poorly ventilated, and had no fixed berths, so in some cases this journey could take up to six days. In most cases, little attempt had been made to accommodate the basic needs of those who needed to be transported to one or other of the base hospitals at Scutari. Hospital ships were available elsewhere, and there is some discussion as to whether these were indeed requisitioned.

Smith, when interviewed by the Roebuck Committee, claimed that he had requested hospital ships in May 1854, but the Admiralty denied this. According to their spokesman, "had a requisition been made I certainly should have taken steps to have had hospital ships fitted up. . . . I must acknowledge that I thought it odd that a requisition was not made. . . . I think that those hospital ships ought to have been fitted up at an earlier date."[45] It is generally believed that the requisition was indeed sent by Smith, but was rejected in either the office of the military secretary, or that of the commander-in-chief, or possibly by the Secretary for War.

In June 1854, Hall had proposed that a ship be made available as a floating hospital. Eventually, the principal naval officer at Constantinople was given permission by the Admiralty to use an old Turkish man-of-war for this purpose. This was to accommodate convalescent patients, and was staffed by two medical officers and a few orderlies. The transports that were used did not in any way resemble the ships that were specially converted for this task.

The medical staffing on these transports tended to be limited, and only the vessels with large complements of sick and wounded had two, or occasionally more, often very junior medical officers on board. It was not uncommon for urgent surgical problems to arise, and only rarely were competent surgical staff available to deal with them. While there was meant to be a ratio of one doctor for each hundred sick or wounded on board, it was only in exceptional cases that this ratio was achieved.

Difficulties were particularly encountered in September, when total admissions to all hospitals in the East amounted to 5,334 men, and exceeded 22% of strength. This included 1,232 admissions and 575 deaths from cholera alone. Almost 1,000 fever cases required admission. To prevent overcrowding in the regimental hospitals in Balaklava, many of the sick were evacuated to Scutari, including many of the cholera cases that were least able to withstand the journey. During the month of October, there was no overcrowding at Scutari, although there was a great shortage of medical stores. Only from December 1854 were medical orderlies assigned to the transports. These individuals were often of poor ability. Each transport was meant to have a complement of twelve medical orderlies to care for the needs of the sick and wounded.

The sick and wounded often had to wait for long periods at the harbor at Balaklava, usually in unsheltered conditions, before they could be transferred to the ships for the journey to Scutari. In the winter months, the inclement weather had a dramatic impact on the mortality rates. Almost all of the men who survived the journey were in a far worse state of health when they arrived there compared to their state of health when they left the harbor at Balaklava. The overall death rate on board these vessels during the three-month period between October and December 1854 was in the region of 7%, with 549 deaths out of a total of 7,682 patients transported to Scutari. In the previous month, the rate was nearer to 11%, due to the additional deaths from cholera.[46]

As there was no harbor close to the base hospitals at Scutari, all of those transported had to be transferred to small boats when they reached their destination, and then ferried ashore. Often the small boats were unavailable for this purpose. There were often insufficient beds available to accommodate the incoming casualties; the less serious cases in the base hospitals had to be moved to the various convalescent homes in order to make room for the more serious cases on board ship. It was often necessary for the men to be kept on board ship for several additional days before the congestion in the hospitals was alleviated. In bad weather, the swell was such that the small boats could not be used because of the risk of them capsizing, and then the men had to be landed elsewhere, at an even greater distance from the hospitals. If the weather was particularly poor, then the roads from these ports were almost impassable to the few wagons that could be requisitioned to undertake this task.

Although large volumes of vital stores and bedding were sent from Britain, much either was lost in transit or arrived at the wrong location and was not distributed to where it was urgently required. Numerous complaints along these lines reached the commander-in-chief. Apart from setting up the occasional inquiry, or requesting in the strongest of terms the dismissal of the individual blamed for the incident, whether wrongly or rightly, there is little evidence that the commander-in-chief investigated any of these cases in any depth. Most of the difficulties encountered seemed to arise from problems that the individual medical officers on the spot were powerless to remedy.

While Raglan was apparently happy to blame all the problems encountered both in the hospitals and on the transports on the medical officers, many of his attacks were seen to be unjustified. Raglan was also criticized for his persistent failure to acknowledge the dedication of the vast majority of the medical staff who got on with their duties as best as they were able.

FLORENCE NIGHTINGALE AND HER NURSES

Florence Nightingale, born in 1820 into a respectable middle-class background, at an early age determined to devote her life to the care of the sick. After considerable opposition from her parents, she gained nursing experience in the Institution of Deaconesses at Kaiserwerth, an organization established by a Protestant pastor, Theodore Fliedner, and located in a small town on the Rhine in Germany. This was a recognized school for training nurses, and in all Miss Nightingale spent three months there. While she gained relatively little practical experience, her stay at Kaiserwerth convinced her that nursing was to be her vocation. She made up for any deficiencies in her knowledge by avidly reading as much as she could locate on the topic.

After reading an item in the *Times* newspaper from their correspondent in the Crimea, in October 1854, suggesting the need for British nurses in the base hospitals at Scutari, Miss Nightingale investigated the matter further. She contacted senior members of the government, and gained the approval of Lords Palmerston and Clarendon. She then contacted and gained the approval of Dr. Andrew Smith, as well as the enthusiastic support of Mr. Sidney Herbert, Secretary-at-War, with whom she was to frequently correspond when she was in the Crimea. She was invited to organize and superintend the nursing staff at Scutari. She was to be designated the "superintendent of the female nursing establishment of the military hospitals in Turkey," and was also to be directly responsible locally to the chief medical officer at Scutari.

The possibility of employing female nursing staff had been considered before the outbreak of the Crimean War, but had been rejected by the military authorities because previous experience had been unfavorable. These nurses had often been addicted to drink, and were often less sympathetic to the suffering of the men than were male ward orderlies. However, due to the constant complaints of the visitors from Britain, and items in the press, the decision was reconsidered and, largely on the advice of Herbert, eventually reversed.

The nursing posts were advertized, and a total of 38 were eventually selected to join Miss Nightingale.[47] While a few had a similar social background to herself, the majority were of much humbler origin, were middle-aged, and had little nursing experience. The professional nurses were particularly difficult to recruit, and it was suggested at the time that those who applied were more interested in the salary offered than in the opportunity to nurse the sick troops in the Crimea. Twenty-four had been recruited from various religious orders; 10 were Sisters from Catholic orders, and 14 were Anglican Sisters. Miss Nightingale and the first party arrived at Scutari at the end of October, and were accommodated in one of the towers in the Barrack Hospital. Out of the 38 nurses, Miss Nightingale considered that only 16 of them could be considered as in any way efficient. While some of the professional nurses were often both drunk and promiscuous, they were at least happy to look after the physical needs of the patients; those from religious orders were often more interested in their souls than their bodies.[48]

Within a few months the conditions in the hospitals gradually improved, as did the diet of the patients. After dressing the wounds and nursing and feeding the most seriously ill patients (see Figure 4.2), Miss Nightingale then turned her attention to the cleaning of the wards. She purchased scrubbing brushes and sacking for this work, and succeeded in shaming the orderlies into undertaking this task. She next investigated the cooking arrangements, and began to provide special diets for those most in need of them, and these were thereafter provided on a regular basis. Attention was then paid to the laundering of the patients' shirts and other washing, and after the necessary equipment was hired, this activity was also running efficiently within a couple of weeks. While there was a contract for the washing of the bedding and general clothing, the men would not allow their shirts to be washed, as they were afraid that these items would not be returned to them. When Miss Nightingale obtained the services of some of the soldiers' wives, this fear was allayed, and over 600 shirts were washed and returned to their owners within a fortnight.[49]

The conditions and atmosphere in the General Hospital were always superior to those in the Barrack Hospital, and this undoubtedly greatly increased the chances of the men's recovery and return to their regiments (see Figure 4.3). Shortly after his arrival at the Barrack Hospital, the Rev. Mr. Osborne was distressed to see the conditions there, and reported his reservations in this regard to the Roebuck Committee. His visit to the hospital had coincided with the arrival of a transport with about 500 casualties from the Battle of Inkerman. With less than 30 minutes' warning of the landing of these wounded men, it is not altogether surprising that the scene appeared, at least superficially, to be a little disorganized. Within about eight hours, all of the men were cleaned, and fed, and their wounds attended to, and all were put to bed on clean mattresses. Osborne vastly exaggerated what deficiencies there were. He also refused to withdraw his allegations, despite the fact that the purveyor and all of the medical

Figure 4.2. Miss Nightingale and the Nurses in the East

Showing a medical officer taking the pulse of a patient.

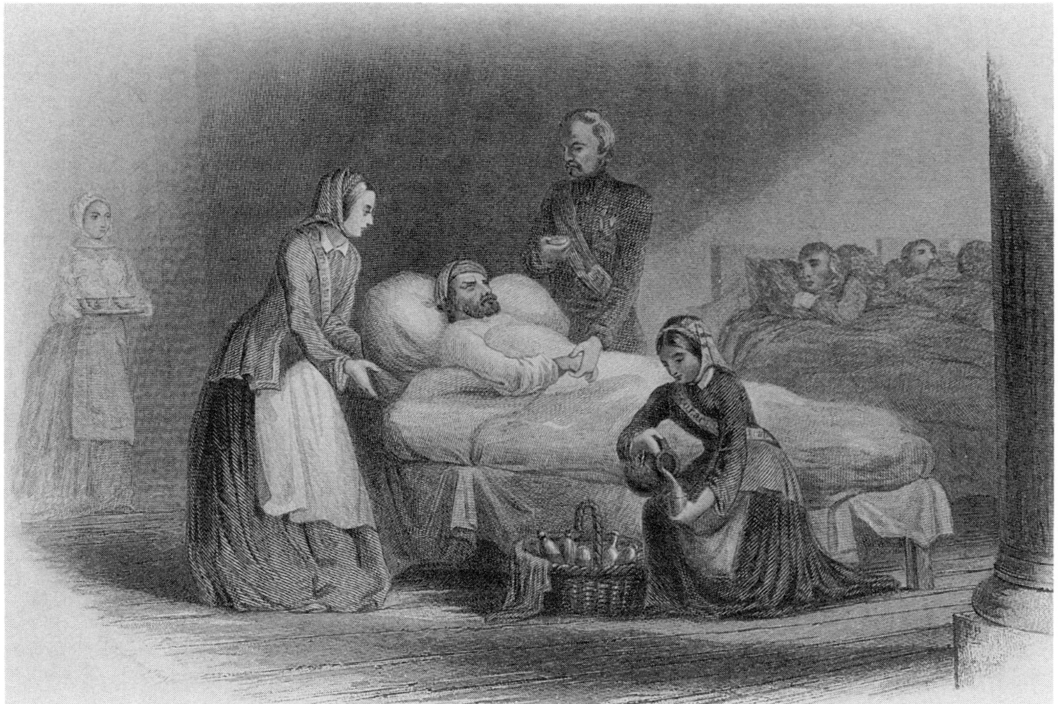

From: E.H. Nolan, 1855-57. *The Illustrated History of the War against Russia*. 2 Volumes (London: James S. Virtue) [Volume 1, 1855; Volume 2, 1857] [Volume 1, Figure opposite p. 706, engraving by Charles Armytage].

Figure 4.3. One of the Wards at the Hospital at Scutari

Said to be a ward in the Barrack Hospital a week after the battle of Inkerman. The artist has included Miss Nightingale in discussion with a medical officer. Sick and sleeping patients are shown in their beds, while convalescent patients are shown sitting near to the wood-burning stove at the centre of the ward. Note the absence of privacy for the patients.

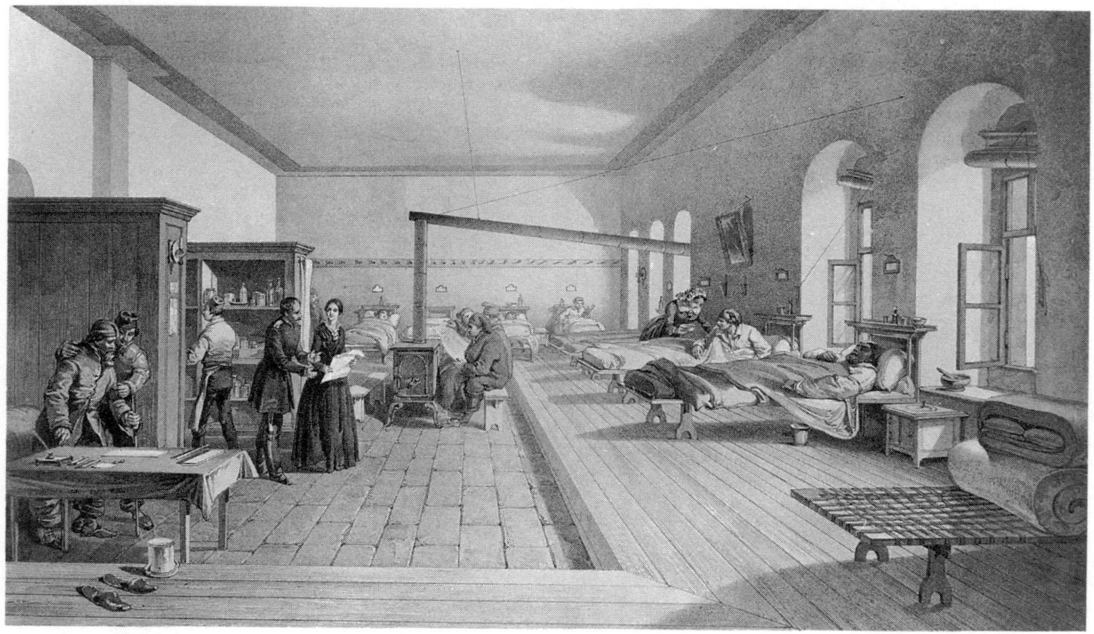

From: W. Simpson, 1855, 1856. *The Seat of War in the East*. In 2 Volumes (London: Paul and Dominic Colnaghi & Co.) [Volume 1, 1855, Plates 1–40; Volume 2, 1856, Plates 1–41 [Volume 1, Plate 34; W. Simpson del., E. Walker, lith.].

and nursing staff emphasized that all necessary items of equipment, dressings, and medicines were available.

Purchasing essential items from the chemists in Constantinople made up all shortfalls during the period between September and January following the loss of the *Prince* with its considerable supplies of stores. Other complaints about the Barrack Hospital—its lack of an operating table and lack of privacy on the wards—while fully justified, were tolerated by both the doctors and the patients. Osborne also contended that some of the men had died from lack of food, but this was strongly refuted by Miss Nightingale and the medical staff.[50]

Because so many of the admissions in November were for diarrhea and other bowel conditions, the drugs used for their alleviation ran into short supply, and additional supplies were ordered by Miss Nightingale and paid for by Mr. MacDonald, the representative from the *Times* fund. While Miss Nightingale worked closely with the local medical staff, if difficulties arose she wrote directly to Herbert in London, and his approval was always forthcoming. It was suggested that a second group of nurses should be sent out to join the first party. While the idea had the approval of Herbert, Miss Nightingale had not been consulted, and was particularly distressed when she heard that the group of 47 nurses were already on their way. She was annoyed to find that she was expected not only to organize their accommodation, but also to administer their activities and maintain discipline.

The second party of nurses reached Scutari on December 17. It contained Catholic Sisters, Irish nurses under the authority of their Mother Superior, and a mixed collection of trained and untrained nurses. Some were sent to the naval hospital at Therapia, others later went to Kuleli (Koulali or Kulalee) Hospital that had only opened in January 1855, and the number based at Scutari was increased to fifty. Despite reservations from many of the doctors and the inevitable tensions between the different religious groups, the presence of Nightingale's nurses appeared to be working well. A considerable number of the medical staff, however, expressed the view that the duties performed by the nurses could, and more appropriately should, have been performed by well-disciplined male hospital orderlies. Unfortunately many of the latter found it difficult or even impossible to obey orders, were often drunk on duty, were a hindrance to good military discipline, and in some cases were a liability to the welfare of the patients.

Miss Nightingale observed numerous examples of military incompetence where, for example, adequate stores in the form of clothing and food, including lime-juice, had been sent out from Britain and were disembarked, but were retained in warehouses in Balaklava and not distributed to the troops. Fresh vegetables arrived from Varna, but were thrown overboard because no individual from the commissariat was prepared to accept responsibility for the consignment because of inadequate paperwork at the port of embarkation. Enormous amounts of hospital stores and medical comforts were lost in transit, such as blankets, port, and brandy. Some materials that should have been landed at Varna were unloaded at Gallipoli or Constantinople. These, and numerous other examples, were cited in her extremely critical *Evidence Given to the Royal*

Commissioners on the State of the Army in 1857, which was published a few years after the end of the war.[51]

What greatly assisted Miss Nightingale was that she had at her disposal large sums of money that had been subscribed by private individuals. If she was unable to obtain items through the normal channels, she had no qualms about purchasing them from either the bazaars at Constantinople or wherever else they could be found. The War Office had also authorized that they would cover the cost of her nurses' salaries and lodging expenses. Her freedom to act independently was also enhanced with the arrival of Mr. MacDonald of the *Times* fund, who also had access to large sums of money, to be used by him to improve the general living conditions of the men. By early February 1855, most of the supplies and equipment had arrived in the Crimea, and it was no longer necessary for these deficiencies to be made up from either Miss Nightingale's or Mr. MacDonald's private resources.

THE CONDITIONS IN WHICH THE MEN LIVED DURING THE FIRST WINTER (1854–1855)

The conditions in the trenches in the Crimea during the first winter were very similar to those in the First World War, though with fewer of the creature comforts that eventually became a feature of the trenches during the 1914–1918 War. Sentry duty occupied up to two nights out of three, and when completed, the soldiers returned to their quarters to prepare their food and then retired to their canvas tents, with no opportunity for either a change of clothing or relief from the cold.

Of those admitted to the regimental hospitals, about 12% died there, and about one-third needed to be transferred to the base hospitals at Scutari. In many of the regiments, during the first winter, between half and two-thirds of their strength were hospitalized at any one time; in some regiments, less than a quarter were fit for military duty. In other regiments, 40–60% of those admitted to the hospital died, and this was largely attributable to the poor physical condition of the new recruits sent out from Britain to make up the numbers of those hospitalized due to sickness. The high losses could probably be accounted for by the absence of spare clean and dry clothing, the poor diet of the men, inadequate cooking facilities, and lack of waterproof accommodation. The lack of weatherproof footwear was also a major problem, although a few managed to obtain these items from plundering the bodies of dead Russians. The officers, who were able to obtain fresh meat and vegetables from the flourishing black market at Balaklava, did not encounter these problems. They also had servants to attend to their needs, and fuel and utensils with which to cook their food.

The fact that the men's diet tended to be deficient in fresh vegetables inevitably led to a high incidence of overt or subclinical scurvy among the troops. In the few regiments where supplies of fresh vegetables or lime- or fruit juice were obtained, the level of ill health among the men tended to be considerably lower than the average. Vegetables were never a popular item in the men's diet, and were not issued as part of the men's rations;[52] if the men had meat and bread, they were content.

In mid-December 1854, with the publication of a general routine order from the commander-in-chief, the troops were no longer required to pay for their own vegetables. This effectively stopped the then-prevalent practice of the men spending their money on drink rather than on vegetables. Regular messing was also introduced following a general order of December 20, and was associated with the arrival of adequate stocks of canteens for cooking the men's meals. As a result of these two measures, no further cases of scurvy were reported. Scurvy also led inevitably to difficulties in wound healing. One of the other consequences of scurvy was ulceration, particularly of the legs, and this sometimes led to gangrene of the affected part. If this sequence of events occurred, then amputation had to be carried out to save the life of the individual.

Because of the difficulty in keeping fires going in the very windy conditions during the winter, many of the men failed to get regular cooked meals, and the salted meat, in particular, often had to be eaten cold. Only when this was fully appreciated were substantial cookhouses built of stone provided, and most of the men were then able to obtain three hot meals each day. This alone was associated with a considerable reduction in hospitalization and mortality among the troops.

Many of the items of clothing requested had in fact been sent out, but due to incompetence on the part of the Commissariat Corps had failed to be distributed to where they were most needed. Hutted accommodation came out too late in the winter to be of much value, and, in any case, Lord Raglan had instructed that these were to be provided for the horses and mules before being provided to the troops. In many of the camps, poor hygiene alone undoubtedly played a substantial part in maintaining the high level of sickness and diarrhea that was then prevalent among the troops.

Between December 1854 and March 1855, the conditions in the Crimea were so dreadful that all thoughts of military activity on both sides all but ceased. To prevent the Russians from breaking out from Sebastopol and attacking the British base at Balaklava, the Allied lines were spread over a distance of about 12 miles, and were heavily supported by artillery. The greatest problem encountered by the Russians came from the threat to their supply lines from the Turkish forces under Omar Pasha.

The British component of the Allied army was reduced in number during the winter months by sickness from a fighting force of over 30,000 men to a force of less than 10,000. The poor sanitary arrangements and the swarms of flies, particularly in October, led to new outbreaks of diarrhea, with 3,782 cases and 115 deaths, and by the end of December, over 25,000 cases of bowel diseases had been admitted to the hospitals since the beginning of the campaign. There were also over 500 recorded cases of dysentery, but a reduction in the cholera cases to 445, with 273 deaths. During October, 1,400 sick and wounded men were transferred from the regimental hospitals to Scutari.

During the first half of November, the weather was mild, but on the 14th a gale force wind did immense damage. Many vessels were destroyed, including the steamship *Prince* that was at anchor off Balaklava with her full cargo of warm clothing for the men. She was lost with all of her crew and passengers. Most of the tented and hutted accommodation was either destroyed or severely damaged. As the weather deteriorated, so did the living conditions of the men. Cooking facilities were severely restricted, and scurvy began to reappear. By December, nearly 30% of the strength needed to be hospitalized, and deaths rose to over 1,200. The principal problem was diarrhea which accounted for 2,633 admissions and 233 deaths. In some of the regiments, about 75% of those admitted with cholera during December died.

New recruits sent from Britain made up some of these deficiencies, but they were more susceptible to cholera, and many succumbed to this condition shortly after their arrival. In December, there were 838 cases reported, with 423 deaths. Many of these recruits should never have been sent out East, as Ballingall had repeatedly drawn attention to the futility of recruiting individuals who were still only in their teens.[53] They were soon exhausted from the hardship of the conditions and had little resistance to disease. The French, in contrast, whose force was in any case considerably larger than their British counterpart, continuously replaced their losses due to sickness by seasoned troops, and consequently encountered far fewer health problems.

The warm clothing that was lost when the *Prince* went down was meant to supply all of the force, and was only made up several months later when vessels arrived with replacement stores, although this was too late to be of value against the harsh winter conditions. Some warm clothing was in store in Balaklava unissued, having arrived during November and December. Twelve thousand greatcoats arrived at the beginning of December, but 9,000 were left in store, and an additional 7,000 were retained in store at Scutari. The coats were apparently not issued because the regulations in force at that time only authorized their issue to the men once every three years. Ten thousand rugs had arrived by early December, and the number had increased to over 25,000 by January, but of these, only 800 were ever issued. At an early stage in the campaign, many regiments replaced the men's Shakos with forage caps. In the winter months, these were in turn replaced by knitted helmets, or "balaklavas," that were much warmer, and covered the entire head.

In January many of the sentries suffered from swollen and numb feet. If they removed their boots when they came off duty, they were often unable to put them on again. In those soldiers already debilitated with dysentery, diarrhea, and exhaustion, this tended to progress to gangrene. When the men were admitted to the regimental hospitals, their condition deteriorated despite the fact that the temperature in the tents was often well above freezing. The cause was in fact peripheral vascular failure in individuals with little physical resistance. Where the gangrene was associated with dysentery, the combination was often fatal.

During the early part of 1855, 35% of the total strength was hospitalized; of the 3,168 deaths, only 119 succumbed due to the secondary consequences of wounds. In nearly 50% of those that died, it was due to bowel disease, with gross inflammation of the bowel followed by ulceration and fatal perforation. Though admissions from cholera fell dramatically in the colder weather, the mortality from this condition was still close to 70%. When the necessary support for the medical staff was not forthcoming, many of the medical officers resigned their commissions and returned to Britain, as there was no order that could prevent this. Furthermore, out of an initial strength of 469, including apothecaries, dispensers, and dressers, 29 had died, and 38 had to be invalided out of the service.[54] It was also particularly difficult to find replacements for those experienced medical officers that had died or been invalided out of the service.

Many of the medical officers did not fully appreciate that it was essential for them to requisition all items of medicine, clothing, and bedding; otherwise it remained in the stores in Balaklava unused. No supplies of knives, forks, spoons, cups, and plates were ever issued, though there were plenty in the stores. By the end of January, however, with the arrival of several supply ships and the distribution of their contents, the conditions in the hospitals gradually improved. Two issues of underclothing had been distributed to all of the men, and they were also supplied with winter coats. While it was still often difficult to obtain certain medical supplies, some of the medical comforts at least could still be purchased in the markets of Constantinople, as could, when necessary, supplies of opium.

In the absence of supplies of soap, the men did not wash. When soap eventually arrived, the men were often so exhausted and apathetic that they continued to remain unwashed. As the men also failed to change their underclothing for weeks on end, many were alive with lice and other vermin, and all attempts to increase the level of personal hygiene failed. It was only when a series of recommendations was made to the commander-in-chief that more time was made available to allow them to wash and change their clothing. The activity of the divisional medical officers was strongly supported by the arrival during early March of the Sanitary Commission, who had the authority to implement changes; they had engineers on their staff, and had the funds to employ local labor.

MEDICAL CONDITIONS DURING THE SPRING MONTHS (1855)

By mid-March, the number of admissions to the regimental hospitals had fallen dramatically, from 4,000 in January to 2,000 in February and 1,000 in March, and this closely reflected the total hospital admissions for these three months. In January, it had accounted for almost 35% of the strength, but by March it had fallen to just under 20%, and in April it was nearer to 14%. By March, a Land Transport Corps was established, divided into two wings, each with its own hospital. This Unit absorbed the drivers and wagons of the Ambulance Corps. Despite repeated pleas by Smith and his successors in office throughout the 19th century for this corps to be put under the control of the PMO, this idea was always rejected, and the corps was retained under military rather than under medical control.

Because of the scarcity of medical staff for the transports and consequent high death rates on board these vessels, hutted accommodation was built in Balaklava for about 600 men. Attempts were made to requisition some of the huts used to shelter the commissariat's mules, but these requests were overruled by the commander-in-chief. The opening of the Kuleli Hospital in January relieved the pressure on the Barrack Hospital, but of the almost 800 patients admitted there, the mortality rate was almost 45%. In April, for the first time, there were about 1,000 vacant beds in Scutari. With an army strength of 44,000 in April, the percentage of bed cover was now at about 20%.

After an inordinate delay between the director-general's request for a body of 1,000 hospital attendants to undertake the duties of hospital orderlies (600 men) and similar activities in the field (400 men), the plan was approved in principle. The men in the latter group would supplement the regimental stretcher-bearers and assist in the evacuation of the casualties to the ambulance wagons and to the regimental hospitals. A Medical Staff Corps was formed by royal warrant in June 1855, but it was then agreed that they would only undertake hospital duties. As the number of ward orderlies was insufficient for the task at hand, another royal warrant was issued in September which authorized the increase in the establishment from 1,000 to 1,200. Individuals could either be recruited directly from civilian life or be transferred from line regiments. They wore a distinct gray uniform, but did not wear the conventional signs of rank. They were given only two weeks of special instruction at the depot at Chatham before their embarkation to the East, and it was hoped that their instruction would be continuous and on the job.

THE FALL OF THE BRITISH GOVERNMENT

The critics of the war effort in the British press were soon reflected in the hostile activities of the opposition in Parliament, and inevitably the government under Lord Aberdeen fell, on January 23, 1855. Lord Palmerston succeeded Lord Aberdeen as Prime Minister, and Sidney Herbert, the Secretary-at-War, was in turn replaced by Lord Panmure, who felt that he should take a less sympathetic line than his predecessor had with the director-general. The fall of the government had been stimulated by the activities of John Roebuck, M.P., who had called for a Commission of Enquiry into all aspects of the running of the war, and constituted a vote of no confidence in the activities of the Prime Minister and his administration.

As part of the director-general's means of appeasing Lord Panmure, he agreed to accept the presence of senior civilian doctors in the Crimea. Very generous rates of pay were to be provided for experienced physicians and surgeons. Not surprisingly, this change of policy regarding salary stimulated much interest in the London medical community, and a considerable number of experienced doctors were appointed and sent to the East.

Improvements in the conditions in the British camps largely appeared to coincide with the appearance of the reports from the various Commissions of Enquiry set up by the government. When, after the War, blame was directed toward the medical staff, Hall, the senior medical officer of the army in the East, was able to demonstrate that whenever he had attempted to institute changes to improve the standard of hygiene in the camps and elsewhere, his actions had invariably been thwarted by the military authorities. When, for example, the suggestion was made to the officer in charge of the region around the harbor of Balaklava that the area should be cleared of the half-buried bodies of the Turkish dead and animal carcasses, as these acted as a constant source of disease, no action was taken. Most of their other requests along similar lines were also ignored.

This generally negative attitude of the executive staff toward any advice given by their medical staff was typical of the hostility that the doctors often received from that quarter. Medical officers had always encountered difficulties when attempting to offer advice on, for example, the optimal siting of camps, means of improving the standard of hygiene in barracks, reducing the spread of infectious diseases, and offering suggestions regarding the most suitable clothing of troops for particular climatic conditions. While McGrigor had been able to recommend to Wellington the appointment of senior medical staff with expertise in these areas for this very purpose, Dr. Andrew Smith had not been similarly successful. The dire consequences were as might have been predicted.

ACTIVITIES OF THE COMMISSIONS AND THE SELECT COMMITTEE

Between November 1854 and April 1855, no less than four commissions and one select committee were established to investigate the conditions in the Crimea, and, with the exception of the select committee, their reports were all published after their individual investigations had been completed. Either all or some of the members of the four commissions traveled to the Crimea to determine how improvements could be made, and in some instances even initiated reforms on their own. The select committee (also termed the Roebuck or Sebastopol Committee) published their findings while the committee was still sitting and taking evidence. Their principal function appears to have been to apportion blame on specific individuals for each and all of the episodes of mismanagement and deficiencies encountered. Evidence was received from doctors, military personnel, politicians, and civilians, all of whom were in some way or another involved in the war effort.

The Hospital Commission was established in November 1854, at the instigation of Dr. Andrew Smith, to investigate the state of the medical services in the East, and to confirm or refute the statements that had appeared in the press, most of which had been of a detrimental nature. The Duke of Newcastle, the former Minister of War, chaired the commission, and its membership included individuals who Smith trusted would provide him with the unvarnished truth, good or bad. Soon after its establishment, the commission was put under government control, and reported directly to the War Office rather than to the Medical Department of the Army, as Smith had intended. Their remit was to investigate the conditions under which the sick and wounded were managed, the state of the hospital accommodation, and all aspects of the medical services in the East. Two medical men, deputy inspector-general Cumming and staff surgeon Laing, assisted by Mr. Maxwell, were sent to the Crimea to obtain appropriate evidence. Their preliminary report was submitted in February 1855, and their definitive report was published in June 1855.

Their principal recommendations were as follows:

1. That the employment of untrained soldiers as ward orderlies was entirely unsatisfactory, and should cease, and that they should be replaced by an intelligent and trained body of men who would be competent to undertake their duties. They recommended the establishment of a hospital Ambulance Corps, with trained staff, and adequate transport in the form of ambulance wagons, as had previously been requested by Smith, and recommended by many others since the Peninsular War.
2. That the duties undertaken by the Purveyor's Department should be undertaken by the Commissariat Department, such as the provision of equipment, clothing, food, and comforts and the undertaking of the laundry. Furthermore, they should maintain a clothes store within each hospital, so that any clothing deficiencies could be made up with minimal difficulty and without the need for requisitions.
3. They recommended that the number of medical officers in regimental hospitals should be reduced in order to increase the number of doctors at the base hospitals.

While the information gathered and published in the report of the first commission was useful, its principal function was superseded by the activities of the Roebuck Committee. Minimal useful information was offered to the first commission by the various commanding officers, as it was clearly apparent that their knowledge of the organization of the medical services was very limited. Miss Nightingale was also interviewed, as were a number of her ex-patients. The end result was that the report was essentially ignored, as were their suggestions for improving the medical services that were included in the report. The definitive report was presented to both Houses of Parliament in June 1855, and while it was widely circulated, it probably achieved very little, apart from providing the medical staff with a public forum for voicing their opinions.

The Roebuck Committee was more effective because of the aggressive personality of its chairman. Its principal aim was to direct blame against specific individuals, possibly to distract public opinion away from blaming the government and previous administrations for their policies since the Peninsular War, in withdrawing funding from the medical services. All evidence was taken in London, and no experts were sent to the Crimea to establish the situation there and verify or negate the material published in the newspapers. Only those that were, for one reason or another, no longer in the Crimea were invited before the committee.

Two of the witnesses who gave evidence before the committee were the Hon. and Rev. Godolphin Osborne and Mr. Augustus Stafford, MP. Both visited the Crimea with the self-appointed task of investigating the conditions themselves following what they had read in the newspapers. Neither had consulted with the director-general, although Mr. Osborne had discussed his mission with Mr. Sidney Herbert, and went with his permission. He made his reports behind the backs of the commander-in-chief, Lord Raglan, and Dr. Hall. As a civilian, with no experience of military medical organization, he expected that the hospitals would be equipped and staffed to the same high standard as in the larger civilian hospitals in the major cities in England.

It was only when Florence Nightingale returned to Britain from her first visit to the hospitals at the Crimea that her attention was drawn to the very unhygienic conditions in some of the voluntary hospitals where the poor were cared for in London. She noted that the conditions in them were about the same, certainly no better, than at Scutari, and her criticisms of the poor standard of treatment of the men in the Crimea mellowed somewhat. This was certainly a great shock to her, and after the war led to the implementation of various measures to dramatically improve the standards in the voluntary hospitals in Britain.

In the majority of the workhouses at that time there was no privacy for the inmates. In the infirmaries associated with these workhouses, there were often minimal facilities for the treatment of the sick, and an almost complete absence of skilled nursing. The few doctors who were associated with these institutions were poorly paid, and often unsympathetic to the provision of any semblance of creature comforts for the poor, as it was generally felt that these only encouraged malingering.

Both visitors were critical of the hospital administration, and informed the committee that there were shortages in all areas. The director-general refuted many of their criticisms. Osborne led the committee to believe that no improvements had been made in the hospitals unless he had suggested them. Both Smith and Mr. Maxwell, the legal member of the Special Hospital Commission, refuted many of his statements.

Evidence was also taken from the Duke of Cambridge, who had commanded the First Division since 1854, Lord Cardigan, who had commanded the Light Brigade, and Lord Lucan, who had commanded the cavalry. Evidence was also taken from other high-ranking military men, all of whom believed that it was not the business of the medical staff to advise on the location of military bases or hospitals - such decisions were made by the commanding officer or by his staff officers. Brigadier General Lord William Paulet was appointed commandant of the General Hospital at Scutari a matter of days before Osborne left Scutari for Britain on December 19. Osborne provided him with suggestions as to how the conditions in the hospital might be improved. He was courteously thanked for his efforts, and informed that all would be done to see that they were implemented.

When the Roebuck Committee interrogated Smith, he indicated that he had little influence on the situation in the Crimea, although he always responded immediately to any problems drawn to his attention by those on the spot. He indicated that he had to work through five different departments in the War Office, and that this had proved to be an administrative nightmare. On hearing this, the Secretary for War authorized Smith to purchase items of medical comforts directly from the contractors, rather than through the commander-in-chief or the Admiralty. Shortly afterward, the Commissariat Department was removed from Treasury control and placed under War Office control, and Smith was largely exonerated of blame for the deficiencies in the medical services in the Crimea.

The first Roebuck report was presented before Parliament on June 18, 1855, and the findings were discussed at length. Despite the difficulties they had encountered, the Army Medical Department largely escaped criticism from the Roebuck inquiry. Many unjust criticisms had been directed at it, particularly from the unqualified "visitors": it was generally felt that the Army Medical Department had escaped with minimal criticism. "Dr. Smith has obtained a victory over his foes, and it is declared that he did everything a man in his situation could have done."[55]

The committee had not only failed to force Smith's resignation, but had also to acknowledge the administrative handicaps under which Smith was forced to work, and the rebuffs he had received to so many of his proposals. No censure of Smith appeared in their final report. Others had criticized the Army Medical Department by detrimentally comparing it with the French medical organization, but this contention was strongly refuted by Bryce, who was keen to draw attention to the considerable talents of the director-general.[56] Bryce had been one of the civilian physicians attached on special service to Kuleli Hospital at Scutari, where he had been in charge of 100 beds.

In the spring of 1856, Bryce joined a party of British surgeons who attended the French patients when they were particularly short of doctors, and remained with them for over a month, an example of the *entente cordiale médicale* which existed between the various Allied armies. In his monograph, he compared the sanitary state of the English and French hospitals at the close of the war. He wished to exonerate the director-general and the Army Medical Department from blame for the administrative problems encountered and the detrimental effect this had had on the medical conditions and treatment of the sick and wounded. He believed that the British press exaggerated the horrors of the sanitary state of the British troops, while the French press kept quiet about the sanitary state of their forces. Bryce also pointed out that "the French surgeon is not answerable for the cleanliness of the sick, beds, wards &c. and of the *dépendances de l'établissement*, all of which duties belong *à l'officier comptable d'administration*."[57] With his experience of working in the French as well as British hospitals, he felt that he had a balanced view of the situation, and was, almost uniquely, qualified to write on the topic.

The principal criticism leveled against the Roebuck Committee was that it appeared happier receiving statements from civilian experts who had often only briefly visited the Crimea than from medical and military officers who had served in the war zone on a full-time basis. In the end, the Roebuck Committee had relatively little impact on the position in the Crimea, because the government had, by the time it reported, set up several other commissions, each with powers to act locally, without the need to refer back to Parliament. These were the Sanitary, Supplies, and Pathology Commissions.

The principal remit of the Sanitary Commission, headed by three of the most senior and experienced medical officers of health and assisted by three sanitary inspectors, was to investigate the conditions in the Crimea and in Constantinople and, where possible, to secure reforms. They were given authority by the Minister to instruct the local authorities as to how and where conditions should be improved. They indicated the means of implementing their suggestions, and also supervized the work until it had been successfully completed. The commissioners also inspected the transports, the state of the harbor at Balaklava, and the condition of the camps and regimental hospitals in the surrounding area.

The commissioners and their staff arrived early in March 1855, and immediately visited the hospitals and the surrounding area. By the middle of the month they recommended the essential changes that urgently needed to be undertaken. Almost all of the work that they recommended was speedily carried out, and ongoing reports were sent to the minister, Lord Panmure. The changes they recommended undoubtedly had a dramatic effect on reducing the mortality in the hospitals and improving the conditions of the sick and wounded in the camps, regimental hospitals, transports, and base hospitals. As well as cleaning the wards, installing new lavatories, and arranging the supply of clean water in the hospitals, they also condemned the use of the two convalescent hulks, and these, in due course, were returned to the navy. The commissioners later visited the Civil Hospital at Smyrna and made similar improvements there. The changes that they recommended also had an effect on the way that the Army Medical Service functioned in the long term. Miss Nightingale believed that "It was this commission that saved the British Army."[58]

It was clear that the peacetime ordering systems employed by the Commissariat Department were unable to cope with wartime situations. Because it was obvious that the Commissariat Department bore a substantial responsibility for the gross mismanagement in the distribution of supplies in the Crimea, the government decided to establish the Supplies Commission,[59] whose principal remit was to inquire into the management of that department. They investigated how the transfer of provisions, essential equipment, clothing, and forage for the horses was organized. They also ascertained how supplies and other essentials were sent to the Crimea and how they were distributed once they reached the harbor at Balaklava.

While the commissioners' criticisms were not directed toward specific individuals, their findings confirmed that members of the Commissariat Department had lacked both initiative and imagination. They recommended that the Commissariat Department be put under the control of the War Office. They also questioned the competence and judgment of a number of members of the high command. This caused a sensation when the findings were made public, and deep resentment in certain circles in the War Office. Those criticized argued that they had not had an opportunity to discuss the contents of the report before it was published. A board of general officers (also termed the Chelsea Board, because the inquiry was held at the Royal Hospital, Chelsea) was established with the consent of the Queen, and as a result, all of those in the high command who had been criticized were completely exonerated. Equally, the Commissariat Department escaped censure, all of the blame for the administrative deficiencies being directed toward the Treasury. The final report emphasized the difficulties the Army Medical Department had encountered. The Chelsea Board itself did not escape public criticism, and their findings were also severely criticized by Miss Nightingale.

The final commission to be established, toward the end of March 1855, was the Pathology Commission. Their remit was to investigate the various diseases to which the men had been exposed during the Crimean campaign.[60] Dr. Lyons, the head pathologist, was instructed to undertake detailed postmortem examinations and "to demonstrate the morbid appearances discovered to such medical officers as may feel disposed to attend." Dr. Lyons was instructed to examine British and French patients, as well as Russian prisoners-of-war, but not to interfere with their medical treatment. Dr. Lyons was particularly directed to take sections of the diseased tissues and subject them to detailed histological examination, as well as retaining specimens for future analysis.

Dr. Lyons was not a good choice as commissioner, and failed to get on with the local military medical officers, the senior military personnel, and even his colleagues on the Commission.[61] He failed to keep his colleagues in his confidence. When he eventually departed to take up the Chair of Medicine and Pathology in the School of Medicine at the Catholic University of Dublin, his junior colleagues Drs. Aitken and Doyle were left to pick up the pieces.

The Commission's final report was extremely disappointing, as it contained no statistical information on the diseases that had so greatly contributed to the loss of life among the troops. The only long-term gain was the improvement that occurred in the establishment of better facilities for conducting postmortem examinations, and the useful feedback that this provided to the physicians. Another long-term gain was the keeping of accurate mortality statistics. Aitken's reputation was considerably enhanced by his work in the Crimea and, on Miss Nightingale's insistence, he was appointed to the Chair of Pathology at the newly created Army Medical School at Fort Pitt in 1860, remaining in this post until his death in 1892.

RESURGENCE OF HOSTILITIES (1855)

With the improvement in the weather, in the early spring of 1855 there was the distinct likelihood that active hostilities would commence, such as an assault on Sebastopol or a Russian attempt to break the siege. With this in mind, both the director-general and Hall actively investigated the fate of the 200 litters and chairs that had been ordered as a matter of urgency the previous November. By mid-March 1855 only about 20 had been supplied, and it was not until March 1856 that all of the items requested had been received. These items were to have been used for the immediate treatment and movement of the likely casualties to the regimental hospitals, to restock the ambulance wagons, and to replenish the mule litters. By the middle of March, only 20 ambulance wagons, 40 ambulance carts, and 500 stretchers were available to cope with any outbreak of hostilities. Toward the end of May 1855, there were only 15 serviceable ambulance wagons and carts available for use in the Crimea, and the full number requested, 20 wagons and 64 carts, did not reach the Crimea until December of that year. With regard to stretchers, Hall's request for 4,000 stretchers was met only in 1856; by April 1855, only 1,300 had been delivered.

Hall sent a requisition directly to the director-general for hospital comforts. While a great deal could be obtained in the markets in Constantinople, demand was beginning to exceed supply. He requested 60,000 bottles of wine, brandy, porter, and ale, 80,000 tins of tinned food, tons of preserved vegetables, sago, arrowroot, and other foodstuffs to be supplied on a monthly basis. By the autumn of 1855, all restrictions were removed from expenditure. One thousand tons of ice were shipped out from Britain until the PMO at Scutari informed the director-general that any quantity of ice could be obtained for $2^1/_2$d a pound from the slopes of Mount Olympus close by.[62]

The Allies commenced the bombardment of Sebastopol and it continued unabated, night and day, from April 9 until April 25. The assault had to be delayed until the railway line from Balaklava had been completed, to allow adequate supplies of ammunition to reach the Allies' batteries. The bombardment had, in any case, to be suspended because the Allies ran out of ammunition. The majority of the casualties were looked after locally in hutted hospitals sited just behind the lines, rather than being transported elsewhere, where in any case there was minimal spare capacity. Over 400 cases were dealt with in these hospitals, although the hospitals could cope with almost 1,000 casualties. These men certainly benefited from the presence of the railway, which was far more efficient and less injurious to their health than the poorly sprung ambulance wagons.

Another bombardment was initiated on June 6, and was followed up the next day by an assault carried out by the French. The French succeeded in capturing the Mamelon redoubt, while the British captured the Quarries. The Russians counterattacked, and the British sustained over 500 casualties. On June 18, the Allies attacked the more formidable fort known as the Redan, but were repulsed, and sustained about 2,000 casualties. After their wounds had been dressed in field hospitals located just behind the front line, the men were transported in mule chairs and litters to the regimental hospitals. This arrangement had the great advantage over the previous system where the men's wounds were treated in the regimental hospitals that often also contained large numbers of fever patients. It allowed the wounded to be treated rapidly and effectively, with minimal risk of their being exposed to contagious diseases.

With the advent of the warmer weather, increasing numbers of cases of cholera appeared, and this soon developed into an epidemic. The epidemic continued for several months, with 1,600 deaths and a mortality of close to 60%. The cholera appeared to have a predisposition toward the newly arrived recruits, and most of the medical staff believed that it was due to the unfavorable environment. Suggestions to the director-general that providing supplies of pure water might control the condition were rejected, and again many unnecessary lives were lost.

It is now believed that most of the cholera cases were acquired in the drink shops and cafés in Balaklava. The onset of symptoms was often sudden, and death usually occurred within 24 hours of diagnosis.[63] When the epidemic was at its worst, it jeopardized the long-term presence of the army in the East, and accounted for the death of a number of senior military and naval figures. The commander-in-chief suffered from an abdominal complaint, and died a few days after its onset. During the summer months, epidemics of diarrhea and fever raged in the camps, and resulted in high rates of hospital admissions. Between July and August, about 4,000 men per month were admitted with diarrhea, and about 7,000 per month with fever, amounting to between 24 and 28% of strength during these months. From April onward, no more than 1,000 patients were transferred to Scutari.

THE CIVILIAN DOCTORS WHO VOLUNTEERED FOR SERVICE IN THE CRIMEA

One particular group received relatively little recognition for their services in the Crimea. This was the group of civilian doctors who volunteered to serve either in close association with some of the regiments or in one of the civil hospitals that were later established. Because their salaries had to be paid from army funds, the majority of these volunteers were appointed to the lowest possible rank, assistant surgeon, whatever their previous experience. This alone actively discouraged more senior medical men from joining the Army Medical Service. A few civilians got permission to visit the war zone, and either acted as observers or worked as unpaid volunteers for a month or more in the hospital at Scutari.

Later in 1854, a number of civilian doctors, all of whom had been qualified for at least 12 years, and therefore had ample professional experience, were allowed to work at Scutari or in the Crimea. While retaining their civilian status, they received the food allocation and allowances of an army captain. These doctors were generally greatly resented by their military medical colleagues, principally because they received a higher rate of pay than did their military colleagues, but also because they were less encumbered by military red tape.

A considerable number of medical students who were exclusively in the clinical years of their course were allowed to attend the hospitals as dressers. Most worked at Scutari, while others spent some or all of their time elsewhere, usually for three to six months, although a few spent up to a year in the war-zone.

Despite the various commissions of enquiry into the medical conditions in the East, little mention was made of the value of the civil hospitals and the activities of the civilian doctors who worked and occasionally died in them. A few of those who volunteered to work in the Crimea were recognized by the award of the Crimean Medal, but most went unrewarded and unrecognized.

THE CIVIL HOSPITAL AT SMYRNA

During the early months of 1855, plans were made for the establishment of a few civil hospitals, to be entirely staffed by civilian doctors. The presence of these doctors was particularly resented because it was rumored that their presence blocked the promotion of their military colleagues.

To reduce the pressure on the beds at Scutari, it was proposed that a convalescent hospital be established at Smyrna, on the Mediterranean coast of Turkey, about a day and a half from Scutari and about four days by steamer from the Crimea. The government proposed that all of the clinical staff would be civilian. It was initially rumored that most of the doctors had been recruited from the London hospitals, but this turned out not to be the case. Over 300 applications had been received for the 25 or so clinical posts. Those who were eventually selected turned out to be a particularly gifted group, with many going on to hold high office in the profession.

The fabric of the hospital was in reasonable order, although it had previously been a barracks complex with inadequate drainage and sanitation. There was a considerable degree of overcrowding even before the arrival of the civilian doctors. Initially, the military authorities supplied a senior physician, two senior surgeons and five assistant surgeons, assisted by a few military nurses and orderlies, to look after about 600 patients. The mortality rate during the first few months was in the region of 13%, extremely high for a convalescent hospital, and this was undoubtedly due to the overcrowding, the very unhygienic conditions in the area around the hospital, and the inhospitable climatic conditions. Only in March 1855 did the civilian medical staff arrive to take over their clinical responsibilities, and consisted of a medical superintendent (the only military appointment), 3 physicians, 3 surgeons, 6 assistant physicians, 10 assistant surgeons, and a resident medical officer. A secretary, 9 dispensers, and a civil engineer were also appointed. Each was contracted to work at the hospital for twelve months, at the termination of which they were to receive a bonus of half their annual salary.

Almost 100 of the original patients who had been transferred to the hospital in February died from a particularly virulent form of typhus. As a consequence of the high patient losses, the numbers admitted there soon diminished, to such an extent that some of the doctors left because they considered that their load was too light. Some took posts elsewhere in the Crimea, while others were so disillusioned that they returned home. A considerable number of nurses and civilian orderlies were also sent to Smyrna, and the high standard of their work was universally complimented. Nearly 2,000 patients were admitted to the civil hospital at Smyrna between February and November 1855, though hostilities ceased in October 1855, with most being admitted between February and May, of whom about 8% died. Of the total admitted, about 20% were due to fever, and slightly less because of bowel complaints (of whom about 20% died). Most of the rest consisted of cases of frost-bite (9%), scurvy (7%), and rheumatic diseases (6%), and only 32 patients had been wounded in action.

The civil hospital at Smyrna functioned sufficiently well to convince the authorities that the troops could just as satisfactorily be treated in a civilian as in a military hospital. Accordingly, plans were activated by the government to build a second large civil hospital. The idea was mooted that this should consist of prefabricated units constructed in England, which could then be assembled at a suitable site in the East. Isambard Kingdom Brunel[64] was selected to design the units and draw up plans for the hospital complex. Within a very short space of time, not only were the units designed, but a considerable number were built and shipped out to the most favored site, at Renkioi, on the southwest shores of the Dardanelles, and about 100 miles from Scutari.

In Brunel's original plan, there were to be a total of 34 hutted units, erected in two parallel lines, but one of the few surviving photographs, dating from March 1856, appears to indicate that only 15 huts had been assembled at that time. As each hut was designed to accommodate two wards, each containing 26 beds as well as a nurses' room, surgery, lavatories, and wash spaces, this would seem to indicate that the hospital at that time could only accommodate, at full bed occupancy, about 780 patients. Additional kitchen units and a laundry were also provided. According to the medical superintendent,[65] accommodation for 300 patients was available by July 1855, for 500 by August, and for 1,500 by January 1856, and when the hospital was finally closed in March 1856, it could accommodate more than 2,000 patients. At that time, the hospital possessed three kitchens, two laundries, and separate quarters for the doctors and the nurses.

The second civil hospital opened in August 1855. While about 1,300 patients were admitted to Renkioi between October 1855 and June 1856, the number admitted between March and June 1856 was only 50. Over the entire intake, only about 7% of the patients had been wounded in action, and the remainder consisted of medical cases. As there was likely to be a considerably greater number of medical compared to surgical cases, the medical staff were selected to reflect this ratio. Consequently, while there were 2 senior physicians and 2 senior surgeons in addition to the medical superintendent, there were 15 assistant physicians and 11 assistant surgeons appointed to the staff, assisted by one apothecary.

About 25% of the patients were admitted to Renkioi because of bowel complaints, and a similar proportion with fever. About 15% were admitted with chest complaints of various types, and a similar proportion with rheumatic complaints. About 45% of the deaths that occurred there were due to typhus or typhoid, and a further 30% died from chronic dysentery. From April 1856, only about 100 patients were admitted per month, and no patients were admitted after June 1856; the last patient was discharged from the hospital in July, and the hospital was finally closed in November. The hospital was then handed over to the Swiss Legion, and the civilian staff transferred from Renkioi.

By the time that the second civil hospital had been built and was ready to receive patients, the pressure on the beds was largely resolved, because far fewer men were being evacuated from the Crimea than formerly. Thus, in October 1855, of the 3,400 available beds, only 1,000 were in fact occupied, and the bed occupancy dropped rapidly from then on. The War Office handed over Kuleli hospital to the German Legion, and all of the remaining patients were transferred to Scutari. The civilian medical specialists were largely idle, and instead of being sent the acute cases they had expected, they received only chronic cases and convalescents. The civilian medical staff complained that they had been promised 18 months on full pay, followed by 12 months' pay as a gratuity; instead, the hospital had closed after only 10 months, and accordingly they were to receive no gratuity or financial compensation. In retrospect, it was probably unjustified to establish new civilian hospitals when the numbers admitted at Scutari were diminishing. While these hospitals might have served a useful purpose as convalescent hospitals, the considerable cost of the highly qualified medical and surgical staff was now seen to be unjustified.

When, in 1856, the efficiency of both of the civil hospitals was considered by the Select Committee of the Medical Department of the Army, a group consisting entirely of regular army medical officers, they were universally critical of the experiment. Considering the criticisms previously raised by the military doctors against their civilian colleagues, this was entirely predictable.

THE FINAL STAGES OF THE CRIMEAN WAR: THE FALL OF SEBASTOPOL

From April until September 1855, the conditions in the British camps improved considerably. With the improved hygiene in the camps and increased rations, fewer succumbed to disease. Nearly all of the regiments had been brought up to strength, and time spent on duty could be reduced. This consequently diminished the level of exhaustion previously encountered during the winter months.

By the end of the summer all of the men could be accommodated in huts, and most of the men had either beds or cots. In the hotter weather, the sick tended to be nursed in tents, because of the increased ventilation these allowed. Most of the huts had, in fact, reached the Crimea by the end of December 1854, but were not distributed for many months because of difficulties with local transport. While a railway line was eventually constructed, principally to carry ammunition to the front line from the harbor, most of the officers would have preferred the provision of a good road system.

As there were insufficient troops to mount a frontal assault on Sebastopol, and in any case the Russian defensive fortifications were strongly supported by large numbers of cannon, it was suggested that the only approach that might prove effective was by cutting off the main supply route to the enemy. All attempts to break out of their position, and attack Balaklava, were successfully repulsed, and the Russians became increasingly demoralized at the stalemate.

The bombardment of Sebastopol was recommenced on September 7, and the French attacked with great strength and succeeded in gaining the Malakoff fortification; they flew the Tricolor from its heights. The British, misreading the significance of the signal, assaulted the walls of the Redan across a region of open country where they were exposed to fierce Russian crossfire. After suffering more than 2,000 casualties, they were forced to withdraw. On the night of September 8, the Russians blew up their magazines in the Redan and withdrew, leaving Sebastopol ablaze. Only the sick and dying were left behind. An armistice was eventually declared on February 29, 1856, and peace declared on March 30, 1856, with the signing of the Treaty of Paris.[66] Despite the Russian withdrawal in September, they retained a large army just to the north of the

Crimea. This necessitated the Allies retaining their armies in the Crimea through the winter of 1855–1856, to prevent the possibility of a Russian counterattack.

CONTRIBUTION OF THE NAVY TO THE CRIMEAN CAMPAIGN

The state of the British navy was far superior to that of the army at the onset of the Crimean War, because the fleet based in Malta, consisting of about 16,000 men, had been in a state of readiness for over a year. Other components of the navy had successfully blockaded the Gulf of Finland, impeded the movement of Russian naval forces, and restricted that country's trade. While no major naval engagements took place during the Crimean War between the British and Russian fleets, the British navy played a significant part in the campaign by their efficient transportation of troops and supplies across the Black Sea. The small naval force of marines that was based on shore near Sebastopol made a considerable contribution to the war effort during the siege of that city.

The navy's principal role during the six months of the siege of Sebastopol was the manning of the gun emplacements and the trenches. In the first few weeks of the campaign, seamen manned 40% of the guns involved in the siege, and they were also involved in all of the major assaults on the fortifications of that city. During the latter activity, the casualty rates were high. During the entire War period, the sick rate in the Naval Brigade was 10.5%, of which 7% were due to wounds. The figures were far lower than comparable rates for the army, particularly the infantry and cavalry units who were involved in similar activity to those in the Naval Brigade, where the respective figures were 24% and 15%. This was probably because they were better clothed and far better fed than were their army colleagues.

The medical record of the navy was also better than that of the army. The ships were better equipped and victualed for a long period of service. Considering the size of the entire naval force, with about 62,000 men in 1855, the Naval Medical Board consisted of only 308 surgeons and 25 assistant surgeons. Despite this paucity of men, they were still able to offer assistance to their colleagues in the army when required to do so.

Only 144 deaths from disease occurred out of the 18,000 officers and men in service in the Baltic fleet during 1855, and about 1,900 men were listed as sick during this period.[67] As there was a considerable shortage of assistant surgeons in the Baltic fleet in 1855, the Admiralty wrote to all medical schools to inform them that medical students who were advanced in their clinical studies would be eligible to serve as dressers, and would serve with the rank of acting assistant surgeon. This offer was generally unfavorably viewed by both the medical students and by the medical press. Despite this, 67 students served in the Baltic fleet during 1855, as much for adventure as for clinical experience, and all are believed to have returned to their medical studies.[68]

During 1855–1856, the Black Sea fleet completely dominated the seaways—the Russians had scuttled their fleet at the entrance to the harbor at Sebastopol. They were principally involved in the transfer of troops by sea from one site of activity to another, as well as being involved in the transportation of supplies and the sick and wounded troops from the battle zone.

At all times during the war, the medical complement of the fleet was below the recommended level, principally because of the slowness of the Admiralty to deal with the complaints of their junior medical staff. The problems of low pay, poor conditions of service, and lack of comparability of pay with their army colleagues were not resolved until after the war, and was the cause of the very poor morale seen in the Naval Medical Service at that time. Most of the transports had an inadequate medical or nursing complement, and many had neither on board. Not surprisingly, the mortality rates on board these ships could be as high as 10%, despite the fact that the journey between Balaklava and Scutari often took only 36 hours.

The conditions in the naval hospital at Therapia were initially extremely poor, but they gradually improved. The hospital was well equipped and reasonably well staffed. In January 1855, the medical complement was increased due to the arrival of the Rev. John Mackenzie, his wife (a trained nurse, who subsequently acted as the matron) and a party of ladies and nurses. Mr. Mackenzie also acted as unofficial chaplain in the absence of an Anglican chaplain in residence. Mrs. Mackenzie was so highly regarded that she was made an honorary member of the officers' mess, an honor never bestowed upon Miss Nightingale. While it is not possible to compare the activities in this relatively small hospital with that in the much larger establishments at Scutari, it worked well and efficiently.

The total number of deaths that occurred in the Baltic and Black Sea fleets was 2,009, of whom 1,574 died of disease and 228 from accidental injuries or drowning, and 227 from wounds in action. This last figure includes the deaths incurred by the Naval Brigade and marines during their land-based activities in the Crimea.[69] The fleet was fortunate in that it was not subjected to a series of extremely damaging commissions of inquiry, and the censure of the press and Miss Nightingale as were their military colleagues. The navy, however, benefited from the reforms that were instituted in both services shortly after the end of the Crimean War.

THE FATE OF DR. (LATER SIR) ANDREW SMITH

During his tenure of office as commander-in-chief, Raglan did not recommend any medical officers for gallantry awards, though a few were "mentioned in dispatches" after the Redan battle. The names of six medical men were subsequently drawn to the attention of the War Office for their courage, coolness, and professional skill. In February 1856, Hall was awarded the K.C.B. (Knight Commander of the Order of the Bath), and C.B.s (Commander of the Order of the Bath) were awarded to deputy inspector-generals Dumbreck, Linton, Forrest, Alexander, Taylor, Gordon, and Mouat. Hall and 16 others received the French Legion of Honor. It is curious that the inspector-general did not receive his K.C.B. (Civil) until more than two years later, on his retirement from that post in July 1858. This award was not well received by the *Times*, and in an article on July 14 they continued to attack him, as they had throughout the

Crimean War, concluding, "He is to be shelved at last, and to be consigned to a splendid insignificance."

The *Lancet*[70] was particularly incensed, and wrote in response to the item published in the *Times*, that this newspaper "Continues to hold Dr. Smith responsible for events which were wholly beyond his control, and for misfortunes which he had predicted, but was not permitted to avert. Subsequent investigations have crowned him with the honour due to foresight and have vindicated fully his claims to the respect and goodwill of his countrymen."

General Peel, the Secretary of State for War, wrote to him shortly after he resigned, acknowledging "The zeal and devotion to the Public Service which you have always evinced in the discharge of your duties and of the most laborious and anxious character of those services at times of unexampled difficulty."[71]

Shortly after he retired, he donated 3,500 of his 15,000 natural history specimens to the University of Edinburgh, and his generosity to his alma mater was duly acknowledged when they awarded him an honorary degree of LL.D. He devoted his last years to his scientific pursuits.[72] He died at the age of 75 in 1872. His notes on the races and tribes of South Africa were gathered together after his death, but were never published.[73]

CONCLUDING OBSERVATIONS REGARDING THE CRIMEAN WAR

The reason that this chapter would appear to be disproportionately long is because the Crimean War was the first war that took place in the public arena. Representatives of the press were quick to draw attention to the deficiencies in the management of all aspects of the campaign, particularly the poor conditions of service of the men. All of those who took part were ultimately held to be accountable for their deficiencies, and those who held the highest offices in the service and in the government were publicly denounced for their failings. Few who took part survived unscathed from the onslaught of the various commissions of inquiry, except perhaps for the ordinary soldiers who had little or no say in the proceedings.

The recriminations that followed the Crimean War led to a complete reevaluation of the roles of everyone from the government down to those in the armed services, not only in times of war, but also in periods of peace. In the interwar period following the Peninsular War, little attention had been paid by the government to the funding of the army and to the maintenance of a high standard of military morale, when other activities were perceived to require a higher level of priority. The price that was paid for these failures was considerable.

When it became obvious that a great war was imminent in the East, there was, at least initially, little appreciation of the number of combatants who would be involved or the magnitude of the losses that would be encountered on all sides. This was particularly the case on the British side, where many died as a consequence of the inadequate state of preparedness of the army to combat the inhospitable conditions they were to encounter in the siege of Sebastopol. Deaths from sickness had always outnumbered those from military combat in previous wars. This was a difficult lesson for the public to appreciate, until the raw figures of the huge number of the fighting force who died in the base hospitals from cholera, typhus, and dysentery were made known on an almost daily basis.

The poor state of preparedness of the army medical services was also clearly apparent. Little funding had been spent over the years on the two Regius Chairs of Military Surgery, in Edinburgh for fifty years, and for only a few years in Dublin. Following the Commission of Enquiry, the government promised that they would support the establishment of an Army Medical School, run along professional lines, instead of the amateurish effort that had previously been made to educate medical officers for the army and the navy.

APPENDIX: BRITISH, FRENCH AND RUSSIAN CASUALTIES DURING THE CRIMEAN WAR

Figures have been published of army losses during the Crimean War, but as they were so great, there is no uniformity of agreement between the different sources. The estimates given here (Table 4.1) are from Lloyd and Coulter,[74] where it is noted that some authorities believe that the Russian figure may be exaggerated, as they never, at any time, had more than 150,000 troops in the field.

Table 4.1
Casualty Rates Incurred by the Principal Combatants during the Crimean War

	Total casualties	Deaths	
	(approximate)	Killed in action	Died of disease
British	96,000	11,848	17,799
French	309,000	11,000*	21,000
Russian	500,000		

*Killed in action, or died of wounds

These figures for the British component of the Allied force are at considerable variance with those reported in Cantlie[75] (Table 4.2).

Table 4.2
Casualty Rates Incurred by the British during the Crimean War

Total hospital admissions from April 1854 to June 1856	167,786
Admissions for disease*	155,825 (includes injuries)
Admissions for wounds	11,961 (includes incised wounds)
Total deaths	18,058 (disease, 16,334; wounds, 1,724)

*Of the chief diseases, the figures cited are as follows:

	Admissions	Deaths	%
Diarrhea	44,164	3,651	8.3
Dysentery	7,882	2,543	32.3
Cholera	7,575	4,513	59.6

Statistics for wounded: Total 12,094 (Officers, 579; Other ranks, 11,515)

While the number of men who died from wounds and diseases of all causes are fairly similar to those quoted by Bryce,[76] the other figures he quotes are quite different. According to Bryce:

The total strength of the British force of soldiers, exclusive of officers, originally embarked for the East, and added to during progress of the war, up to date of evacuation of Crimea		93,959
Reduced by deaths: killed in action (1,788) and died of wounds (2,658)*	4,446	
Reduced by deaths from disease	16,298	
Reduced by invaliding	12,903	
Total reductions	33,647**	
Remaining effective strength of Crimean army, noncombatants exclusive, at end of war		60,312

*These numbers are supplied from a Parliamentary return quoted in the *United Service Magazine*.
**Total *hors de combat* at close of war 35.81%.

The equivalent figures for the French force are also supplied by Bryce,[77] and are also very different from those quoted above (Table 4.1). The French figures were originally cited in the *Moniteur* of October 23, 1856, and were prepared by Marshal Vaillant at the express request of the Emperor (Table 4.3). They are as follows:

Table 4.3
Casualty Rates Incurred by the French during the Crimean War

The effective strength of the French troops embarked for the East		309,268
Reduced by deaths from all causes, killed in action included	69,229	
Invalided singly, and allowed to leave on furlough during the war	65,069	
Recalled during war	20,390	
Unaccounted for	1,781	
Total number returned to France and Algiers		227,135
Ditto, after signature of Peace		141,676

Summary:

Taken to the East	309,268
Lost there	69,229
	240,039
Reentered France and Algeria	227,135
Difference*	12,904

*According to Bryce, "This item disturbs all calculations."

In a later section of his book, Bryce quotes figures for the French losses that he believed were more realistic than those presented to the Emperor.[78] He was of the view that these figures (Table 4.4) represented the lowest summary of French losses. These figures were prepared by M. Baudens.

Table 4.4

Amended, Possibly More Accurate, Casualty Rates Incurred by the French during the Crimean War

Deaths—killed in action	8,750
Deaths—ambulance service, from wounds and disease	31,000
Deaths—Constantinople hospitals	32,000
Deaths—Dobrudscha expedition	6,000
Deaths—on passage from Crimea to Constantinople	7,500
Deaths—Gallipoli, Varna, and elsewhere	3,000
Deaths—of invalids on passage from Turkey to France; and of sick and invalids, ditto, on evacuation of Crimea	5,000
Total deaths	93,250

Amputations carried out on British troops: Out of over 12,000 wounded, primary amputations were performed in 1,027 cases, and of these 287 died (28%).
Mortality (indicated in percent who died) according to site of amputation: hip joint (100); thigh—according to site (56–87); knee joint (55); leg (35); shoulder (33); arm (26); foot and ankle (14–16); forearm (5).

NOTES

1. E. H. Nolan, 1855–1857. *The Illustrated History of the War against Russia.* 2 Volumes (London: James S. Virtue) [Volume 1, 1855; Volume 2, 1857], Volume 1, pp. 32–33.

2. Cinchona (syn. Chinchona, Peruvian or Jesuit's bark) was long known in South America as a cure for fever. Named by Linnaeus in 1742 after the Countess of Chinchón who, when vice-queen of Peru, was cured of a fever by Peruvian bark, and afterward brought a supply of it into Spain. It is the source of many alkaloids, including quinine, quinidine, cinchonine and cinchonidine. See: Anon., 1973. *The Shorter Oxford English Dictionary on Historical Principles.* 3rd Edition. In 2 Volumes (Oxford: Clarendon Press). Peruvian bark was first enthusiastically used in the British army by John Ranby, principal serjeant-surgeon to His Majesty, for the treatment of large lacerated gunshot wounds. He believed that this agent was "a medicine, which no human eloquence can deck with panegyric, proportionable to it's [sic] virtues. Of such incomparable benefit it is to mankind." See: J. Ranby, 1760. *The Method of Treating Gun-shot Wounds.* 2nd Edition (London: Robert Horsfield), pp. 35–42 [for use of Bark in treatment of gunshot wounds; for quotation, p. 36; first edition , 1744].

3. Anon., 1854. The cholera. *Lancet* **II**, 345.

4. N. Cantlie, 1974. *A History of the Army Medical Department.* 2 Volumes (Edinburgh and London: Churchill Livingstone), Volume 1, pp. 454–493.

5. C. Messenger, 1986. *History of the British Army* (London: Bison), pp. 77–83.

6. M. Windrow and F. K. Mason, 1975. Raglan, Fitzroy James Henry Somerset, 1st Baron (1788–1855), Field-Marshal. In: *A Concise Dictionary of Military Biography: Two Hundred of the most significant names in land warfare, 10th–20th century* (London: Purnell Book Services), pp. 236–238.

7. Nolan, *War against Russia*, Volume 1, pp. 544–545: "Lord Raglan wishes the cavalry to advance rapidly to the front, to follow the enemy and try to prevent the enemy carrying away the guns. Troop of horse-artillery may accompany; French cavalry is on your right. *Immediate*."

8. J. Macdonald, 1984. *Great Battlefields of the World* (London: Michael Joseph), pp. 82–85; Messenger, *History of the British Army*, pp. 80–81; Nolan, *War Against Russia*, Volume 1, pp. 532–567; J. W. Fortescue, 1899–1930. *A History of the British Army*. 13 Volumes (London: Macmillan & Co.), Volume 13, see pp. 100–110; J. Shepherd, 1991. *The Crimean Doctors: A History of the British Medical Services in the Crimean War*. 2 Volumes (Liverpool: Liverpool University Press), Volume 1, pp. 216–226.

9. P. Mercer, 1998. *Inkerman 1854: The Soldiers' Battle* (London: Osprey Military Publishing).

10. Shepherd, *Crimean Doctors*, Volume 2, pp. 381–395.

11. Shepherd, *Crimean Doctors*, Volume 2, pp. 395–401.

12. Shepherd, *Crimean Doctors*, Volume 2, pp. 401–404.

13. Shepherd, *Crimean Doctors*, Volume 2, pp. 405–409.

14. According to their report, "It would seem that your visits to the camp were few and far between, and your staff seems to have known as little as yourself on the conditions of your gallant men."

15. Anon., 1872. Sir Andrew Smith, K.C.B. *Lancet* **II**, 244–245; Anon., 1959–1960. Smith, Sir Andrew (1797–1872). *Dictionary of National Biography* **18** (Oxford: Oxford University Press), 423.

16. A. Peterkin, and W. Johnston, 1968. *Commissioned Officers in the Medical Services of the British Army 1660–1960*. 2 Volumes. Vol. 1, 1660–1898, 638 pp., Vol. 2, 1898–1960, 452 pp (London: Wellcome Historical Medical Library) [This volume is sometimes referred to as: "Drew, R. (Editor)," with the same details], Reference Number 3998, pp. 266–267.

17. Anon., 1959–1960. Hennen, John, M.D. (1779–1828). *Dictionary of National Biography* **9** (Oxford: Oxford University Press), 424.

18. Anon., 1851. *Lancet* **I**, 163 [Editorial relating to the pay of Dr. Andrew Smith on his appointment as successor to Sir James McGrigor as director-general of the Army Medical Department]: "We observe that the post so long and so honourably occupied by Sir James MacGrigor [sic], as the head of the army medical department, and from which he retired some time ago, has been filled up by the appointment of Dr. Andrew Smith, Inspector-General of Hospitals, by whom a large portion of the duties of the office have been ably performed for several years past. We regret, however, to state, that the office has, as we feared several months ago, been restricted in its importance, and the salary reduced from £2,000 to £1,200 a-year. The country will find, to its cost in case of war, that it is not in the underpaid and undervalued medical department that such reductions of power and emolument can be made. We fear that for a paltry saving of £800 per annum, and the acquisition of a little patronage by the Government, a considerable injury has been inflicted upon the medical department of the army."

19. Cantlie, *Army Medical Department*, Volume 2, p. 3.

20. Harrison, 1858. *Medical and Surgical History of the British Army in the War Against Russia 1854–6*. 2 Volumes. Volume 1, Preface (Cited by Cantlie, *Army Medical Department*, Volume 2, p. 7).

21. D. J. Larrey, 1812–1817. *Mémoires de Chirurgie Militaire, et Campagnes*. 4 Volumes (Paris: J. Smith), Volume 1, Plates III–VIII; J. H. Dible, 1970. *Napoleon's Surgeon* (London: William Heinemann Medical Books Ltd.), pp. 16–17.

22. Cantlie, *Army Medical Department*, Volume 2, p. 175.

23. Cantlie, *Army Medical Department*, Volume 2, p. 72.

24. Regulations affecting the Sanitary Condition of the Army, Appendix LXXIX, Letter 16, Eyre & Spottiswoode, 1858 (Cited by Cantlie, *Army Medical Department,* Volume 2, p. 19).

25. Anon., (Special Correspondent). 1854. The War. *Lancet* **I**, 202–203, p. 203: "The order from England for wearing the moustache was issued to the troops at Monastère this day (August 7th, 1854). It has been already, for some time past, adopted in other divisions,—it is presumed, with the sanction of the general commanding them. That part of the order which enjoins the under lip, chin, and upper part of the throat to be shorn, as well as a fixed space on each side of the angle of the mouth, will present a fair test of the advantages which were anticipated, in a medical point of view, from the growth of the hair in this situation, whether as a respirator affecting the air passing to the lungs, or as an external protection under all circumstances of exposure to the upper part of the throat. . . . It is reported that the commander of the forces will, for the present, dispense with the use of the razor altogether. . . . Few can doubt that the growth of hair on the lower part of the face and upper part of the throat would be a valuable protection. But whether this growth can be permitted without detracting from that propriety of appearance and uniformity which the military eye requires . . . is a matter which must be settled elsewhere." The moustache at that time was also thought to be of value in malarial country.

26. G. J. Guthrie, 1854. On the Medical Service of the British Army. *Lancet* **I**, 237–240.

27. Losses sustained during the First Burma War, 1824–1826, provide typical figures for the mortality and morbidity of the British forces who were involved in the colonial wars undertaken between 1824–1853: out of a strength of 2,716, 1,215 died of disease, 60 were killed in action and 30 died of wounds (Cantlie, *Army Medical Department*, Volume 1, p. 459).

28. G. J. Guthrie, 1853. *Commentaries on the Surgery of the War in Portugal, Spain, France, and the Netherlands, from the Battle of Roliça, in 1808, to that of Waterloo, in 1815, Showing the Improvements made during and since that period in the great art and science of surgery on all the subjects to which they relate.* 5th Edition (London: Henry Renshaw).

29. Anon., 1854. Mr. Guthrie's directions to army surgeons (Extracted from his *Pamphlet on the Hospital Brigade*). *Lancet* **II**, 155–157.

30. Guthrie, *Commentaries on Surgery*, 1853. The only reference to anesthetic agents in this book occurs in the final paragraph on the last page of text (p. 585), and this states as follows: "423. Chloroform, which has been recommended in all the great operations as a general rule, sometimes proves fatal, when incautiously administered as to quantity, or its use is too long continued. In America chloric ether has been found equally efficient and less dangerous. It should, therefore, be brought into more general use, and its qualities fully determined."

31. G. J. Guthrie, 1855. *Commentaries on the Surgery of the War in Portugal, Spain, France, and the Netherlands, from the Battle of Roliça, in 1808, to that of Waterloo, in 1815, with Additions Relating to those in the Crimea in 1854–55, Showing the Improvements made During and Since that Period in the Great Art and Science of Surgery on all the Subjects to which they Relate.* 6th Edition (Revised to October 1855) (London: Henry Renshaw).

32. For section on amputations, see: G. Ballingall, 1852. *Outlines of Military Surgery.* 4th Edition (Edinburgh: Adam & Charles Black), pp. 386–416. For observations on diagnosis of a patient with a fictitious illness using chloroform, p. 586.

33. First reports appeared in the *Lancet* of January 2, 1846 to draw attention to the earlier American report of Dr. H. J. Bigelow on "the anodyne effects of the inhalation of the vapour of sulphuric ether." This had been communicated to the editor by Dr. F. Booth

(*Lancet* **I**, 1847, pp. 5–8). According to Liston, writing in a letter to Dr. Booth dated December 21, 1846, an abstract of which was published here, "I tried the ether inhalation today in a case of amputation of the thigh . . . with the most perfect and satisfactory results." (*Lancet* **I**, 1847, p. 8).

34. R. Liston, 1824. Observations on amputation. *Edinburgh Medical and Surgical Journal* **21**, 42–46.

35. J. Syme, 1824. Successful case of amputation at the hip-joint. *Edinburgh Medical and Surgical Journal* **21**, 19–27; J. Syme, 1824. Remarks on amputation. *Edinburgh Medical and Surgical Journal* **21**, 27–42.

36. J. Y. Simpson, 1847. A new anaesthetic agent, more efficient than sulphuric ether. *Lancet* **II**, 549–550.

37. Anon., *Guthrie's directions to army surgeons*. According to Guthrie: "32. Chloroform may be administered in all cases of amputation of the upper extremity and below the knee, and in all minor operations; which cases may also be deferred, without disadvantage, until the more serious operations are performed. 33. Amputation at the upper and middle parts of the thigh are to be done as soon as possible after the receipt of the injury. The administration of chloroform in them, when there is much prostration, is doubtful, and must be attended to, and observed with great care. The question whether it should or should not be administered in such cases being undecided."

38. Guthrie, 1855. Military Surgery in the Crimea. A Lecture delivered at the Royal College of Surgeons of England, on Saturday, April 14, 1855. *Lancet* **I**, 413–417, pp. 414–415.

39. Guthrie, *Commentaries on Surgery, 1855*, pp. 37, 40, Addenda pp. 617–619.

40. Guthrie, *Commentaries on Surgery, 1855*, Addenda, p. 619.

41. T. Wakley, 1848. A record of one hundred experiments on animals, with ether and chloroform. *Lancet* **I**, 19–25.

42. Cantlie, *Army Medical Department*, Volume 2, p. 125.

43. Cantlie, *Army Medical Department*, Volume 2, p. 129.

44. Cantlie, *Army Medical Department*, Volume 1, p. 336. The chief items included in the panniers were lint, surgeon's tow, sponges, linen—both loose and in rollers, silk and wax for ligatures, pins, tape, thread, needles, adhesive plaster—ready spread and in rolls, opium—both solid and in tincture, submuriate of mercury, antimonials, sulphate of magnesia, volatile alkali, and oil of turpentine. There was in addition a capital case of surgical instruments. Medical comforts were also kept in the panniers, and included tea, chocolate, portable soup, lemon juice, and sometimes wine.

45. Roebuck Committee, 16556–16561, cited by Cantlie, *Army Medical Department*, Volume 2, p. 54.

46. Shepherd, *Crimean Doctors*, Volume 1, p. 158.

47. This number was selected by Miss Nightingale to allow two and a half to three nurses for every 100 bed cases. See: Cantlie, *Army Medical Department*, Volume 2, p. 91.

48. Cantlie, *Army Medical Department*, Volume 2, p. 91.

49. Cantlie, *Army Medical Department*, Volume 2, pp. 96–97.

50. Cantlie, *Army Medical Department*, Volume 2, pp. 97–98.

51. F. Nightingale, 1859. *Notes on Hospitals: Being Two Papers read before the National Association for the Promotion of Social Science, at Liverpool, in October 1858. With Evidence Given to the Royal Commissioners on the State of the Army in 1857* (London: J.W. Parker & Son); E. Cook, 1913. *The Life of Florence Nightingale*. In 2 Volumes (London: Macmillan & Co.) [Volume 1, 1820–1861; Volume 2, 1862–1910]; C. Woodham-Smith, 1950. *Florence Nightingale 1820–1910* (London: Constable); Z. Cope, 1958. *Florence Nightingale and the Doctors* (London: Museum Press).

52. Cantlie, *Army Medical Department*, Volume 2, p. 81.

53. G. Ballingall, 1823. *Practical observations on fever, dysentery, and liver complaints, as they occur amongst the European troops in India; illustrated by numerous tables and cases. To which is annexed an essay on syphilis*. 2nd Edition (Edinburgh: Adam Black; London: T & G Underwood; Dublin: Hodges & McArthur); G. Ballingall, 1855. On the too early enlistment of recruits. *Lancet* **I**, 78–79.

54. Cantlie, *Army Medical Department*, Volume 2, p. 132.

55. S. M. Mitra, 1911. *The Life and Letters of Sir John Hall M.D., K.C.B., F.R.C.S.* (London: Longmans, Green & Co.), see p. 386.

56. C. Bryce, 1857. *England and France before Sebastopol, looked at from a medical point of view* (London: J. Churchill), pp. (b) and 2.

57. Bryce, *Sebastopol*, p. 45.

58. Cantlie, *Army Medical Department*, Volume 2, p. 145.

59. The two commissioners were Sir John McNeill, a doctor by training who had for 24 years been Chargé d'Affaires in Teheran, and had then been appointed chairman of the Board of Supervision administering the new Poor Law in Scotland. The other commissioner was Colonel Alexander Tulloch, a regular army officer with a considerable interest and knowledge of statistics. They traveled to Scutari, where they took evidence from a substantial number of witnesses of all ranks. Their fine work was eventually acknowledged in that McNeill was made a member of the Privy Council, and Colonel Tulloch was knighted. It was generally accepted that the commission's findings, which were in any case already in the public domain, stood the test of time, and the changes in military administration recommended by them were, in the long term, largely implemented.

60. Miss Nightingale, in a letter to Sidney Herbert, had drawn attention to the fact that since so few postmortem examinations had been carried out on those who had died, virtually no information was available on the principal causes of death, other than the diagnoses made by the attendant medical officers, many of which were either vague or nonexistent (cited by Shepherd, *The Crimean Doctors*, Volume 2, p. 405).

61. Shepherd, *Crimean Doctors*, Volume 2, pp. 406–408.

62. Cantlie, *Army Medical Department*, Volume 2, p. 153.

63. Cantlie, *Army Medical Department*, Volume 2, p. 160.

64. Engineer of the Great Western Railway and the Rotherhithe Tunnel under the Thames.

65. Shepherd, *Crimean Doctors*, Volume 2, p. 439.

66. J. W. Fortescue, 1899–1930. *A History of the British Army*. Thirteen Volumes (London: Macmillan & Co.), Volume 13, p. 227; Cantlie, *Army Medical Department*, Volume 2, p. 183.

67. Shepherd, *Crimean Doctors*, Volume 2, p. 540.

68. Shepherd, *Crimean Doctors*, Volume 2, p. 542.

69. The detailed breakdown of the various diseases that led to the death of seamen in the Baltic and Black Sea fleets is provided by C. Lloyd and J.L.S. Coulter, 1963. *Medicine and the Navy 1200–1900*. Volume 4—1815–1900 (Edinburgh and London: E. & S. Livingstone Ltd.), see p. 152.

70. Anon., 1858. The Distinction Conferred on Dr. Andrew Smith. *Lancet* **II**, 69 [brief editorial].

71. Michie, 1877. *Memoirs of Sir Andrew Smith* (Alnwick: Blair), p. 15 (cited by Cantlie, *Army Medical Department*, Volume 2, p. 214).

72. A. Smith, 1849. *Illustrations of the Zoology of South Africa Consisting Chiefly of Figures and Descriptions of the Objects of Natural History Collected During an Expedition into the Interior of South Africa, in the years 1834, 1835, and 1836; fitted out by "The Cape of Good Hope Association for Exploring Central Africa"* (London: Smith,

Elder & Co.) [In 5 Volumes: Mammalia, Aves, Reptilia, Pisces, and Invertebratae. Note that these volumes are unnumbered and, apart from the prefaces, the pages in these books are also unnumbered].

73. Cantlie, *Army Medical Department*, Volume 2, p. 215.
74. Lloyd and Coulter, *Medicine and the Navy*, p. 153.
75. Cantlie, *Army Medical Department*, Volume 2, p. 185.
76. Bryce, *Sebastopol*, pp. 10–11.
77. Bryce, *Sebastopol*, p. 10.
78. Bryce, *Sebastopol*, p. 34.

5

EDUCATION OF MEDICAL OFFICERS DURING THE POST–CRIMEAN WAR PERIOD

THE ESTABLISHMENT OF THE ARMY MEDICAL SCHOOL AT FORT PITT, CHATHAM (1860), AND ITS RELOCATION AT NETLEY (1863)

One of the consequences of the Crimean War, highlighted by the public's alarm at the poor medical services and terrible treatment of the sick and wounded, was the appointment by the government, in 1857, of a Royal Commission. Its specific remit was to inquire into "the regulations affecting the sanitary condition of the army, the reorganization of military hospitals, and the treatment of the sick and wounded." The president of the commission was the Right Honourable Sidney Herbert, and one of the members was Sir James Ranald Martin, physician to the Secretary of State for India. The commission reported back to Parliament early in 1858. One of its principal proposals was the establishment of an Army Medical School, along similar lines to those suggested toward the end of the previous century by John Bell, and by McGrigor during his appointment as director-general of the Army Medical Services. The Royal Commission recommended: "That, after the first, or Entrance examination, candidates for commissions should be sent to a military general hospital, there to go through a course of instruction in military hygiene and in clinical military medicine and surgery, for which purpose the necessary professional chairs, in lieu of the two now existing in Edinburgh and Dublin, should be instituted at the principal general hospital in England."

This would clearly involve the expenditure of large sums of public money on the building of a purpose-built postgraduate institute with its own teaching hospital with direct access to suitable clinical material and adequate research facilities. Medical officers who planned to enter one of the services, such as the army, navy, or Honourable East India Company, would be sent there for usually three to six months of intensive postgraduate training. They would be exposed to the typical problems that they would be likely to encounter in their respective service, as well as being introduced to the rigors of military discipline. Their studies would be undertaken in an academic environment, and their teachers would be both specialists within their respective disciplines and, just as important, experienced in active service in the field.

Previously, only negligible sums of money had been expended in Edinburgh and later in Dublin in supporting the salary of two academic appointments, any other expenditure being offset by students' fees, with additional indirect administrative and other support from the host institutions. While this approach clearly served a useful purpose in introducing a small selection of medical students who happened to be studying in Edinburgh or Dublin to the possibility of a career in the military medical service, it could only be, at best, an interim solution.

After a delay of over 60 years since its first conception by Bell,[1] the Army Medical School was eventually established at Fort Pitt, Chatham, toward the end of March 1860, when its senate or governing body was appointed. Jackson[2] had recommended the establishment of an "army medical practical school," indicating, in considerable detail, the subjects which he considered ought to be taught in it. What had particularly depressed many serving medical officers during the late 18th and 19th centuries was the knowledge that on the Continent schools had long been established for the advanced training of military and naval medical officers. This was particularly the case in France, where as early as 1747 schools of military surgery and medicine had been established in connection with army hospitals in large garrison towns such as Metz, Strasburg, Toulon, and Lisle. Later, in 1852, the training of army medical officers was concentrated in the great military medical school at Val-de-Grâce, near Paris.[3] Naval medical schools had also been established at Toulon, Brest, and Rochefort, the latter as early as in 1722.

McGrigor established a specialist institute at Fort Pitt, Chatham, where postgraduate military medical studies could be undertaken in 1817, which had both a museum and library facilities. New recruits into the medical service of the army would, immediately after their acceptance into the service, spend a period of time at Chatham before joining a regiment. Here they could benefit from the excellent academic facilities, complemented by access to clinical cases at the local military hospital at Haslar and specialist lecturers with a wide experience in the service in both local and foreign stations.

Seven members of the senior medical staff who were appointed in 1860 to oversee the teaching at the postgraduate institute consisted of three senior administrators and four professors:

Inspector-General	Gibson	Director-General, Army Medical Department
Inspector-General	J. R. Martin	Physician to the Secretary of State for India
Inspector-General	J. R. Taylor	Inspector-General, Army Medical Department, at Chatham
Surgeon-General	Sir Thomas Longmore	Professor of Military Surgery (1860–1891)
Surgeon-Major	C. Morehead	Professor of Military Medicine (1860–1861)
Surgeon-General	W. C. Maclean	Professor of Military Medicine (1861–1886)
	Dr. E. A. Parkes	Professor of Military Hygiene (1860–1876)
	Dr. (later Sir) William Aitken	Professor of Pathology (1860–1892)

Drs. Longmore and Parkes were retired officers of the Army Medical Department, Dr. Morehead belonged to the Indian Medical Service, and Dr. Aitken had served as pathologist to the army in the Crimean War. Surgeon-major Morehead resigned in March 1861, and was succeeded by surgeon-major (hon. surgeon general) W. C. Maclean, who remained in office until 1886.

Mr. Tufnell, who had lectured on military hygiene and military surgery in Dublin since 1846, had collected a substantial museum consisting principally of models of appliances for the transport and treatment of the wounded. These items were subsequently transferred to Netley in 1863.

The school was originally constituted to train 45 candidates every six months for entry into the Army Medical Department. The course itself was to last for only four months. All of the candidates were admitted following a competitive examination, and all possessed appropriate medical qualifications. The parliamentary committee had decided that candidates henceforth "had to possess qualifications equal to those of civil doctors entering practice." This meant that candidates had to not only possess the Diploma of the Royal College of Surgeons, but also be licentiates of the Royal College of Physicians.[4] Before commissioning, candidates had to have attended courses of instruction in military medicine, surgery, and hygiene. The committee also decreed that these courses had to be given in a military hospital. This inevitably led to the establishment of the Army Medical School, and brought an end to the support provided by the government for the Regius Chairs of Military Surgery in Edinburgh and Dublin. Many candidates at that time were reluctant to return to school, despite not having previously been exposed to the specialist subjects to be taught at the Army Medical School.

From 1863 to 1865, only those candidates who had been selected for service in the Army Medical Department attended the School. It was only from 1871 that naval candidates also attended Netley. In order to accommodate the special needs of the naval candidates, an additional Chair of Naval Hygiene was established. In 1880, with the establishment of the Naval Medical School at Haslar Hospital, at Gosport, those officers entering the Naval Medical Service were then taught at Haslar. The last group of military medical officers (Royal Army Medical Corps) attended Netley in 1902, when the new Army Medical School and Staff College were opened at Millbank. After 1902, candidates for both the Army Medical Service and those intending to enter the Indian Medical

Service were sent to the new school for a period of two months. Those destined for the Royal Army Medical Corps were then transferred to Aldershot, while those intending to enter the Indian Medical Service went to Netley for an additional period of two months of instruction in military medicine and military surgery.

During the period between 1863 and the beginning of the 20th century, the Army Medical School encountered numerous difficulties. In 1876, the government decided that the cost of training candidates for the Army Medical Service should no longer be a charge on the State. Some Members of Parliament considered that it was no longer possible to justify the 4-month period of training, when this was only associated with the 10-year "short service" commission. It was only when the senate of the Medical School provided a lengthy report in which they justified the retention of the School's existence that the proposal to close the School was withdrawn.

The School soon demonstrated that it was a model on which schools in other countries should be based, and officers from several of the Continental armies attended its courses. Calls were again made for its closure in the 1880s, again on the grounds of its unjustified expenditure.

After the South African War, the government decided that the Army Medical School should be relocated in London, to be closer to the other institutions of medical learning already established there. In May 1907, the Royal Army Medical College, as it was then styled, opened in well-equipped premises at Millbank, in London, with a commandant and Director of Studies who was responsible to the director-general, rather than a senate. The school at Netley finally closed in 1905, after which time the candidates attended the school at Millbank, with additional periods of instruction at Aldershot.[5]

THE HOSPITAL TO BE ASSOCIATED WITH THE ARMY MEDICAL SCHOOL

The clinical (practical) component of the course was initially taught at Fort Pitt, as this was the only establishment with adequate numbers of convalescent patients from abroad. The very poor standard of the sanitary arrangements there was not considered conducive to the teaching of the principles of hygiene. The Army Medical School remained at Fort Pitt for three years until it moved to Netley, when it became associated with the Royal Victoria Hospital.

With the opening of the Royal Victoria Hospital at Netley in 1863, all the invalids from abroad were now directed here instead of to Fort Pitt. Queen Victoria had laid its foundation stone in May 1856, and it was originally designed as an invaliding hospital, without any intention of having an Army Medical College grafted onto it. Queen Victoria believed that the sick and wounded of her army should have the healthiest and best accommodation that money and skill could procure. The Queen had visited the General Hospital at Fort Pitt, Chatham, on four occasions during the Crimean War when it was being used as the principal hospital for receiving those who had been invalided during the war.

During one of her early visits, she drove from the Brompton Barracks Hospital to St. Mary's Hospital, where she inspected more than 600 convalescent soldiers all drawn up in line.[6] All had a label indicating their name, rank, nature of their injury, and where the injury had been sustained. After inspecting these men, the Queen and her party walked across to see the Casement Barracks, and were quite horrified at the conditions there. "Are these really the barrack-rooms of these invalids?" The medical officer who accompanied the royal party, deputy inspector-general of hospitals George Dartnell, said, "Yes, indeed, they are Your Majesty," and Prince Albert, looking over toward the splendid convict prison recently built in view of the Casement Barracks, said, "Well, it seems very extraordinary that there should be no difficulty in obtaining money to erect a magnificent building like that for convicts, and that it should be impossible to find the means of building a commonly comfortable barrack for our convalescent soldiers."

It is said that both Queen Victoria and Prince Albert took a personal interest in the selection of the site, and the subsequent planning of the hospital.[7] The building was completed in April 1863, and received its first intake of soldiers who had been invalided during service in India and in the Colonies. While it had accommodation for 1,000 patients, the number of inmates often fell far short of this. During the South African War, the hospital was full to overflowing, and huts were set up in the grounds to accommodate the overflow.

THE DIFFICULTIES ENCOUNTERED BY MEDICAL OFFICERS IN THE THREE BRANCHES OF THE SERVICE, THE ARMY, NAVY, AND INDIAN MEDICAL SERVICE, DURING THE PERIOD BETWEEN THE CRIMEAN WAR AND 1879

By far the most detailed and accessible account of the state of the medical services in the Army, Navy, and Indian Medical Service between the Crimean War and 1879 is to be found in Rivington.[8] This encyclopedic monograph discussed all aspects of the medical profession in Britain at that time. It also detailed the mode of entry into these various branches of the service, their pay structure, mechanism of achieving promotion, the grades structure, and, particularly, the conditions of service. Details of the various warrants that governed all aspects of the pay and conditions of service of these officers are provided, and how these either bettered or worsened their conditions of service.

What was also emphasized were the difficulties medical officers invariably encountered in relation to obtaining parity with other officers of nominally similar rank within the same service or between the different services. While the conditions of service in the Army Medical Department over this period were poor, and the chance of promotion limited, becoming increasingly so over the relatively brief period considered, the situation in the navy was in all regards far worse. Not surprisingly, this information reached the medical student population, and for many individual years during this period the number of candidates seeking entry into this service were often far fewer than there were places available to fill.

It is therefore appropriate to consider why the conditions were often so poor that the quality of the entry, even into the Army Medical Department, was, in the opinion of the senior medical staff, almost invariably associated with second-rate candidates. Of those who successfully gained entry into the service during this period, the majority were in fact trained in Ireland. This situation had never previously been encountered during the pre–Crimean War period.

ENTRY REQUIREMENTS INTO THE DIFFERENT BRANCHES OF THE SERVICE

After the establishment of the Army Medical School, the mode of entry into all three medical services was by competitive examination. Candidates for commission into the army medical branch had to be between 21 and 32 years of age, free from physical defect or constitutional disease, and with vision that was sufficiently good that the individual could perform surgical operations without glasses. The age range for entry into the naval branch was 21–28, and for the Indian Medical Service was 22–28. The entrance examination took place over a period of six days. Candidates were initially examined in anatomy, physiology, medicine including therapeutics, diseases of women and children, surgery, chemistry, and pharmacology, and practical knowledge of drugs. Each of these subjects carried a maximum mark of 1,000.

The examinations in medicine and surgery were partly of a practical nature, and included operations on the dead body, application of surgical apparatus, and the examination of medical and surgical patients at the bedside. The candidates could also be examined in a series of additional voluntary subjects, such as French, German, or Hindustani (for the Indian Medical Service only), each of which carried a maximum mark of 150, while the examination in natural sciences carried a maximum mark of 300. The eligibility of candidates into the service was determined on the basis of the marks in the compulsory subjects, but marks from the voluntary subjects were added in order to determine the "order of merit."

The successful candidates then underwent a four-month probationary period at Netley Hospital, near Southampton. They also had to attend one course of practical instruction in the following subjects: hygiene, clinical and (naval and) military medicine, clinical and (naval and) military surgery, pathology of diseases, and injuries incident to military service. The military surgery component of the course paid particular attention to gunshot wounds and the duties of army surgeons on active service and in the field.

Full details of the equivalent ranking structure between individuals in the various medical branches and the field and wardroom ranks is then discussed, with details of their appropriate salaries.

CONDITIONS OF SERVICE IN THE ARMY MEDICAL DEPARTMENT DURING THE EARLY POST–CRIMEAN WAR PERIOD

Rivington[9] draws attention to the average death rate of medical officers at various times during the pre- and post–Crimean War period, and compares these figures with those of individuals in civilian occupations (per 1,000 adult males in England at that time). The information is as follows:

Average annual death rate per 1,000	adult males in England	9–10
–ditto–	army officers (excluding medical officers)	15
–ditto–	army medical officers (1839–1854)	34
–ditto–	army medical officers (during the Crimean War)	67
–ditto–	army medical officers (since the Crimean War)	20

The death rate of members of the Army Medical Department was 44% higher than that of males of all social classes, in civilian occupations, and 75% higher than that of males of the same social class.

There was considerable concern within the civilian medical community, many of whom felt that the constraints imposed on their colleagues in the medical service of the army did not allow them to express their concern as freely as they might wish. A deputation from the Parliamentary Bills Committee of the British Medical Association whose president, in 1874, was Sir William Fergusson, sergeant-surgeon to the Queen, the director-general of the Army Medical Service, Sir William Muir, accompanied by a considerable delegation of distinguished doctors, went to see the Secretary of State for War, Mr. Gathorne Hardy, at the War Office. Mr. Ernest Hardy, chairman of the parliamentary committee summarized the concerns of the military medical officers in an article in the *British Medical Journal*.

There was "very wide dissatisfaction in the Army Medical Service, . . . disappointment, . . . some felt that they were not being justly dealt with. Especially in junior ranks, but it pervaded the entire service. Most important issue, complete stagnation of promotion." Mr. Hart drew attention to the fact that "In 1859, for instance, the average general service in the junior rank, without promotion, was 7 years; in 1860, it was 8 years; then, in 1862, it had risen to 9 years; in 1864, it had risen to 10 years; in 1866, it had come to 12 years; in 1868, it had come to 13 years; and from 1870 to 1874, it had been 15 years." This contrasted with the situation in the IMS, "where it was established that, after 12 years' service, the medical officer was to receive promotion." He continued, "The present Director-General . . . was promoted to be Deputy Inspector-General after 16 years of service; but under the present state of things, he would have had to serve for 16 years before he was promoted out of the junior rank; and it would now take a man as long to reach the rank of Surgeon-Major, as it took Sir William Muir to reach the position of Deputy Inspector-General."[10]

In 1878, the number of candidates was entirely insufficient to fill the vacancies in the service; moreover, the standard of candidates was falling on a regular basis. The committee of 1878 admitted that "the diminished supply (of good candidates) has necessitated the employment of medical men lower and lower down the pass lists, although even then the establishment has not been kept up." In some of the home stations, the pressure had been so great that the deficiencies had had to be made up by employing civilian medical practitioners.

CONDITIONS OF SERVICE IN THE NAVAL MEDICAL DEPARTMENT

Rivington also considered the grievances of the medical officers in the navy in considerable detail.[11] Possibly the most contentious issue relating to the conditions of service in the navy was due to the failure of implementation of the order in council of George III of 1805, obtained by Lord Melville, through the good offices of Lord Nelson. This order of council conferred on naval medical officers "similar rank with the officers of the same class in His Majesty's Land Service." From 1805 until 1859, this order was not implemented by the Lords of the Admiralty, despite intermittent efforts, for example, in 1839–1840, by parliamentary committees set up specifically to investigate grievances in the service, and empowered "to make recommendations for its improvement." Some changes were brought about with respect to salary, but assistant-surgeons, who were not considered wardroom officers, were still relegated to the cockpit.

A resolution was eventually carried, in opposition to the wishes of the government of the day, that "the accommodation provided for the assistant-surgeons on board Her Majesty's ships of war is inadequate and insufficient for securing the full benefit of their professional services." The Lords of the Admiralty, however, insisted that assistant-surgeons were not permitted in the wardroom until they had been three years in the service, and attained the rank of surgeon. With the outbreak of the Crimean War, in 1854, the right of entry to the wardroom was finally granted to medical officers immediately on their entry into the service.

For the first time, in 1869, examiners from the Army Medical Department conducted the examination for the admission of candidates into the navy. From 1871, an arrangement between the Admiralty and the War Office allowed candidates for the Naval Medical Service to attend the courses of professional instruction at Netley. This led to an increase in the number of good candidates offering themselves for the Naval Service and in 1873 more candidates came forward than there were places for them in the service. Sixteen out of the total of 19 candidates who were accepted were the products of the Irish medical schools.

Considering the number of warrants that were issued during the post–Crimean War period, and the abject failure to address the resentment felt by medical officers in both the army and navy, it is only possible to draw two conclusions: (1) that the lines of communication between those in the two services and their political masters were at all times grossly impaired, and (2) that the generals in the War Office and admirals in the Admiralty were completely out of touch with the groundswell of opinion in the medical branches of the two services. What clearly did not help the situation was the behavior of their lordships in the

Admiralty, who persisted in holding the view that medical officers were socially inferior to executive officers and should not be admitted to the wardroom. Slightly less extreme views were also held in the army, but these nevertheless still severely hampered social integration between medical and field officers in that service.

THE EVOLUTION OF THE ARMY MEDICAL CORPS

There was a universal acceptance that the system employed by the French since the end of the 18th century, as proposed and implemented by Baron Larrey, provided an excellent solution to the problems encountered in the rapid and efficient evacuation of casualties from the battlefield. It was also agreed that the provision of a corps of appropriately trained staff who would be available to assist the medical officers in their duties was an excellent idea. Despite this, there appears to have been an unwillingness to implement such a plan in the British army, principally because the regiments were reluctant to release fit men for noncombatant duties. By contrast, in the French army, because of conscription, there was no shortage of able-bodied recruits who could be assigned to these duties.

While Wellington acknowledged the value of an efficient Army Medical Department, because it significantly increased the number of combatants available to him, he was not prepared to release fit men for noncombatant duties. The effect of this policy was obvious in the Peninsular War, and similar problems were encountered in the Crimean War. It was clearly apparent that little purpose was to be served by supplying individuals from the regiments who were physically, educationally, and psychologically unfit for military duties to assist the medical staff in their activities.

When such individuals were assigned as drivers in the Peninsula, for example, they were often so drunk as to be entirely incapable of carrying out their duties. Similarly, when they were assigned to regimental or general hospitals as ward orderlies, their behavior more often than not meant that they were a danger to the well-being of their charges. In the campaign in the West Indies, toward the end of the 18th century, it was generally considered a blessing when their lives were cut short by drunkenness and yellow fever.[12]

The Hospital Corps, which briefly existed in the West Indies, survived for only about six months, while the Corps that had been proposed by van Millingen[13] failed to become a reality. During the Crimean War, a Hospital Conveyance Corps was established, with recruits from military pensioners and other groups of largely ineffective and often dysfunctional noncombatants. They acted as stretcher-bearers on the battlefield, supplied drivers for the transport of the sick and wounded, and worked as servants for the medical officers as well as ward orderlies in the hospitals. As in previous campaigns, the system was a complete failure, principally because of the unsuitability of the men delegated to undertake these duties. For a time, the Land Transport Corps organized the transport of the sick and wounded to the hospitals after they had been removed from the battlefield.

It was only in June 1855, following the issuing of an appropriate royal warrant, that the first Medical Staff Corps was established. This initially consisted of 9 companies, each containing 78 men; these were assigned exclusively to hospital duties. It contained only one officer, for the general management of the corps, and he was based at their depot initially at Chatham, but in 1863 was moved to Netley. In 1873, its headquarters moved to London, while its depot moved from Netley to Aldershot in 1875. When the men were assigned to hospital duties, they were put under the command of the principal medical officer and the purveyor. Their noncommissioned officers (NCOs) bore no military badges of rank, but ranked as equivalent to the different NCO grades.[14]

By September 1855, a further royal warrant was issued which increased their strength to 10 companies, each consisting of 120 men. Despite high expectations, the corps was a failure. This principally was because of the absence of any military structure in its organization. The recruits were all volunteers from other line regiments, but had no special training, and were often poorly educated. This deficiency was soon recognized, and a new royal warrant was issued in August 1857 which established "a new corps of attendants at Military Hospitals . . . which shall be called *The Army Hospital Corps*." When associated with hospitals, they were put under the control of the principal medical officer of each station, or senior medical officer of each regiment. The members of the corps initially wore a gray uniform, but in 1861 this was changed to a blue uniform with gray facings, and later this was amended to scarlet facings.[15] The uniform of the officers was changed from scarlet to blue to be similar to that of the men they commanded. Only toward the end of the century did those of a dull cherry replace the scarlet facings.

All of the men had to be of good character, had to be able to read and write, and had to be recommended by their commanding officer. They served on probation for six months before they were transferred to the corps. In August 1877, another royal warrant decreed that the director-general of the Army Medical Department was to be in overall charge of the administration of the corps. A number of additional royal warrants were issued during the 1880s, and these dealt specifically with the conditions of pay within the service and the designation of its officers and NCOs. By a royal warrant of June 23, 1898, all officers of the army medical staff below the rank of surgeon-general, and the warrant-officers, NCOs, and men of the Medical Staff Corps were united to form the Royal Army Medical Corps.

CHANGES BROUGHT ABOUT TOWARD THE END OF THE 19TH CENTURY WITH THE ESTABLISHMENT OF THE ROYAL ARMY MEDICAL CORPS IN 1898

Reference to Blair's recent *History of the Royal Army Medical Corps* reveals many examples which confirm that it was again the stimulus of the British Medical Association that pressed the Secretary of State for War, Lord Lansdowne, to bring in long-needed reforms.[16] Their principal concern was the very low morale of officers in the Army Medical Department. Negotiations continued for some considerable time, until the Queen agreed that the new corps should be called the Royal Army Medical Corps, and Royal Warrant Army Order 93 of 1898 confirmed the foundation of the Royal Army Medical Corps. With this warrant, the Medical Staff Corps was abolished.[17]

NOTES

1. J. Bell, 1798. *Memoir on the Present State of Naval and Military Surgery. Addressed to the Right Honourable Earl Spenser [sic], First Lord of the Admiralty* [21 pp. Yarmouth, January 20, 1798].

2. R. Jackson, 1805. *A System of Arrangement and Discipline for the Medical Department of Armies* (London: J. Murray).

3. J. H. Dible, 1970. *Napoleon's Surgeon* (London: William Heinemann Medical Books Ltd.).

4. N. Cantlie, 1974. *A History of the Army Medical Department*. 2 Volumes (Edinburgh and London: Churchill Livingstone), Volume 2, p. 202.

5. K. MacLeod, 1906. Netley. *Caledonian Medical Journal* **6**, 379–390; D. G. Crawford, 1914. *A History of the Indian Medical Service 1600–1913*. 2 Volumes. Volume 1, 529 pp; Volume 2, 535 pp. (London: W. Thacker & Co.; Calcutta & Simla: Thacker Spink & Co.), Volume 1, pp. 524–528.

6. G. R. Dartnell, 1904. Notes of Queen Victoria's visit to Fort Pitt and Chatham. Parts I and II. *Journal of the Royal Army Medical Corps* **3**, 87–92, 191–196, pp. 91–92.

7. Crawford, *Indian Medical Service*, Volume **1**, 524–528; MacLeod, *Netley*, p. 379.

8. W. Rivington, 1879. *The Medical Profession: being the Essay to which was awarded the First Carmichael Prize of £200 by the Council of the Royal College of Surgeons, Ireland, 1879* (Dublin: Fannin & Co.; London: Longmans & Co.; Baillière, Tindall, & Cox; Edinburgh: Maclachlan & Stewart), pp. 208–239.

9. Rivington, *Medical Profession*, pp. 210–211.

10. Anon., 1874. The Association and the Army Medical Officers. *British Medical Journal* **1**, 622–624, p. 622.

11. Rivington, *Medical Profession*, pp. 232–237.

12. J. Fergusson, 1846. *Notes and Recollections of a Professional Life, by the Late William Fergusson, Esq. M.D. Inspector General of Military Hospitals. Edited by his son, James Fergusson* (London: Longman, Brown, Green & Longmans).

13. J. G. van Millingen, 1819. *The Army Medical Officer's Manual upon Active Service; Precepts for his Guidance in the Various Situations in which he may be placed; with Observations on the Preservation of the Health of Armies upon Foreign Service* (London: Burgess & Hill) [According to F. Smith, 1929. *A Short History of the Royal Army Medical Corps* (Aldershot: Gale & Polden Ltd.), this volume was first published in 1805, and reprinted in 1819].

14. W. Johnston, 1917. *Roll of Commissioned Officers in the Medical Service of the British Army who served on full pay within the period between the Accession of George II and the Formation of the Royal Army Medical Corps 20 June 1727 to 23 June 1898. With an Introduction Showing the Historical Evolution of the Corps, by W. J., Ed. by H.A.L. Howell* (Aberdeen: University Press), pp. lx–lxiii.

15. Smith, *Royal Army Medical Corps*, pp. 13, 20–22.

16. J.S.G. Blair, 1998. *Centenary History of the Royal Army Medical Corps (1898–1998)* (Edinburgh: Scottish Academic Press), pp. xviii and xix.

17. Smith, *Royal Army Medical Corps*, pp. 16–52; Cantlie, *Army Medical Department*, Volume 2, pp. 233–235, 354–364.

6

CONCLUSIONS: THE 19TH CENTURY— A CENTURY OF CONFLICT

During this discussion of the role of the Army Medical Department during the second half of the 18th and most of the 19th centuries, numerous examples of tensions between different groups have emerged. Some of the more glaring examples will be considered in this section, because of the light they shed on contemporary attitudes toward the activities of the Army Medical Department during this period.

After the relatively brief period of enlightened leadership provided by surgeon general John Hunter,[1] the Secretary for War decided that it would be advantageous if the duties previously supervised by Hunter were shared among three distinguished civilian clinicians.[2] Sir Lucas Pepys,[3] physician-in-ordinary to the King, was appointed physician-general, Mr. John Gunning, who had recently been Master of the Surgeons' Company, was appointed surgeon general, and Mr. Thomas Keate, a former regimental surgeon to the Foot Guards, was appointed inspector of regimental hospitals. Their activities were to be undertaken on a part-time basis, with a small backup secretarial staff. Their specific remit was to supervise all aspects of the administration of the service, but they still managed to spend much of their time attending to their other clinical activities. Unfortunately, among them they had only a minimal amount of experience of military administration. These deficiencies were clearly evident from some of the decisions made, particularly by Sir Lucas Pepys, the senior member of the Board, shortly after his appointment. Hunter recommended that anyone with adequate military experience gained in any part of the world should be eligible to become a military physician, as this in his view more than compensated for any lack of academic qualifications. This was not a view shared by physician-general Pepys. Pepys indicated that only individuals with an Oxbridge medical degree associated with a diploma from the London College of

Physicians would henceforth be eligible for appointment as physician within the service. This decision alone excluded virtually all serving medical officers, many with considerable military experience, from applying for promotion within the service, and rapidly led to a breakdown in morale in the ranks and an outcry from many quarters.[4]

Considerable difficulties were also encountered when expeditions left British shores, as principal medical officers tended to act autonomously by filling in vacancies when they arose with local candidates of proven ability, rather than awaiting appointees sent out by the Board. These were often returned home on arrival at their destination, as the post they had come to fill was no longer available. Appointments made by the Board were frequently made on the basis of influence rather than on military experience. While the three members of the Board had different but overlapping areas of authority, the system failed because of the incompatible personalities of the three appointees. One in particular, Francis Knight, who had previously served as a regimental surgeon in the Guards but had not held a senior administrative post in the service, was appointed inspector of regimental hospitals in 1801. Knight often acted on his own initiative, and was extremely hostile to the activities of his two senior colleagues. The situation came to a head in 1809 when 4,000 men died from a type of malaria termed "polder" or "Walcheren fever," and another 11,000 had to be invalided out of the service following the expedition to the island of Walcheren. Neither the physician-general nor the surgeon general wished to visit the island to establish the cause of the problem.[5] The commander-in-chief, the Duke of York, was outraged, and a government inquiry with very wide-ranging powers was established. It investigated all aspects of the Board's activities and found little to justify its retention. Evidence of favoritism in medical appointments was uncovered, as well as numerous examples of gross inefficiency and wastage.[6] The Board was accordingly dissolved, and a new Board established consisting exclusively of senior regular military medical officers. The decision was also made that in future, no more part-time civilians would be appointed to the Board.

The lack of military experience displayed by the members of the Army Medical Board eventually led to its downfall. This was in marked contrast to the situation in the Crimean War, where Miss Nightingale's lack of military experience but considerable administrative competence was an undoubted advantage to her. For her first few months in the East, she had the ear and enthusiastic support of Mr. Sidney Herbert, the Secretary-at-War, in London. She could communicate directly with him should the need arise, and was always given a sympathetic hearing. It was with his invitation that she organized and superintended the female nursing activities at the British medical hospitals in Turkey.[7] While her activities in the East were undertaken with the approval of Dr. Andrew Smith, the director-general of the Army Medical Department, she was, however, directly responsible locally to his deputy, the chief medical officer at Scutari. With the financial support of Mr. MacDonald of the *Times* fund[8] she had the resources to act independently of the military hierarchy should the need arise. This proved invaluable in times of difficulty when, for example, individuals in the Commissariat Corps were being particularly intransigent. On such occasions, she had no qualms in purchasing items of stores from the bazaars in Constantinople.

Tensions certainly existed during the Crimean War due to differences between military and civilian ideas of competence and efficiency. This was the case vis à vis the relationship between Dr. Andrew Smith and his medical staff and the members of the military high command. Smith was in charge of the medical staff officers, but had only limited control over the regimental medical officers, as they held commissions in their respective regiments and were under the orders of their commanding officers. The Medical Department was technically a civil department, and this complicated any dealings Smith had with the headquarters staff. Most of the military hierarchy did not accept the need for the existence of an Army Medical Department whose command structure was independent of military control, and any formal requests they made for assistance tended to be ignored or, at best, were only dealt with as matters of the lowest priority. When decisions had to be made, for example, regarding the optimal siting of camps, improving the standard of hygiene of the men, reducing the risk of infection, or the selection of suitable clothing for particular climatic conditions, the medical staff were never consulted.[9] If they offered an opinion, this was invariably ignored. On occasions this led to the death due to illness of large numbers of men, and sometimes to the destruction of whole armies, as occurred in the West Indies toward the end of the 18th century.[10]

Possibly the most glaring examples of military administrative incompetence and inefficiency observed during the 19th century relate to events associated with the Crimean War. Many were drawn to the attention of the nation on an almost daily basis by the various official and in some cases unofficial war correspondents that served in the East.[11] It was frequently claimed, for example, that the poor provision of medical staff, dressers, and ward orderlies, as well as inadequate equipment, occasionally led to untold suffering among the men. While this may only occasionally have been the case, all of the information of this type caused grave public concern in Britain that in the end could not be ignored by the government.[12] Concern was also expressed in the numerous items that appeared in the medical journals, sent from doctors serving at the Front, many of whom thought it expedient to remain anonymous.

One of Smith's greatest causes for concern was the lack of suitable arrangements for rescuing and transporting the wounded from the battlefield. This was associated with the additional problem of transporting the sick to appropriate hospital accommodation, whether locally to the regimental hospitals or via transports to the base hospitals at Scutari or back to Britain.[13] Despite repeated pleas from Ballingall[14] and others[15] to the governments of the day stressing the value of mobile ambulances associated with an appropriately trained ambulance corps,[16] neither the equipment nor the trained staff were either available of immediately forthcoming.

In mid-February 1854, the military secretary to the commander-in-chief asked Smith about his proposed arrangements for the transportation of the sick and wounded. Instructions for the building of appropriate two-wheeled wagons, designed by Smith but clearly based on Larrey's earlier successful model, and a larger, but inevitably less manageable, four-wheeled model, were submitted to the War Office in March 1854. These reached the Crimea in only relatively small numbers, and rather late in the campaign. Despite Smith's good intentions, the mobile ambulance units were a failure, principally because the War Office had insisted that the lightweight wheels stipulated by Smith be replaced by the far heavier artillery wheels. Not only did this make the wagons unstable, but also, due to their increased weight, they tended to get bogged down in the wet and muddy terrain. Even when the relatively few ambulances did arrive, their drivers were unsuitable for the task in hand, principally due to their age, infirmity, and, not infrequently, incompetence. The wagons that were available were not under the control of the Army Medical Department. Complaints were frequently received by the director-general to the effect "that transport for general officers' baggage had invariably been provided before that for the sick or hospitals had been forthcoming."[17] Another problem was that the wagons that were intended to be drawn by four horses with two drivers required six of the small Bulgarian horses to pull them. More drivers were required than were available, and hospital orderlies had to be removed from their other duties and delegated for the purpose, a task for which they were unqualified and for which they had not volunteered. Not surprisingly, the harnesses supplied would not fit, and no specialist staff were available to maintain the wagons or look after the horses.[18]

While adequate volumes of hospital supplies left Britain for the East, because of the often-inclement weather along the route, delays in delivery were inevitable. The lack of tents, for example, led to severe overcrowding. On more than one occasion, items of bedding dispatched three months earlier failed to reach the base hospitals at Scutari. When the situation was investigated, it was revealed that whole cargoes had been unloaded at the wrong destination, and only months later turned up where they should originally have been landed. Other essential items of food and clothing were landed and kept in storehouses, but because of inadequate paperwork at the port of embarkation were not distributed to the men. One of the more distressing incidents was the loss of the cargo ship *Prince*, at anchor off the harbor at Balaklava on November 14, 1854. Her full cargo of warm clothing and all of her crew and passengers were lost in a severe gale. A number of other cargo vessels at anchor were also lost during the same gale, as was much of the hutted accommodation and tenting. It took many months before replacement warm clothing arrived, too late to be of value during the worst of the winter months. Possibly one of the worst examples of incompetence occurred during the winter of 1854–1855, when 16,000 greatcoats remained in store in Scutari and were not issued to the men because no authorization had been received for their distribution. Furthermore, only 800 of over 25,000 rugs that arrived during December were distributed despite the fact that only a few miles away many were dying from the cold.

Other examples emerged when evidence was presented by the witnesses called to speak before the Roebuck Committee, whose principal function would seem to have been apportioning blame on individuals or groups of individuals who displayed obvious evidence of incompetence. The committee was also criticized because they appeared to be happier receiving evidence from so-called experts who had only briefly visited the Crimea, rather than listening to the medical and military men who had served in the war zone. Despite its aggressive chairman, the committee had little effect because its functions were largely superseded by a number of other commissions.[19] These all had the authority to act locally, without needing to refer back to Parliament, when they felt that urgent changes needed to be implemented. The sanitary commissioners played an important part in alleviating the principal problem encountered in the distribution of essential items to the regimental and base hospitals. They confirmed the general impression that while the Commissariat Department might have been able to cope in peacetime the methods they employed were unsuitable in times of war. As they were in charge of the reception and distribution of supplies in the Crimea, they bore a considerable responsibility for the chaos that arose with regard to the transfer of provisions, essential items of equipment, food, and clothing, once they reached the harbor at Balaklava to where they were needed. As the members of the commissariat staff lacked both initiative and imagination in undertaking these essential tasks, the commissioners recommended that their activities should be transferred from the control of the Treasury to that of the War Office.

The commissioners also dared to criticize the competence and judgment of members of the high command. This inevitably caused deep resentment in that quarter,[20] and the independent inquiry that was set up, termed the Chelsea Board, not surprisingly, as it consisted exclusively of senior military officers, made sure that all blame was deflected away from the high command toward the Treasury. The Chelsea Board's own findings did not escape criticism from Miss Nightingale and the public, however, and the changes recommended by the commission were, in the long term, largely implemented.

While Miss Nightingale had scant regard for the way that the military functioned, she had an equally poor opinion of the competence of the majority of her professional nurses, as few with the appropriate qualifications offered themselves for consideration. She was not that impressed with those of her nurses that belonged to the various religious orders, as these often tended to be more interested in the men's souls than in their physical well-being.[21] While Miss Nightingale's approach when she arrived in Scutari caused some concern among both the medical and military hierarchy, it was obvious to all that her first priority was toward the well-being of the men. For this reason her views were highly respected when she presented her testimony both during and shortly after the war. Because she had been in Scutari during most of the war, her views were of paramount importance in the various debates that followed the war. When the changes recommended by the various commissions were in due course implemented, they led to a dramatic increase in the efficiency of the way that the Army Medical Department functioned from that time.[22]

At the beginning of the Crimean War most of the senior medical officers had little or no experience in the use of general anesthetics. The introduction of pain-free surgery into civilian practice during the late 1840s was so revolutionary that those in authority in the Army Medical Department were reluctant to accept its obvious advantages. For example, inspector general Hall cautioned the men against the use of chloroform in patients with severe shock from gunshot wounds. This advice closely followed the views expressed by Guthrie early in the war,[23] despite the fact that most of the younger surgeons had read of its value in allowing capital operations to be performed in anesthetized patients in civilian practice. Its slow introduction in the service should not be altogether surprising. During the early 1850s one of the two standard textbooks in common usage made only a passing mention to chloroform anesthesia, in the section on "Feigned and Factitious Diseases,"[24] while the other textbook made only a cursory mention of anesthetic agents in the final paragraph of the last page of its text.[25] The situation changed only when Guthrie published numerous case reports that confirmed the successful use of general anesthesia by the young surgeons in the East.[26] It is likely that many of these men had attended his lectures on the topic in London, and as a result they created a climate of opinion that stimulated the rapid introduction of general anesthesia into military practice. It is unlikely that many of the medical officers would have had an opportunity to see the section on the use of general anesthetics published in the 6th Edition of Guthrie's *Commentaries on Surgery* while they were still serving in the East, as this appeared late in 1855.[27] This volume contains advice on the mode of administration of general anesthetics and some of their potential hazards.

A similar transition occurred during the Peninsular War with the gradual evolution of ideas regarding the optimal treatment of gunshot injuries to the limbs. Initially, almost all military surgeons accepted the conservative views expressed by John Hunter, who was a strong advocate of undertaking secondary rather than primary amputations.[28] It was only because of the forceful personality of surgeons such as Guthrie that an increasing number of primary amputations were undertaken. By the end of the Peninsular War, while the number of amputations undertaken was far fewer than had earlier been the case, most tended to be of the primary variety. This was principally because the survival rate following this procedure was so much greater and the incidence of complications so much lower than when secondary amputations were routinely performed.[29] Toward the end of the Peninsular War, Guthrie advocated the local excision of joints when these were severely damaged as the procedure of choice rather than amputation of entire limbs. Such conservative procedures had the great advantage that they preserved a degree of limb function.[30] These were only uncommonly performed at that time, and it was to be many years before these procedures became the accepted practice.

It is appropriate to ask why the Treasury funded the establishment of the Royal Military Academy at Sandhurst during the second decade of the 19th century, but provided only derisory funding to support education in the fields of military medicine and surgery during the period between 1806–1860. The simplest answer to this question is likely to be a combination of lack of appropriate patronage, strength of case, and perseverance. While the Royal Military Academy had the support of the commander-in-chief of the forces, the Duke of York, and later that of the King,[31] it was also strongly supported by the majority of the senior military establishment, who were eventually convinced of the value of such an institution.[32] The Treasury eventually relented, and funds were allocated in 1808 to establish an academy for the purpose proposed by Le Marchand. By 1817, all the outstanding construction work was completed.[33] Shortly after the end of the Napoleonic War, the Treasury demanded reductions in its running expenditure, and from 1832 until shortly after the Crimean War it had to be self-funding. It was only after the Crimean War, due principally to the overwhelming influence of public opinion, that public funding was again directed toward the Royal Military Academy. What eventually emerged was an educational institution that provided both military theory and practice at the equivalent of both undergraduate and junior postgraduate level for those who wished to enter the officer corps.

Evidence from all of the other European nations with a professional officer corps had clearly demonstrated the distinct advantage of such an arrangement over the systems then still current in Britain during the 18th and early part of the 19th centuries of purchase and patronage. While such systems had worked with variable degrees of efficiency in a pre–Revolutionary world order, they excluded all but a minute proportion of the population from consideration for the officer corps, those of noble birth and those with extreme wealth. The only European nation where such a system continued into the early part of the 20th century was Russia, where it too was overthrown by the revolutionary zeal of the populace.

The poor status of the military medical officers in the army compared to the executive officers in that service and naval doctors compared to wardroom officers in the navy meant that any attempt on their part to elevate their status was likely to be met with almost overwhelming difficulties. The situation in the Crimean War perpetuated a system that had existed from the previous century when the medical staff in both the army and the navy were considered to be of a lower status than executive officers, being on a par with the tradesmen in the service, such as the engineers and padres. Any advances that were achieved, for example, in improving their status vis à vis their colleagues were achieved only when their conditions of service were so poor that concessions had to be made to encourage candidates to enter the service.[34]

In the navy during the 18th century the executive officers that associated in the wardroom were, to a man, all of aristocratic stock, and brought with them into the service the prejudices acquired during generations brought up on their country estates. During both the 18th and 19th centuries, the younger members of the aristocracy and the sons of the very well-off landowners normally entered the service as midshipmen, often with the intention of spending the rest of their careers on board ship. While the salary must have covered the basic necessities of living at sea, a comfortable existence would not have been possible without a substantial supplement from their own private funds. Because of the frequency of wars during the 18th and first half of the 19th centuries, naval captains and, but to a lesser extent, their officers, could become extremely rich from acquiring bounties while acting in the service of the sovereign. What little was left over was distributed to the warrant officers, including the surgeon and the padre. Possibly more distressing to those who served in the medical branch of the navy was the failure of implementation of the Order in Council of January 1805. This not only accepted that changes had to be made in the service, but also recommended the means by which the quality of the intake might be improved. It was with this order that naval medical officers were first allowed to wear a distinguishing uniform and were given a comparative rank in the service suitable to their station: a similar arrangement was already in force in the Army Medical Department.[35] It was also at about this time that Turnbull[36] indicated, along lines similar to those previously expressed by John Bell, that naval medical officers, once in the service, should be offered specialist postgraduate courses based at the various naval hospitals.[37]

During 1855, when the conditions of service in the navy were so poor that no candidates offered themselves to fill the vacant assistant surgeons' posts in the Baltic fleet, clinical medical students in the final year of their studies were actively encouraged to enter in their place.[38] When this approach was also rejected, the conditions within the service were then improved, and numbers of students then entered as dressers in the fleet. From 1805 until 1859, the Order in Council of 1805 was not implemented by the Lords of the Admiralty, who "were not inclined to obey the order of the Sovereign"[39] despite intermittent efforts, for example, in 1839–1840, by Parliamentary committees set up specifically to investigate grievances in the service, and empowered "to make recommendations for its improvement." Some changes were brought about with respect to salary, but assistant-surgeons, who were not considered wardroom officers, were still relegated to the cockpit. A resolution was eventually carried, in opposition to the wishes of the government, with effect that "the accommodation provided for the assistant-surgeons on board Her Majesty's ships of war is inadequate and insufficient for securing the full benefit of their professional services." This did not meet with the approval of the Lords of the Admiralty, who continued to insist that assistant-surgeons were not permitted in the wardroom until they had been three years in the service and attained the rank of surgeon. Shortly after the outbreak of the Crimean War, in 1855, the right of entry to the wardroom was finally granted to medical officers immediately on their entry into the service. What was not settled at this time was the contentious issue of parity of rank—with surgeons ranking with a commander and above a lieutenant, and at the other extreme, an inspector with an admiral! It was only due to the persistence of the First Lord, Sir John Pakington, that these changes were also implemented in 1859.[40]

It took many years before requests that serving medical officers should be eligible to receive awards for gallantry or bravery were seriously considered.[41] Even when they did become eligible in the Army Medical Department, such awards were never given in proportion to those serving in the medical compared to those in the executive branch of the service. For example, during his tenure of office as commander-in-chief during the Crimean War, Raglan did not recommend any medical officers for gallantry awards, though a few were mentioned in dispatches after the Redan battle. The names of a number of medical men were subsequently drawn to the attention of the War Office for their courage, coolness, and professional skill. In February 1856, inspector general of hospitals John Hall was awarded the K.C.B. (Knight Commander of the Order of the Bath), and a C.B. (Commander of the Order of the Bath) was awarded to seven deputy inspector generals. Hall and 16 others received the French Legion of Honor. It is curious that Smith did not receive his K.C.B. (civil, rather than its military equivalent) until more than two years later, on his retirement from the post of inspector general of the Army and Ordnance Medical Departments, though he was officially styled superintendent general, in July 1858. This award was made despite considerable opposition in many quarters.[42] When the Duke of Wellington died, only regimental medical officers were invited to attend his funeral at St. Paul's Cathedral;[43] pointedly, no members of Smith's Army Medical Department, all of whom were technically civilians and therefore "neither officers nor gentlemen," received invitations.[44] According to the description of the funeral procession in the *Times* of November 19, 1852, one of the first carriages contained "Physicians to the deceased." Behind the carriage carrying "the Corpse" were "Officers and men from every Regiment in the service; consisting of one Captain, a Subaltern, a Sergeant, a Corporal, and five men from every Regiment."[45] As Sir James McGrigor had retired during February of the previous year, it is likely that he attended St. Paul's Cathedral in a private capacity.

One of the principal causes of resentment in the Naval Medical Service during the early post–Crimean War period was that fewer naval medical officers compared to those in the army received honors. During 20 years, a single naval medical officer (an inspector-general) had received a C.B.—and it was generally believed in the service that he should have been awarded a K.C.B. No deputy-inspector in the Naval Medical Service had been awarded a C.B. In contrast, 74 naval captains (i.e., wardroom officers) had been made C.B., and in the Army Medical Department, in 1865 alone, two K.C.B.s and 14 C.B.s had been awarded. While 10 army medical officers had received the V.C. (Victoria Cross), this decoration for gallantry had never been awarded to a naval medical officer.[46]

Unfortunately John Bell's entirely reasonable case, in his memoir of 1798,[47] and later, in a more detailed form in his memorial, of 1800,[48] to Earl Spencer for the establishment of a school of military medicine and surgery to which candidates intending to enter the service of either the Army or Navy Medical Department would attend, was presented to the wrong individual. While the First Lord of the Admiralty was undoubtedly an important individual in the Whig administration, he was subject to the whims of government which, at that time, were not particularly sympathetic to supporting potentially expensive minority causes. While, in theory, the health of the troops and seamen may have been important to an individual force commander, it was never considered to be a matter of national importance. It was generally accepted that the army and navy would always function, as other individuals could always be found to replace those who died either in action or of disease or were invalided out of the service because they were sick or wounded. With the majority of the adult male population to hand, the number that could be called upon, at worst by conscription, was almost limitless. As far as the officer corps was concerned, it was not quite such a simple matter, as it was not possible for them to be replaced with equally skilled individuals, and it would certainly not be appropriate to replace them with immature and inexperienced cadets.[49]

While John Bell and later McGrigor, Ballingall, and others had attempted to influence successive governments as to the importance of providing appropriate advanced training for those that planned to enter the medical branch of one of the armed services, there was clearly insufficient momentum to carry their case forward. They had no single individual with sufficient authority or charisma to champion their cause. Even McGrigor, who was clearly invaluable to Wellington during the latter part of the Peninsular War, had little influence on him during times of peace. It took the shock tactics of the war correspondents during the Crimean War, and Miss Nightingale both during and after the war, to draw attention to the deficiencies that existed in the administrative infrastructure within the army before any action was taken. Lord Aberdeen's government fell in January 1855, and was replaced by the administration of Lord Palmerston, while Sidney Herbert, the Secretary-at-War, was replaced in office by Lord Panmure. Numerous committees of inquiry were set up, and individuals and groups who were perceived to be deficient were named and shamed, principally to allay public concern regarding the terrible treatment of the men in the Crimea. As a direct consequence of all of this activity, proper funding was eventually provided for both the Royal Military Academy and the establishment of an Army and a Naval Medical College. Just over 60 years after John Bell had first indicated the urgent need for "one great School of Military Surgery" the government set up the Army Medical School at Fort Pitt, Chatham, in 1860, which in 1863 moved to Netley. Naval medical candidates were not to receive specialist training until 1871, when they were also allowed to attend Netley, with the appointment of a professor of naval hygiene. It took until 1880 before the Naval Medical School was established at Haslar Hospital, Gosport.[50]

The fact that all of the European nations that maintained armies and navies established appropriate military medical academies at various times during the 18th century had no influence on the situation in Britain, and no comparable institution was established in Britain until some years after the Crimean War. Elsewhere, those candidates who planned to enter the medical service of either the army or the navy received a minimum of several years of specialist training suitable for their future needs in one or other service. The Army Medical School at Fort Pitt, Chatham, was therefore established by the Government between 100 to 150 years after comparable institutions had been established elsewhere in Europe.

Despite all of McGrigor's efforts, and the recommendations of many others, he never succeeded in obtaining a military academy based along similar lines to those established at the Royal Military Academy at Sandhurst during his period as director-general of the Army Medical Department. From about 1817, shortly after his appointment as director-general, he established a museum and a library at Fort Pitt, Chatham,[51] but few already in the service had the opportunity to spend much time there. Because of the severe financial constraints imposed on the system by the government during the post–Waterloo period, relatively few places were available for those who planned a career in the service. Those who were selected, however, spent between four and six months at Fort Pitt before being sent to join their regiment, whether at home or abroad. The value of such an arrangement was therefore somewhat variable, and the facilities offered only fully appreciated by those who were fortunate enough to spend the maximum period of time there. All candidates at Fort Pitt, additionally, had the benefit of seeing patients in the local military and naval hospitals at Haslar and Portsmouth. While the library, museum, and hospital facilities there were second to none, there was little in the way of formal teaching available, or guidance from appropriately qualified staff. Those who joined the service just before the onset of the Crimean War, however, spent little or no time at Fort Pitt before they were sent out East.

In 1806, when the University of Edinburgh authorities were informed of Thomson's appointment to the newly created Regius Chair of Military Surgery, there was an outcry, but little that they could do.[52] Thomson had been invited to apply to His Majesty's Government for the commission to be professor of military surgery in Edinburgh. The Secretary of State for the Home Department, Earl Spencer, advised His Majesty to create this professorship, and after the most cursory of investigations into his academic background and political affiliations recommended Thomson for the appointment, at a salary of £100 per annum.[53] Thomson had already held the Royal College of Surgeons of Edinburgh Chair of Surgery from 1804,[54] and had a reasonable salary from his private practice. This was clearly not the case in 1822, when Ballingall was appointed to the Regius Chair. He was on the retired list and on half-pay from the army from 1817, and clearly had considerable difficulties in covering his domestic expenses, as he had no other source of income.[55]

The Regius Chair of Military Surgery in Edinburgh, which functioned between 1806 and 1855 and the Regius Chair of Military Surgery in Dublin that functioned between 1855 and 1860,[56] although pathetically funded by government over the years, undoubtedly had a disproportionately valuable effect on the education of a significant number of medical students in these two centers. It should be recalled that these courses were also open to medical officers from the various services gratis,[57] and many military surgeons took leave to attend them with the full blessing of their senior officers. While the military surgery course in Edinburgh and later that in Dublin[58] and Guthrie's lecture courses in London could only provide a limited alternative to full-time postgraduate training, it is clear that they served a particularly useful purpose. Guthrie provided the only postgraduate teaching available in London during the post–Waterloo period, albeit exclusively on topics associated with military surgery.[59] It was only after 1860, with the establishment of the Army Medical School, that experienced specialist staff in a wide range of disciplines could provide a viable alternative system. Such courses as were available during the first half of the 19th century were provided single-handedly in Edinburgh by Thomson and then by Ballingall and later by Tufnell in Dublin.[60]

The maximum that the Treasury was prepared to expend on specialist training in military surgery during the early part of the 19th century was the £100 per annum needed to cover the cost of the Regius Chair of Military Surgery established in Edinburgh in 1806.[61] Funds for the Edinburgh Chair were eventually withdrawn early in 1856.[62] A similar outlay was expended in Dublin, from 1855 to 1860, to cover the stipend of Mr. Tufnell's Regius Chair in that city.[63] All candidates for the Edinburgh Chair were expected to have been retired military surgeons on half-pay who would, in due course, probably also obtain or already have obtained a part-time clinical appointment in the Royal Infirmary. It is of interest to reflect that the government and/or university might reasonably expect to get a respectable candidate to apply for this post when it was only associated with such a derisory stipend. It was clearly their belief that the post was such a prestigious one that there would be no shortage of appropriately qualified candidates. When, in due course, the vacancy arose, only two serious candidates with the appropriate qualifications applied.[64]

While it might reasonably be argued that the Army Medical School professionalized the training of military medical personnel, the opportunity to expose impressionable medical students to the glamour of the military life was lost when the government withdrew funding for the two Regius Chairs of Military Surgery in Edinburgh and in Dublin. While the information is not available to estimate what proportion of the candidates who entered the army, navy, or Indian Medical Service attended the courses provided in Edinburgh and Dublin, all the evidence so far available strongly suggests that in this regard they both fully justified their existence. These were, after all, the only institutions in Britain until the establishment of the Army Medical School where both undergraduate medical students and medical officers from the army, navy and Indian Medical Service could receive both theoretical and practical instruction in all aspects of military medicine, surgery, and hygiene.

NOTES

1. Despite his limited military experience, he was an extremely able military administrator. He had been recalled from half-pay to be appointed deputy surgeon general from 1786–1790, and surgeon general from 1790 until his death in 1793. See: J. Hunter, 1794. *A Treatise on the Blood, Inflammation and Gun-Shot Wounds, by the late John Hunter. To which is prefixed, a short account of the author's life, by his Brother-in-Law, Everard Home* (London: George Nicol) [The account of John Hunter's life appears on pp. xiii–lxvii]; Anon., 1908. John Hunter (1728–1793). *Dictionary of National Biography* **10** (London: Smith, Elder & Co.), 287–293; H.A.L. Howell, 1912. John Hunter, F.R.S., Surgeon-General and Inspector-General of Hospitals. *Journal of the Royal Army Medical Corps* **19**, 143–150.

2. With the inevitability of a major conflict with France looming, and the substantial increase in the work load that this was likely to bring with it, it was believed that the load would be too great for one individual. See: N. Cantlie, 1974. *A History of the Army Medical Department.* 2 Volumes (Edinburgh and London: Churchill Livingstone), Volume 1, pp. 170–209.

3. Sir Clifton Wintringham died shortly after taking up the appointment as physician-general, and was replaced by Sir Lucas Pepys.

4. J. Fergusson, 1846. *Notes and Recollections of a Professional Life, by the Late William Fergusson, Esq. M.D. Inspector General of Military Hospitals. Edited by his son, James Fergusson* (London: Longman, Brown, Green & Longmans), pp. 56–58.

5. J. W. Fortescue, 1899–1930. *A History of the British Army.* 13 Volumes (London: Macmillan & Co.), Volume 10, 1920, p. 195.

6. W.F.P. Napier, 1828–1840. *History of the War in the Peninsula and in the South of France, from the Year 1807 to the Year 1814.* 6 Volumes (London: Thomas & William Boone), Volume 5, 1836, Book 19, p. 250.

7. The War Office covered the cost of her nurses' salaries and lodging expenses.

8. Mr. MacDonald, the representative of the *Times* newspaper, had access to large sums of money donated by private individuals which he was allowed to spend, usually on the advice of Miss Nightingale, on purchasing supplies and equipment for improving the general living conditions of the men.

9. This contrasts with the situation in civilian practice where, during the various outbreaks of cholera in Britain during the 1830s and later, doctors with military experience were often called upon to advise the civilian medical authorities on the containment of the disease and in other urgent public health measures.

10. Fergusson, *Recollections*, pp. 67–68.

11. Such as Mr. William Howard Russell, the official war correspondent of the *Times* newspaper.

12. The Roebuck Committee was set up in the spring of 1855 to specifically investigate all aspects of the organization of the army in the Crimea, including that of the Army Medical Department. See: J. Shepherd, 1991. *The Crimean Doctors: A History of the British Medical Services in the Crimean War.* 2 Volumes (Liverpool: Liverpool University Press), Volume 2, pp. 381–395.

13. It was proposed that the most seriously wounded casualties and men that were only fit enough to be invalided out of the service were to be repatriated back to Britain.

14. G. Ballingall, 1833. *Outlines of the Course of Lectures on Military Surgery, delivered in the University of Edinburgh* (Edinburgh: Adam Black; London: Longman, Rees, Orme, Brown & Green), pp. 94–108.

15. For the detailed proposals of van Millingen, see: J. G. van Millingen, 1819. *The Army Medical Officer's Manual upon Active Service; Precepts for his Guidance in the Various Situations in which he may be placed; with Observations on the Preservation of the Health of Armies upon Foreign Service* (London: Burgess & Hill); for additional observations, see: J. Hennen, 1818. *Observations on Some important points in the Practice of Military Surgery, and in the Arrangement and Police of Hospitals. Illustrated by Cases and Dissections* (Edinburgh: A. Constable & Co.; London: Longman, Hurst, Rees, Orme & Brown; Dublin: J. Cumming), p. 23.

16. Along the lines pioneered by Larrey and employed by the French during the Peninsular War. See: D. J. Larrey, 1812–1817. *Mémoires de Chirurgie Militaire, et Campagnes.* 4 Volumes (Paris: J. Smith) [Volume 1, 1812; Volume 2, 1812; Volume 3, 1812; Volume 4, 1817]. Volume 1 contains a series of fine plates. Plate III shows the 2-wheeled horse-drawn wagon, Plate IV shows a sectional view of the 2-wheeled wagon with an amputation patient on board, Plate V shows the 4-wheeled wagon, Plate VI shows the Ambulance du Baron Percy, with three soldiers on board, Plates VII and VIII show two views of a pannier being carried by a camel, one showing an amputation patient in one of the panniers; J. H. Dible, 1970. *Napoleon's Surgeon* (London: William Heinemann Medical Books Ltd.).

17. Cantlie, *Army Medical Department*, Volume 2, p. 175. This example bears comparison with the order given by Lord Raglan with regard to the priority for usage of the hutted accommodation which, in any case, arrived too late in the winter to be of maximal value to the troops. The huts were to be provided, in the first instance, for the horses and mules rather than for the accommodation of the troops.

18. Shepherd, *Crimean Doctors*, Volume 1, p. 79.

19. It should be noted that between November 1854 and April 1855, the government established four commissions and a select committee (also termed the Roebuck or Sebastopol Committee) in order to investigate the conditions in the Crimea. The first commission to be established was the Hospital Commission, and this was followed by the Sanitary, Supplies, and Pathology Commissions.

20. They argued that they had had no opportunity of defending their decisions before the commission's findings were made public.

21. Out of a total of 38 nurses that were eventually selected to join Miss Nightingale, 24 came from various religious orders: 10 were Sisters from Catholic Orders, and 14 were Anglican Sisters. All of the nurses were middle-aged, and most had little nursing experience.

22. F. Nightingale, 1859. *Notes on Hospitals: Being Two Papers read before the National Association for the Promotion of Social Science, at Liverpool, in October 1858. With Evidence Given to the Royal Commissioners on the State of the Army in 1857* (London: J. W. Parker & Son); F. Nightingale, 1858. *Notes on Matters Affecting the Health, Efficiency and Hospital Administration in the British Army*. Printed Privately (London: Harrison & Sons) (cited by J. B. Neal, 1957. The history of the Royal Army Medical College. *Journal of the Royal Army Medical Corps* **103**, 163–172).

23. Anon., 1854. Mr. Guthrie's directions to army surgeons (Extracted from his *Pamphlet on the Hospital Brigade*). *Lancet* **II**, 155–157.

24. This relates to a patient with rigid stiffness of the elbow joint of no known cause. After consultation, the decision was made to excise the elbow joint to restore flexibility to the joint. The patient was anesthetized with chloroform, and with some difficulty the joint was brought to "a state of semiflexion." The operation was consequently abandoned. See: G. Ballingall, 1852. *Outlines of Military Surgery*. 4th Edition (Edinburgh: Adam & Charles Black), p. 586. There is no mention of the use of anesthetic agents for capital surgery in the 5th Edition of this book. See: G. Ballingall, 1855. *Outlines of Military Surgery*. 5th Edition (Edinburgh: Adam & Charles Black; London: Longman & Co.).

25. G. J. Guthrie, 1853. *Commentaries on the Surgery of the War in Portugal, Spain, France, and the Netherlands, from the Battle of Roliça, in 1808, to that of Waterloo, in 1815, Showing the Improvements made during and since that period in the great art and science of surgery on all the subjects to which they relate*. 5th Edition (London: Henry Renshaw), p. 585.

26. Guthrie, 1855. Military Surgery in the Crimea. A Lecture delivered at the Royal College of Surgeons of England, on Saturday, April 14, 1855. *Lancet* **I**, 413–417; G. J. Guthrie, 1855. Surgical Practice in the Crimea. *Lancet* **I**, 544 [A brief letter]; G. J. Guthrie, 1856. Cases in Military Surgery Occurring in the Crimea. Communicated by G. J. Guthrie, Esq., F.R.S. *Lancet* **I**, 65–67.

27. Guthrie, G. J. (1855). *Commentaries on the Surgery of the War in Portugal, Spain, France, and the Netherlands, from the Battle of Roliça, in 1808, to that of Waterloo, in 1815, with Additions Relating to those in the Crimea in 1854–55, Showing the Improvements made During and Since that Period in the Great Art and Science of Surgery on all the Subjects to which they Relate*. 6th Edition. (Revised to October 1855) (London: Henry Renshaw).

28. Hunter, *Inflammation*.

29. G. J. Guthrie, 1815. *On Gun-Shot Wounds of the Extremities, Requiring the Different Operations of Amputation, with their after-treatment: Establishing the Advantages of Amputation on the Field of Battle to the Delay usually recommended, &c. &c. With Four Explanatory Plates* (London: Longman, Hurst, Rees, Orme & Brown) [2nd Edition, 1820; 3rd Edition, 1827].

30. G. J. Guthrie, 1838. *Clinical Lectures on Compound Fractures of the Extremities, on Excision of the Head of the Thigh-Bone, the Arm-Bone, and the Elbow-Joint: On the Diseases of the Peninsula, and on Several Miscellaneous Subjects. Delivered at the Westminster Hospital* (London: John Churchill).

31. According to the King: "I consider the Military College an object of the deepest national importance . . . you will all the time be raising a race of officers, who will make our army the finest in Europe." See: A. Shepperd, 1980. *Sandhurst: The Royal Military Academy Sandhurst and its Predecessors* (London: Country Life Books), p. 36).

32. As a result of the personal enthusiasm and initiative of Captain Le Marchant, plans were drawn up for improving, initially, the swordsmanship in the cavalry. He also found time to draft a series of manuals covering all aspects of cavalry training, as well as means of improving the efficiency of the Home Guard. He soon became convinced that the efficiency of the army itself could not be improved without first improving the training of its officers. His outline plans met with the approval of the Duke of York, and gradually became the accepted view. See: D. Le Marchant, 1841. *Memoirs of the Late Major General Le Marchant* (London) (cited by Shepperd, *Sandhurst*, pp. 22–24).

33. Shepperd, *Sandhurst*, pp. 32–44.

34. Over the years before the Crimean War, Thomas Wakley, editor of the *Lancet*, was particularly vociferous with regard to drawing attention to the poor conditions of service within the Naval Medical Department. See: Anon (1964–1965). Wakley, Thomas (1795–1862). *Dictionary of National Biography* **20** (London: Oxford University Press), 461–465. Spencer Wells, editor of the *Medical Times and Gazette*, was equally distressed about the poor conditions of service in both the Army and Navy Medical Departments. See: Shepherd, J.A. (1965). *Spencer Wells: The Life and Work of a Victorian Surgeon* (Edinburgh: E. & S. Livingstone Ltd.), pp. 27–33.

35. This Order in Council conferred "similar rank with the officers of the same class in His Majesty's Land Service."

36. W. Turnbull, 1806. *The Naval Surgeon; Comprising the Entire Duties of Professional Men at Sea. To which are Subjoined, a System of Naval Surgery, and a Compendious Pharmacopoeia. The Whole Illustrated by Plates* (London: Richard Phillips & B. McMillan).

37. "Would it not, therefore, after a student has acquired some general knowledge of the extent of the service, be proper to limit his views, in the finishing part of his studies, to the Naval Department alone; and, instead of wasting his time in attending on the common Medical and Surgical Lectures, that an institution should be formed, by the appointment of Government, for completing the instruction of all such whose practice is afterwards to be devoted to the Naval Department." See: Turnbull, *Naval Surgeon*, pp. xxxiv–xxxv.

38. They were to serve as acting assistant surgeons from April until October 1855, so that they could return to their studies during the winter session. The rate of pay was 2/- per diem, and a gratuity of £25 was to be paid at the end of their period of service. This offer was generally unfavorably viewed by both the medical students and the medical press. Despite this, 67 students served in the Baltic fleet during 1855, and are all believed to have returned to their medical studies. See: Shepherd, *Crimean Doctors*, Volume 2, p. 542.

39. W. Rivington, 1879. *The Medical Profession: being the Essay to which was awarded the First Carmichael Prize of £200 by the Council of the Royal College of Surgeons, Ireland, 1879* (Dublin: Fannin & Co.; London: Longmans & Co.; Baillière, Tindall & Cox; Edinburgh: Maclachlan & Stewart), p. 229.

40. With the Naval Medical Warrant of May 30, 1859. See: Rivington, *Medical Profession*, pp. 232–237.

41. Sir George Ballingall had written to General Sir George De Lacy Evans with regard to his campaign in Parliament in support of the award of military honors to military medical officers. See: G. Ballingall, 1844. Letter addressed by Sir George Ballingall, M.D. to Sir De Lacy Evans on the subject of the right of military surgeons to military honors. *Lancet* **II**, 215–216.

42. See, for example, the *Times* of July 14, 1858, in an article that concluded with the following remark: "He is to be shelved at last, and to be consigned to a splendid insignificance." The *Lancet* published a strongly worded editorial in his defense. See: Anon., 1858. The Distinction Conferred on Dr. Andrew Smith. *Lancet* **II**, 69.

43. Wellington was buried in St. Paul's Cathedral with great pomp and ceremony on November 18, 1852. See: Anon., 1964–1965. Wellesley, Arthur, first Duke of Wellington (1769–1852). *Dictionary of National Biography* **20** (London: Oxford University Press), 1081–1115.

44. Cantlie, *Army Medical Department*, Volume 2, p. 3.

45. For a report of the funeral procession, see the *Times* of November 19, 1852.

46. Rivington, *Medical Profession*, p. 233.

47. J. Bell, 1798. *Memoir on the Present State of Naval and Military Surgery. Addressed to the Right Honourable Earl Spenser [sic], First Lord of the Admiralty* [21 pp. Yarmouth, January 20, 1798].

48. J. Bell, 1800. *Memorial Concerning the Present State of Military and Naval Surgery. Addressed Several Years ago to the Right Honourable Earl Spencer, First Lord of the Admiralty; and now Submitted to the Public* (Edinburgh: Longman & Rees; London: Cadell & Davies) [41 pp.].

49. C. Duffy, 1987. *The Military Experience in the Age of Reason* (London and New York: Routledge & Kegan Paul).

50. K. MacLeod, 1906. Netley. *Caledonian Medical Journal* **6**, 379–390; Neal, *Royal Army Medical College*; Cantlie, *Army Medical Department*, Volume 2, pp. 217–233.

51. In 1833, the museum contained over 14,000 preparations of comparative anatomy, natural history and pathology, as well as maps and a wide variety of drawings and paintings. See: Anon., 1833. *Catalogue of Preparations, &c. in Morbid, Natural, and Comparative Anatomy, Contained in the Museum of the Army Medical Department, Fort Pitt, Chatham* (London: Richard Taylor). The number of pathological preparations dramatically increased over the period between 1833 and 1845. See: G. Williamson, Ed. 1845. *Catalogue of Preparations &c. in Morbid Anatomy and Experimental Physiology, Contained in the Museum of the Army Medical Department, Fort Pitt, Chatham* (London: Smith, Elder & Co.); the collection of 450 human crania in the museum was also substantial, and the curator's detailed catalog of this collection provides one of the first works on the ethnological implications of craniometry. See: G. Williamson, 1857. *Observations on the human crania contained in the Museum of the Army Medical Department, Fort Pitt, Chatham* (Dublin: McGlashan & Gill).

52. A. Miles, 1918. The Chair of Military Surgery. In: *The Edinburgh School of Surgery before Lister* (London: A. & C. Black Ltd.), pp. 108–120.

53. *Town Council Minutes, Edinburgh*, November 8, 1806. When William III established the first Regius Chair, in 1694, the salary at that time was £100 for the proposed Regius Professor of Divinity and Ecclesiastical History in Edinburgh, to be paid "out of the royal grant in perpetuity from the Bishop's rents." This first appointment was made to John Cumming, and he received his commission from the crown in 1702. When Monro primus was appointed to the Chair of Anatomy, in 1720, the annual salary was £15, and the annual salary for this chair was only raised to £50 in 1798 (See: R. E. Wright-St. Clair, 1964. *Doctors Monro: A Medical Saga* (London: Wellcome Historical Medical Library), p. 78). When James Russell was appointed to the Regius Chair of

Clinical Surgery in 1803, he received a crown endowment of £50 per annum as salary. See: J. D. Comrie, 1932. *A History of Scottish Medicine*. 2nd Edition. 2 Volumes (London: Baillière, Tindall & Cox), Volume 2, p. 503; Anon., 1963–1964. Russell, James (1754–1836). *Dictionary of National Biography* **17** (London: Oxford University Press), 439–440.

54. J. Thomson, 1826. *Hints Respecting the Improvement of the Literary and Scientific Education of Candidates for the Degree of M.D., &c. with Observations prefixed, addressed to the Royal University Commissioners*. (Edinburgh). See: J. Thomson, 1859. *An Account of the Life, Lectures, and Writings of William Cullen, M.D., Professor of the Practice of Physic in the University of Edinburgh. 2 Volumes. Volume 1. First Published in 1832. Now re-issued along with the second volume, and having pre-fixed to it a biographical notice of the author* (Edinburgh and London: W. Blackwood & Sons) [For biographical notice of Dr. John Thomson, see pp. 5–84]; D. C. Simpson, 1977. The Chairs of Surgery at Edinburgh. *Journal of the Royal College of Surgeons of Edinburgh* **22**, 91–102.

55. Before his retirement from the army and being appointed to the Regius Chair, he matriculated at the University of Edinburgh during the 1816–1817 session and attended both chemistry and military surgery, in order to be eligible to submit his M.D. thesis. He also wrote and submitted a dissertation for his fellowship diploma of the Royal College of Surgeons of Edinburgh, and published a few clinical case reports. This would probably not have left him with much time to undertake locum clinical posts to supplement his half-pay.

56. Two sources indicate that Thomas Jolliffe Tufnell was appointed Regius Professor of Military Surgery at the Royal College of Surgeons of Ireland, from 1851–1860. See: Anon., 1963–1964. Tufnell, Thomas Joliffe (1819–1885). *Dictionary of National Biography* **19** (Oxford: Oxford University Press), 1220–1221; A. Peterkin & W. Johnston, 1968. *Commissioned Officers in the Medical Services of the British Army 1660–1960*. 2 Volumes (London: Wellcome Historical Medical Library), Volume 1, Reference Number 4649, p. 315; this information contrasts with that in a copy of a letter from Peel to Tufnell dated August 19, 1855, written on behalf of Lord Panmure, which notified Tufnell of his appointment to the Regius Chair of Military Surgery in Dublin. See: Letter in Special Collections Section, Edinburgh University Library, from the War Office, MS. Ref: 3082.3 Fol. 7.

57. As was Thomson's lecture course on military surgery delivered during his tenure of the Royal College of Surgeons of Edinburgh's Chair of Surgery.

58. Both of which covered a much wider range of topics than might be assumed from the respective titles of the Edinburgh and Dublin Regius Professorships.

59. Guthrie, *Clinical Lectures*. For a compendium of his former published work, see: Guthrie, *Commentaries on Surgery*.

60. While he held the posts of surgeon to the City Hospital and to the district military prison in Dublin, he set up a classroom, in 1846, and lectured on military hygiene.

61. The stipend of £100 per annum in 1822 amounted to just over £4,400 in present day terms, and should only be considered an honorarium, rather than a salary, as it would have required the holder to find the majority of his income from other sources.

62. Following Ballingall's death in December 1855.

63. According to Tufnell's letter of appointment from Lord Panmure, the full quotation is as follows: "I am directed by Lord Panmure to acquaint you that he has appointed you to be Regius Professor of Military Surgery at Dublin, with a salary of £100 per annum, for the purpose of giving lectures on Military Hygiene." See: Letter in Special Collections Section, Edinburgh University Library, from the War Office, MS. Ref: 3082.3 Fol. 7.

64. The two serious candidates were Ballingall and Dr. David Maclagan, both were Fellows of the Royal College of Surgeons of Edinburgh and supported by the College. A third candidate was Dr. Borthwick, who was the brother-in-law of one of the Town Council, and his recommendation for the post was made at the personal request of the Lord Provost, rather than in his formal capacity.

SELECTED BIBLIOGRAPHY

JOURNALS CITED

British Medical Journal

Caledonian Medical Journal

Edinburgh Medical and Surgical Journal

Edinburgh Medical Journal

The Gentleman's Magazine: and Historical Chronicle

History Today

Journal of the Royal Army Medical Corps

Journal of the Royal College of Surgeons of Edinburgh

Journal of the Royal Naval Medical Service

Lancet

London Medical Gazette

London Medical Journal

Medical History

Medico-Chirurgical Review

Philosophical Transactions (Royal Society of London)

Proceedings of the Royal Society of Medicine

Scottish Medical Journal

BOOKS CITED

Alcock, R. 1838. *Notes on the Medical History and Statistics of the British Legion of Spain; Comprising the Results of Gun-Shot Wounds in Relation to Important Questions in Surgery*. London: J. Churchill.

Ballingall, G. 1823. *Practical observations on fever, dysentery, and liver complaints, as they occur amongst the European troops in India; illustrated by numerous tables and cases. To which is annexed an essay on syphilis*. 2nd Edition. Edinburgh: Adam Black; London: T & G Underwood; Dublin: Hodges & McArthur.

Ballingall, G. 1833. *Outlines of the Course of Lectures on Military Surgery, delivered in the University of Edinburgh*. Edinburgh: Adam Black; London: Longman, Rees, Orme, Brown & Green [This is the 1st Edition of Ballingall's *Outlines of Military Surgery*; 3rd Edition, 1844; 4th Edition, 1852; 5th Edition, 1855].

Bell, C. 1814. *A Dissertation on Gunshot Wounds*. London: Longman, Hurst, Rees, Orme & Brown.

Bell, J. 1798. *Memoir on the Present State of Naval and Military Surgery. Addressed to the Right Honourable Earl Spenser [sic], First Lord of the Admiralty* [21 pp. Yarmouth, January 20, 1798].

Bell, J. 1800. *Memorial Concerning the Present State of Military and Naval Surgery. Addressed Several Years ago to the Right Honourable Earl Spencer, First Lord of the Admiralty; and now Submitted to the Public*. Edinburgh: Longman & Rees; London: Cadell & Davies. [41 pp.]

Blair, J.S.G. 1998. *Centenary History of the Royal Army Medical Corps (1898–1998)*. Edinburgh: Scottish Academic Press.

Blanco, R. L. 1974. *Wellington's Surgeon General: Sir James McGrigor*. Durham, N.C.: Duke University Press.

Blane, G. 1799. *Observations on the Diseases of Seamen*. 3rd Edition. London: Murray & Highley [The 1st edition was published in 1785, the 2nd in 1789, and the 3rd edition is the much enlarged version].

Bynum, W. F. and R. Porter, eds. 1993. *Companion Encyclopedia of the History of Medicine*. 2 vols. London and New York: Routledge.

Cantlie, N. 1974. *A History of the Army Medical Department*. 2 Volumes. Edinburgh and London: Churchill Livingstone.

Chambers, R. ed. 1854. *A Biographical Dictionary of Eminent Scotsmen*. New Edition. 4 Volumes (in 9 Divisions). London: Blackie & Son [New Edition, Revised, 1864. 5 Volumes].

Comrie, J. D. 1932. *A History of Scottish Medicine*. 2nd Edition. 2 Volumes. London: Baillière, Tindall & Cox.

Cope, Z. 1958. *Florence Nightingale and the Doctors*. London: Museum Press.

Dible, J. H. 1970. *Napoleon's Surgeon*. London: William Heinemann Medical Books Ltd.

Dictionary of National Biography. London: Oxford University Press (various editions).

Fergusson, J. 1846. *Notes and Recollections of a Professional Life, by the Late William Fergusson, Esq. M.D. Inspector General of Military Hospitals. Edited by his son, James Fergusson*. London: Longman, Brown, Green & Longmans.

Fortescue, J. W. 1899–1930. *A History of the British Army*. 13 Volumes. London: Macmillan & Co.

Gordon-Taylor, G. and E. W. Walls, 1958. *Sir Charles Bell: His Life and Times*. Edinburgh and London: E. & S. Livingstone.

Gore, A. 1879. *The Story of Our Services under the Crown. A Historical Sketch of the Army Medical Staff*. London: Ballière, Tindall & Cox.

Gurwood, [John]. 1834–1838. *The Dispatches of Field Marshall The Duke of Wellington K.G during his various Campaigns in India, Denmark, Portugal, Spain, The Low Countries, and France. From 1799–1818. Compiled from Official and Authentic Documents.* 12 Volumes, and Supplement to the 1st, 2nd, and 3rd Volumes relating to India 1799–1818. London: John Murray.

Guthrie, G. J. 1815. *On Gun-Shot Wounds of the Extremities, Requiring the Different Operations of Amputation, with their after-treatment: Establishing the Advantages of Amputation on the Field of Battle to the Delay usually recommended, &c. &c. With Four Explanatory Plates.* London: Longman, Hurst, Rees, Orme & Brown. [2nd Edition, 1820; 3rd Edition, 1827].

Guthrie, G. J. 1838. *Clinical Lectures on Compound Fractures of the Extremities, on Excision of the Head of the Thigh-Bone, the Arm-Bone, and the Elbow-Joint: On the Diseases of the Peninsula, and on Several Miscellaneous Subjects. Delivered at the Westminster Hospital.* London: John Churchill.

Guthrie, G. J. 1853. *Commentaries on the Surgery of the War in Portugal, Spain, France, and the Netherlands, from the Battle of Roliça, in 1808, to that of Waterloo, in 1815, Showing the Improvements made during and since that period in the great art and science of surgery on all the subjects to which they relate.* 5th Edition. London: Henry Renshaw [6th Edition, 1855].

Hamilton, R. 1788. *The Duties of a Regimental Surgeon Considered: with Observations on his General Qualifications; and Hints Relative to a More Respectable Practice, and Better Regulation of that Department. Wherein are Interspersed many Medical Anecdotes, and Subjects Discussed, Equally Interesting to every Practitioner.* 2 Volumes. London: J. Johnson, J. Murray, T. Longman; Ipswich: J. Shave.

Haythornthwaite, P. J. 1994. *The Armies of Wellington.* London: Arms and Armour Press.

Hennen, J. 1818. *Observations on Some important points in the Practice of Military Surgery, and in the Arrangement and Police of Hospitals. Illustrated by Cases and Dissections.* Edinburgh: A. Constable & Co.; London: Longman, Hurst, Rees, Orme & Brown; Dublin: J. Cumming.

Hunter, J. 1794. *A Treatise on the Blood, Inflammation and Gun-Shot Wounds, by the late John Hunter. To which is prefixed, a short account of the author's life, by his Brother-in-Law, Everard Home.* London: George Nicol.

Jackson, R. 1791. *A Treatise on the Fevers of Jamaica, with some Observations on the Intermitting Fever of America, and an Appendix Containing Some Hints on the Means of Preserving the Health of Soldiers in Hot Climates.* London: J. Murray.

Jackson, R. 1805. *A System of Arrangement and Discipline for the Medical Department of Armies.* London: J. Murray.

Jacyna, L. S. 1994. *Philosophic Whigs: Medicine, Science and Citizenship in Edinburgh, 1789–1848.* London: Routledge.

Johnston, W. 1917. *Roll of Commissioned Officers in the Medical Service of the British Army who served on full pay within the period between the Accession of George II and the Formation of the Royal Army Medical Corps 20 June 1727 to 23 June 1898. With an Introduction Showing the Historical Evolution of the Corps, by W.J. Ed. by H.A.L. Howell.* Aberdeen: University Press.

Larrey, D. J. 1812–1817. *Mémoires de Chirurgie Militaire, et Campagnes.* 4 Volumes. Paris: J. Smith.

Lind, J. 1753. *A Treatise of the Scurvy. In Three Parts. Containing an Inquiry into the Nature, Causes, and Cure, of that Disease. Together with a Critical and Chronological View of what has been Published on the Subject.* Edinburgh: Sands, Murray and Cochran; London: A. Millar.

Lloyd, C. and J.L.S. Coulter 1961. *Medicine and the Navy 1200-1900*. Volume 3, 1714–1815. Edinburgh and London: E. & S. Livingstone Ltd. [Volume 4, 1815–1900, 1963].

Lonsdale, H. 1870. *A Sketch of the Life and Writings of Robert Knox the Anatomist. By his Pupil and Colleague*. London: Macmillan & Co.

McGrigor, J. 1861. *The Autobiography and Services of Sir James McGrigor, Bart. Late Director-General of the Army Medical Department, with an Appendix of Notes and Original Correspondence*. London: Longman, Green, Longman & Roberts.

Miles, A. 1918. *The Edinburgh School of Surgery before Lister*. London: A. & C. Black Ltd.

Monro, D. 1780. *Observations on the Means of Preserving the Health of Soldiers: and of Conducting Military Hospitals. And on Diseases Incident to Soldiers in the Time of Service, and on the same Diseases as they have appeared in London*. 2 Volumes. Volume 1 and Volume 2 bound together. 2nd Edition. London: J. Murray and G. Robinson.

Napier, W.F.P. 1828–1840. *History of the War in the Peninsula and in the South of France, from the Year 1807 to the Year 1814*. 6 Volumes. Volume 1, 1828 London: John Murray; Volumes 2–6, 1829–1840, London: Thomas & William Boone.

Nolan, E. H. 1855–1857. *The Illustrated History of the War against Russia*. 2 Volumes. London: James S. Virtue [Volume 1, 1855; Volume 2, 1857].

Paterson, R. 1874. *Memorials of the Life of James Syme*. Edinburgh: Edmonston & Douglas.

Peterkin, A. and W. Johnston 1968. *Commissioned Officers in the Medical Services of the British Army 1660–1960*. 2 Volumes. Volume 1, 1660-1898, Volume 2, 1898–1960. London: Wellcome Historical Medical Library [This volume is sometimes referred to as: "Drew, R. (Editor)," with the same details].

Pettigrew, T. J. 1839. *Medical Portrait Gallery. Biographical Memoirs of the most celebrated Physicians, Surgeons, etc. etc. who have contributed to the Advancement of Medical Science*. 4 Volumes (Volumes 1 and 2 bound together; Volumes 3 and 4 bound together). London: Fisher, Son, & Co.

Pringle, J. 1750. *Observations on the Nature and Cure of Hospital and Jayl-fever. In a letter to Doctor Mead, Physician to his Majesty, &c*. London: A. Millar & D. Wilson [52 pp.].

Risse, G. B. 1986. *Hospital Life in Enlightenment Scotland: Care and Teaching at the Royal Infirmary of Edinburgh*. Cambridge: Cambridge University Press.

Rivington, W. 1879. *The Medical Profession: being the Essay to which was awarded the First Carmichael Prize of £200 by the Council of the Royal College of Surgeons, Ireland, 1879*. Dublin: Fannin & Co.; London: Longmans & Co.; Baillière, Tindall & Cox; Edinburgh: Maclachlan & Stewart.

Rosner, L. 1991. *Medical Education in the Age of Improvement: Edinburgh Students and Apprentices 1760–1826*. Edinburgh: University Press.

Shepherd, J. 1991. *The Crimean Doctors: A History of the British Medical Services in the Crimean War*. 2 Volumes. Liverpool: Liverpool University Press.

Shepperd, A. 1980. *Sandhurst: The Royal Military Academy Sandhurst and its Predecessors*. London: Country Life Books.

Smith, F. 1929. *A Short History of the Royal Army Medical Corps*. Aldershot: Gale & Polden Ltd.

Struthers, J. 1867. *Historical Sketch of the Edinburgh Anatomical School*. Edinburgh: Maclachlan & Stewart.

Thomson, J. 1813. *Lectures on Inflammation, exhibiting a view of the General Doctrines, Pathological and Practical, of Medical Surgery*. Edinburgh: W. Blackwood; London: T. Cadell.

Thomson, J. 1816. *Report of observations made in the British Military Hospitals in Belgium, after the Battle of Waterloo; with some remarks upon amputation*. Edinburgh: W. Blackwood; London: T. Cadell & W. Davies.

Thomson, J. 1859. *An Account of the Life, Lectures, and Writings of William Cullen, M.D., Professor of the Practice of Physic in the University of Edinburgh. 2 Volumes. Volume 1. First Published in 1832. Now re-issued along with the second volume, and having pre-fixed to it a biographical notice of the author*. Edinburgh and London: W. Blackwood & Sons.

Turnbull, W. 1806. *The Naval Surgeon; Comprising the Entire Duties of Professional Men at Sea. To which are Subjoined, a System of Naval Surgery, and a Compendious Pharmacopoeia. The Whole Illustrated by Plates*. London: Richard Phillips & B. McMillan.

van Millingen, J. G. 1819. *The Army Medical Officer's Manual upon Active Service; Precepts for his Guidance in the Various Situations in which he may be placed; with Observations on the Preservation of the Health of Armies upon Foreign Service*. London: Burgess & Hill.

Woodham-Smith, C. 1950. *Florence Nightingale 1820–1910*. London: Constable.

INDEX

About the Author

MATTHEW H. KAUFMAN is Professor of Anatomy at the University of Edinburgh. He has taught Anatomy and Embryology for more than 25 years, initially in the University of Cambridge and more recently in the University of Edinburgh. He has published a number of books and numerous papers that include a range of topics associated with the history of medicine.